An Introduction to Medical Spanish

An Introduction to

Medical Spanish

Communication and Culture

FIFTH EDITION

Robert O. Chase and Clarisa B. Medina de Chase

Yale UNIVERSITY PRESS/NEW HAVEN & LONDON

Editor: Sarah Miller
Publishing Assistant: Ashley E. Lago
Manuscript Editor: Deborah Bruce-Hostler
Production Editor: Ann-Marie Imbornoni
Production Controller: Katie Golden

Set by Newgen North America.

Printed in the United States of America.

Library of Congress Control Number: 2018937825
ISBN 978-0-300-22602-7 (paperback : alk. paper)

A catalogue record for this book is available from the British Library.

This paper meets the requirements of ANSI/NISO Z39.48-1992 (Permanence of Paper).

10 9 8 7 6 5 4 3 2 1

We dedicate this book to health care professionals who defy the notion of "language barrier" and skillfully establish helping relationships and effective communication in the linguistic and cultural contexts of their patients; to brave explorers who cross these boundaries to discern, respect, and consider patient views that are accessible only by empathy and language accommodation.

The rich like borders and the poor do not.

To have another language is to possess a second soul.

    — CHARLEMAGNE

Contents

Scope and Sequence

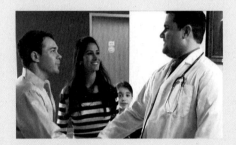
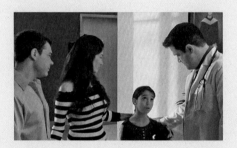

Chapter 3
«¿Qué le pasa?»

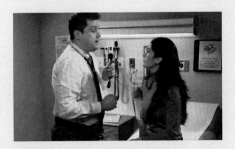

COMMUNICATION GOALS
Discuss Colds and Influenza 62
Ask Whether a Patient Feels
   Comfortable 68
Discuss Pain 80
Diagnose Injuries 82

VOCABULARY
What is the matter? 62
Common Cold and Flu 64
Comfort 68
Parts of the Body 71
Pain 81
Injuries 82

STRUCTURE
The Verb *Tener* 63
The Verb *Doler* 80
The Past Participle 83

CULTURAL NOTE
Expressions for Every Day 90

COMPANION WEBSITE
Video: *¿Qué le pasa?; La comodidad*
Audio: *¿Qué tiene?; La gripe; Las partes del
   cuerpo; El dolor;* Pronunciation of *G, C, J,*
   and *H; Exposición*
Electronic Workbook; Downloadable
   Forms

Chapter 4
El recepcionista

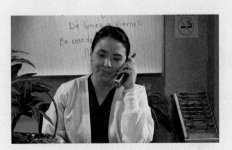

COMMUNICATION GOALS
Tell a Patient His or Her Vital Signs 98
Take a Telephone Message 102
Make Dates for Future
   Appointments 107
Ask and Tell Age 109
Conduct a Registration or Admissions
   Interview 112

VOCABULARY
Numbers from Zero to 1,000 98
The Month, the Date, and the Time 107
Personal Information 112

STRUCTURE
Possession 104
Forming Questions 105

CULTURAL NOTE
What's in a Name? 117

COMPANION WEBSITE
Video: *La recepcionista; Los números de
   teléfono*
Audio: *Los meses del año;* Telling Time; *Los
   datos personales;* Pronunciation of *Ñ, R,
   RR, LL,* and *Y; Exposición*
Electronic Workbook

Chapter 5
La familia

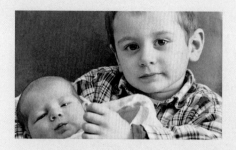

Chapter 6
La farmacia

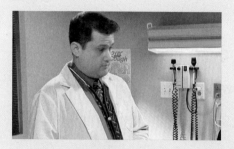

Chapter 7
La nutrición y las dietas

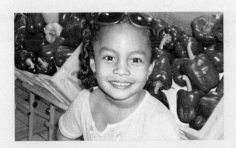

Chapter 8
El examen físico

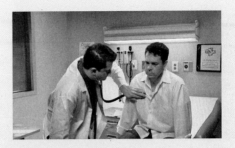

Chapter 9
«¿Qué pasó?»

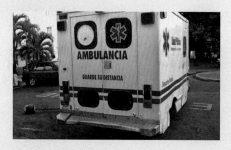

COMMUNICATION GOALS

VOCABULARY

STRUCTURE

CULTURAL NOTE

COMPANION WEBSITE

Chapter 10
Padecimientos e historia médica

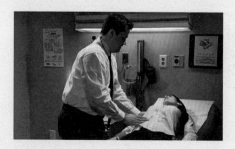

COMMUNICATION GOALS

VOCABULARY

STRUCTURE

CULTURAL NOTE

COMPANION WEBSITE

Chapter 11
Internamientos, odontología y la salud mental

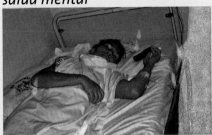

COMMUNICATION GOALS

VOCABULARY

STRUCTURE

CULTURAL NOTE

COMPANION WEBSITE

Chapter 12
Maternidad y protección **sexual**

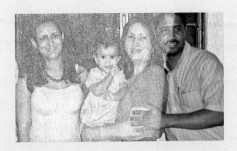

COMMUNICATION GOALS

VOCABULARY

STRUCTURE

CULTURAL NOTE

COMPANION WEBSITE

Preface

Effective communication is essential in health care, and communication is most effective when both parties share a common language. Ideally, patients articulate history, symptoms, and their understanding of diagnosis and treatment recommendations. Health care workers clarify this information, teach patients about treatment options, and obtain informed consent for procedures. In a series of exchanges, the practitioner and patient negotiate not only a correct understanding of factual information, but appreciation for broader issues of roles and expectations as well. This ideal exchange is often challenged by language and cultural differences.

When the patient and the health care provider do not speak the same language, the provider must accommodate the patient. Language accommodation increases health care access for a growing clientele of people with limited English proficiency. Providers who accommodate the patient's language elicit better information for diagnosis and treatment and inspire patients to follow recommendations, thus reducing delays in seeking care, enhancing quality of care, and improving treatment outcomes. When health care providers are able to include family and community members in communication, patients are more able to make use of these informal supports.

Language accommodation, also called language-access services, helps to meet legal requirements and accreditation standards, increases patient satisfaction and retention, and may decrease malpractice claims. Good practice is the best inoculation against malpractice. The angry patient is the most likely to become litigious. Efforts to form satisfying relationships and invest in effective communication may help reduce exposure to costly judicial intervention.

Working in two languages is satisfying to health care givers as well. With more than a competitive edge in the job market, bilingual health care workers gain the ability to communicate directly with patients who otherwise would require an interpreter. Of course, qualified medical interpreters are essential for complex communication tasks that are beyond the language ability of the practitioner. However, in many high-frequency interactions a functionally bilingual professional is able to conduct specific interviews in the patient's language without inappropriately relying on a family member or non-qualified person as interpreter. Nonnative speakers of a second language develop positive attitudes toward the second language and its speakers. They learn to appreciate the challenges and accomplishments of their patients who acquire English as a second language. Bilingual health care workers are more sensitive to cultural nuances that affect communication, relationship styles, and treatment adherence. In addition, studies have shown that bilingualism itself promotes memory and helps postpone age-related cognitive losses.

United States law requires language accommodation. Title VI of the Civil Rights Act of 1964 prohibited the exclusion of individuals from federally funded activities on the basis of race, color, or national origin. Almost ten years later in California, a group of students of Chinese origin raised its concern that inconsistent access to English as a Second Language instruction in the San Francisco Unified School District kept some students from receiving a meaningful education. The United States Supreme Court addressed this (Lau v. Nichols, January 21, 1974) by clarifying that Title VI prohibited conduct that had a disproportionate effect on limited-English-proficiency individuals, because such conduct constituted national origin discrimination.

In the United States, most hospitals and health care providers receive federal money from at least one source. The Civil Rights Division of the United States Department of Justice enforces laws that require taking reasonable steps to provide meaningful access for limited-English-proficiency (LEP) individuals. LEP individuals do not speak English as their primary language and have a limited ability to read, write, speak, or understand English. Many LEP persons are in the process of learning English and have various levels of proficiency. LEP status may be context specific. That is, an individual may have sufficient English skills to communicate basic information but not to communicate detailed medical or affective information in English.

Health care institutions and individual providers are encouraged to identify the extent to which patients from their service area require language accommodation services and to make a plan to address these needs. The plan may include training staff to work effectively with LEP persons, advising patients of the availability of language services, confirming the language skills and role understanding of interpreters and bilingual staff, and providing accurate written translations of important documents.

The Record of Care requirements of the Joint Commission (JCAHO) require hospitals and other providers to identify and document the patient's preferred language for discussing health care. *Preferred language* is similar to *primary language* in the practical matter of assessing the need for language access services. However, the standard of documenting *preferred language* refers to the language that the limited-English-proficiency individual identifies as the language that he or she wants to use when communicating with his or her health care providers. Preferred language takes precedence over primary language. Also, when the patient is a child, then the communication needs of the parents, guardian, or surrogate decision maker must be determined.

The Human Resources requirements of JCAHO include measuring the proficiency of language interpreters. The requirements of the Provision of Care and Rights and Responsibilities of the Individual call for organizations to respect the right and need of patients for effective communication, and require that they provide oral and written communication appropriate to the patient's preferred language.

In many areas, Latinos suffer disproportionately from preventable diseases, late prenatal care, and hospitalization for chronic conditions such as childhood asthma and complications of adult diabetes. Although poverty and lack of insurance can be factors, studies have identified a relationship between level of English proficiency and adverse events resulting in physical harm. Adequately addressing an individual patient's language and cultural needs will improve patient safety, health outcomes, and quality of care.

Practitioners and health care organizations can take various steps toward becoming linguistically competent and accessible. These include hiring clinically, linguistically, and culturally competent bilingual staff; employing qualified interpreters; and providing materials written in the target language. Bilingual employees who work in two languages must be carefully screened for their linguistic proficiency in both languages, rewarded for their important contribution, and given interpreter and cultural competency training. Qualified interpreter agencies are useful when proven bilingual staff is not available, and telephone services should be reserved for emergencies. Professionals who work through interpreters can seek training to learn to use interpreters more effectively.

Monolingualism can be cured. Taking a course based on *An Introduction to Medical Spanish* is a good first step toward acquiring Spanish as a second language for providers who are committed to relating directly with patients seeking health services. Subsequent steps include further course work, regular practice with native speakers, and if possible, an immersion experience in a Spanish-speaking country or community.

Acknowledgments

First, heartfelt thanks to you, the students, professors, institutions, and medical professionals who use this book to enhance relationships and improve communication with patients. This book becomes worthwhile when you speak Spanish with the people you serve.

Thanks to wonderful friends who enrich our lives. Frequently we call upon minuteman wordsmith José Durán Toribio to propose the best word or phrase in a pinch. Other friends are medical dialogue experts from a variety of medical specialties, including Doctor Jorge Amarante, *nutriólogo clínico;* Doctor Josephina Rodríguez R., *fisiatra;* psychiatrist Alexandre Carré, MD; pediatrician Angela Geddis, MD; and general practitioner William F. Jiménez P. They helped with lexical needs assessments so that you learn the Spanish for the words and phrases you most frequently use. In addition, these generous physicians quickly responded to our requests for review of many passages. Frank Dlugoleski of DartZ Business Solutions has been our artist since the first edition appeared in 1998, illustrating language with graphics. Frank and his wife Brenda are valued friends. Our long-time friend, musician Karina Jiménez again blessed us with her beautiful voice to record additions to the audio program.

We are grateful for the many ways in which our *Drama improvisado* practice activities have been inspired by the pioneering work of Viola Spolin, by classes and practice sessions that we have enjoyed with the Sea Tea Comedy Improvisation Troupe of Hartford, Connecticut, and by fellow student improvisers and daring Spanish students. These add fun to your classroom experience and promote more spontaneous thinking and speech.

We send sincere thanks to our development editor, Kris Swanson of Swanson Editorial Services. Kris expertly nitpicked as needed for precision's sake and made sure that we did not skip logical steps in the process of instruction. Kris helped to create the new *Exposición* feature, which deepens subject matter engagement and critical thinking by moving students to the presentational mode of communication. We are grateful to manuscript editor Deborah Bruce-Hostler, who has been a valuable asset since the fourth edition. We acknowledge with thanks our team at Yale University Press, including Sarah Miller, Ash Lago, Ann-Marie Imbornoni, and Internet gurus Thomas Breen and Travis Kimbel.

Contemplating the fifth edition, we sent surveys to a group of professors who had adopted the fourth edition. These professors told us what they liked about the program and contributed ideas for improvement. Then we sent surveys to a group of professors who had used other texts, to learn about their needs and particular situations. After reviewing and synthesizing all responses, we dedicated ourselves to addressing the linguistic needs and pedagogic preferences of as many classrooms as possible.

We thank both groups of professor-collaborators for their time in responding to surveys and for their thoughtfulness in providing constructive feedback. They include Carmen Tarantino, University of Tampa; Diana Aldrete, Goodwin College; Kimberly Vázquez, Spalding University; Giuditta Monterosso, MassBay Community College; Lois B. Cooper, Berkshire Community College; Dr. Elena M. De Costa, Carroll University; Joseph McClanahan, Creighton University; Nataly Tcherepashenets, State University of New York at Empire State College; Irena Stefanova, Contra Costa College; Elena Lattarulo, National University; Juan A. Thomas, Utica College; Araceli Canalini, Chicago State University; María Cristina Campos Fuentes, DeSales University; Cecilia Tenorio, Purdue University; Dana Monsein, Endicott College; Mauricio Almonte, Florida Atlantic University; Kathleen Thompson-Casado, University of Toledo; Angela Helmer, University of South Dakota; Myrta Mathews, Penn State University; Herman Johnson, Xavier University of Louisiana; Ann Ortiz, Campbell University; Robert L. Turner, University of South Dakota; Katie Sinclair, North Carolina Central University; an unnamed professor from the International Languages Department of the Dominican University of California; Maryann Brady, Rivier University; Rafael Pérez, Winston-Salem State University; Margaret A. Morales, Saint Francis University (Pennsylvania); and M. Virginia Braxs, Washington University of Saint Louis.

Introduction

An Introduction to Medical Spanish facilitates better communication between health care providers and the growing Spanish-speaking community in the diaspora. It is not a phrase book or a translator. It is a first course in Spanish, progressively merging conversation and a health care lexicon in various medical contexts. Although it does not call for a prerequisite knowledge of Spanish, this book is also helpful to people who speak limited Spanish and aspire to apply their Spanish in a medical setting. Topics include building the patient-practitioner relationship, the patient's chief complaint, taking medical history, and defining current symptoms. We progress to injuries, pharmacotherapy, diet and nutrition, tests and procedures, diagnoses, and specialized topics such as hospitalizations, dentistry, illnesses, heart disease, tropical and infectious diseases, neurology, mental health and addictions, palliative care, maternity, pediatrics, and sexual protection.

New to the Fifth Edition

Prior to this fifth edition, we solicited comments and suggestions from professors from all over the United States who had adopted the text, and from a group of professors who had not adopted the text. The feedback led to an expanded lexicon to support communication about muscles, heart disease, pediatric and neurologic screening examinations, and emerging tropical and infectious diseases, including zika. We created new illustrations to support the expanded lexicon.

With regard to the larger lexicon, to make longer vocabulary lists less daunting, we divided several into *Palabras de frecuente uso* and *Palabras para completar su léxico*. We considered presenting vocabulary outside of semantically related groups, as some believe this produces learning that is more resistant to interference. However, we maintained the contextual organization in view of the use of the book as a vocabulary reference and in view of the benefits to memory of organizing information to be memorized. We added a vocabulary recap at the end of each chapter, and lengthened the audio program to accommodate much of the newer vocabulary.

With regard to structure, we reviewed grammar explanations for clarity, conciseness, and quick integration into medical dialogue. We added the present progressive tense and the use of direct and indirect object pronouns together.

We created a more robust, interactive, and easier-to-navigate companion website, relocated the video program there, and added an electronic workbook of self-correcting learning activities. Access to the website is free with the purchase of a new book. We updated the audio program on the website to accommodate the expanded lexicon and to include audio comprehension exercises and samples of student presentational mode projects. You'll be able to download helpful graphics such as the skeleton, the pain scale, history-taking forms in Spanish, and the classroom activity sheets that support survey-taking communicative activities. By moving the video program to the website, we created room for additional lexicon in the book and increased the video's accessibility.

The video consists of twenty-four video clips that are brief enough to enhance "replay-ability" and not overwhelm the student. Video segments are called *La trama* (the plot) and *Demostración*. *La trama* is a series of interactions between the Flores family, Dr. Vargas, and nurse Rosmery. These closely follow the lexicon and grammar as they develop in the book. *Demostración* is a segment that demonstrates a specific communication task in health care. For example, in chapter 4, Rosmery demonstrates taking telephone numbers.

We clarified *Drama improvisado* instructions without imposing excessive structure, and many of these were changed to more closely resemble actual, proven improvisation games that are used in theater classes and useful in developing more spontaneous speech. We put these to the test with our students at Tunxis Community College and the University of Saint Joseph, where students enjoyed the creative play and regarded the exercises as helpful.

We added a presentational mode activity called *Exposición,* in which students practice specific linguistic skills by listening to a model reading (found on the companion website), organizing information presented, and creating an analogous presentation. This consolidates vocabulary, stimulates subject matter engagement, promotes critical thinking, enhances student participation, and increases the persistence of new skills.

Pedagogy and Chapter Sections

The crucial precepts of the book are context and communication. Vocabulary is organized by specific medical themes, and grammar lessons support the goal of conversing with patients. The message is first, and the student learns correct speech by using language for a purpose. For this reason, the text is divided into sections that are named for the practical communication goals, such as "Test a Patient's Orientation." This affirms the student's goal of learning the functional language that delivers health care in a patient's preferred language. Grammar appears in the context of specific communication tasks. For example, command forms are taught in the context of giving medication instructions. This is a guided, learn-by-doing approach in which students acquire language while using it in meaningful interaction.

 A soccer goal icon identifies a broad communication goal, and heads a large section of material. This backward design in lesson planning calls for focus on what students soon will know how to do. With a goal in mind, we provide nearly 300 learning experiences in the form of in-class activities that compel students to speak Spanish in the classroom, preparing them for the emotional and linguistic challenges of speaking to native-Spanish-speaking patients. These are organized under the headings *Hacia precisión,* referring to mechanical exercises that promote accurate speech; and *Hacia fluidez,* which signals interaction activities that develop abilities in the interpersonal mode of communication.

A bicycle icon denotes *Ejercicios,* or directed activities that usually have one correct response and are intended to promote accuracy. These are predominant in the first chapter, where everything may be new to you; and in the chapter about pharmacy, where accuracy is critical. You'll find an Answer Key to the *Ejercicios* at the end of the book, and we omitted from the Answer Key those exercises whose responses may vary greatly.

An icon of faces identifies communicative *Actividades,* which are interactive and more open-ended. They call for students to use Spanish to complete a practical task that is typical to a medical setting. These require creating with language. The instructor provides coaching and consultation, and students practice with partners, play roles, and solve problems.

Two Greek drama masks signal unscripted improvisation activities, called *Drama improvisado.* This cross-pollination of theater and language acquisition is a hyperextension of the communicative classroom. Improvisation promotes spontaneous speech and interpersonal communication. During improvisation, you practice the Spanish that you know, and may clarify your message with gestures as needed. This helps to keep your thoughts in the target language and transforms the frustration of being a novice speaker into playful fun. Improvisation exercises help groups of students to become supportive teams. When you improvise, you climb a scaffold of grammar and vocabulary and speak within a loosely prescribed social and lexical context. Of all the risks you'll take as a novice speaker, improvisation may be the most enjoyable. Improvisation is a fun way to build confidence. Of these exercises, one student said, "I like the games. You can talk. You can make mistakes. It is fun. In my English class we just listen."

The girder icon alerts you to a grammar explanation that is peppered with language examples. Grammar should be secondary to immersion and communication, and is a worthwhile shortcut to developing more accurate speech.

When acquiring a second language, it is not possible to review too much. A three-arrow recycling icon appears next to *Reciclaje* activities that consolidate learning by showing new uses for previously learned vocabulary and structures. These first appear in chapter 3 and are placed at the end of each chapter prior to the *Exposición* feature.

 An *Exposición* feature is new to the fifth edition, and guides you into the presentational mode of communication. You'll listen to models and organize information as you plan to present cases and patient education content.

 Earbuds let you know that the identified exercise, conversation, or vocabulary list is available on the website. You can listen online or download audio files to your smart phone or other personal digital audio player. The audio program script may be downloaded from the website as well.

A Cultural Note appears near the end of each chapter. These inform you on matters of immigration, acculturation, worldviews, diverse customs, communication styles, and language accommodation to support your development of an even more culturally competent practice.

The medical information and illustrations included in the text are not intended to diagnose or treat illnesses. Although these dialogues, vignettes, and exercises are derived from lexical needs assessments and the authors' experiences interpreting for and observing diverse practitioners, they are included here for the sole purpose of teaching language.

Chapter 1
«Buenos días, soy médico»

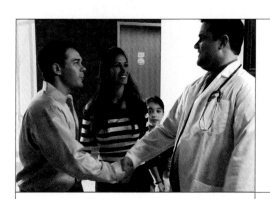

Communication Goals

Greet Your Patient and Introduce
Yourself   2

Ask Your Patient's Name   17

Describe People   19

Vocabulary

Structure

Cultural Note

Website   www.yalebooks.com/medicalspanish

Video   *Trama: Presentaciones y especialidades; Demostración: Presentaciones*

Audio   Greetings and Farewells; Professions; Personal Characteristics; Pronunciation
of Vowels; *Exposición*

Electronic Workbook

By the time you finish this book, you will be able to conduct essential medical interviews in Spanish, including patient registration, history-taking and physical examinations, common procedures, instructions for diet and pharmacotherapy, and health education. You will be able to talk about common illnesses and conditions, tropical diseases, mental health, reproductive care, and safer sex practices. You will be more aware of some cultural dynamics of the healing relationship. With practice and experience, you will be able to communicate effectively in Spanish in your medical setting. By the end of this chapter you will be able to greet patients in Spanish, introduce yourself by name and profession, and describe people.

Greet Your Patient and Introduce Yourself

Diálogo

The earbuds icon signals that you can listen to this portion of text on the website and download it as an .mp3 file

Dr. Vargas: Buenos días. Soy el doctor Vargas.
Sr. Flores: Buenos días, doctor. Soy Francisco Flores.
Dr. Vargas: Mucho gusto.
Sr. Flores: El gusto es mío. ¿Cómo está usted?
Dr. Vargas: Muy bien, gracias, ¿y usted?
Sr. Flores: Bien, bien, gracias.

Vocabulario: Saludos y despedidas (*Greetings and Farewells*)

Hola.	Hello.
Buenos días.	Good morning.
Buenas tardes.	Good afternoon.
Buenas noches.	Good evening; good night.

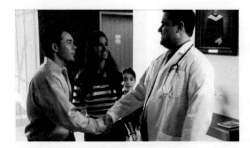
«Mucho gusto».

¿Cómo está usted?	How are you? (formal, use with adults)
¿Cómo estás?	How are you? (informal, use with children and friends)
Estoy bien, gracias.	I am fine, thank you.
Muy bien.	Very well.
Me alegro.	I'm glad.
¿Y usted?	And you?
Estoy mal.	I'm ill.
Lo siento.	I'm sorry.
De nada.	You're welcome.
Mucho gusto.	Pleased to meet you.
Encantado/a.	Pleased to meet you.
El gusto es mío.	The pleasure is mine.
Igual / Igualmente.	Same here.
Adiós.	Good-bye.
Hasta luego.	See you later.

Preguntas útiles

¿Cómo se llama usted?	What is your name?
¿De dónde es usted?	Where are you from?

Expresiones útiles

Soy el doctor Vargas.	I am doctor Vargas.
Soy la doctora González.	I am doctor González.
Me llamo Francisco Flores.	My name is Francisco Flores.
Soy de Puerto Rico.	I am from Puerto Rico.
Soy puertorriqueño/a.	I am Puerto Rican.
Le presento a la doctora García.	I introduce you to Doctor García.
Es cardióloga.	She is a cardiologist.

HACIA PRECISIÓN

1.1 Ejercicio _____

> The bicycle signals a mechanical exercise, usually with one correct answer. Answers to most *ejercicios* may be found in the Answer Key at the end of the book.

Write two of the above expressions for each of the following language functions. Include accents and punctuation marks.

A. Greeting _____

_____

B. Taking leave _____

_____

C. Introducing oneself _____

_____

D. Expressing joy/sympathy _____

_____

E. Responding to an introduction _____

_____

1.2 Ejercicio_____

In this dialogue, Dr. Vargas greets a patient at his clinic. The rest of the lines are out of order. Put them in the correct order by numbering them in the spaces provided. Then with a partner read your finished product to the class.

_1_	Dr. Vargas:	Buenos días. Soy el doctor Vargas.
____	Sr. Flores:	Bien, bien, gracias. Doctor, le presento a mi esposa Marisol García de Flores.
____	Dr. Vargas:	Muy bien, gracias, ¿y usted?
____	Sr. Flores:	El gusto es mío. ¿Cómo está usted?
____	Dr. Vargas:	Encantado.
____	Dr. Vargas:	Soy de Puerto Rico.
____	Sra. Flores:	Igualmente. Usted habla español. ¿De dónde es usted?
____	Dr. Vargas:	Mucho gusto.
____	Sr. Flores:	Buenos días, doctor. Soy Francisco Flores.

HACIA FLUIDEZ

A faces icon marks an activity in which students work with partners. Switch roles often and share your results with the class whenever prompted by the instructor.

1.3 Actividad _____

The instructor will read greetings and farewells to demonstrate pronunciation. After group practice, get up and move around the room, greeting each person. It is customary to shake hands when you greet someone. When finished, volunteer to act out for the class the best of your exchanges.

Note that many people consider *hola* too casual for a first meeting. The letter "h" is silent in Spanish, as in *hola* (OH-la) and *hospital* (os-pi-TAL). There are pronunciation sections at the end of each of the first five chapters, and corresponding recordings are posted on the website.

1.4 Actividad_____

From your places, take turns introducing yourselves to your neighbor by name.

Modelo: Estudiante 1:   Buenas tardes. Me llamo Paul. ¿Cómo se llama usted?
            Estudiante 2:   Buenas tardes. Me llamo Carol.
            Clase: Hola, Carol. ¿Cómo está usted?
            Estudiante 2:   Bien, gracias. (Then to student 3) Buenas tardes. Me llamo Carol. ¿Cómo se llama usted?

Continue in this way until everyone has had a turn.

1.5 Actividad_____

Finish and act out the following conversations with a partner.

A. —Buenas tardes. Me llamo _____ . ¿Cómo se llama usted?

   —Me _____ .

   —Mucho _____ .

   — _____ .

B. —¿Cómo _____ ?

   —Estoy muy bien, gracias.

   —Me _____ .

   —¿Y usted? _____ ?

   —Estoy _____

C. —Hola, me llamo _____ . ¿De dónde _____?

   —Soy _____ .

   —Hasta luego.

   — _____ .

1.6 Drama improvisado _____

Form a circle. Everyone's name is *doctor* or *doctora González.* One student addresses another across the circle and says, *«Buenos días, doctor/a González».* The second student responds, *«Buenos días, doctor/a González».* The first, still addressing the second, gestures to a third student and states, *«Doctor/a González, le presento al doctor / a la doctora González».* The pattern repeats, with the second student addressing the third student, *«Buenos días, doctor/a González»* and the third student replying to the second as the second had to the first. The second then introduces the third to a fourth *doctor/a González.* The game continues and increases in pace. If someone makes an error, the errant person becomes *doctor/a Rodríguez.* From that point on, this student must be addressed with his or her new name. Anyone who calls a *doctor/a Rodríguez* by the name *doctor/a González* or vice versa becomes a *doctor/a Rodríguez.*

 ## Estructura: El género y número de los nombres y artículos definidos (*Gender and Number of Nouns and Definite Articles*)

- In Spanish some nouns are masculine, like *el hospital* (the hospital), while others are feminine, like *la cama* (the bed). With some exceptions, nouns ending in *-o* are masculine, and nouns ending in *-a* are feminine. (*Día* is masculine, so we say ¡Buen día! *Mano* is feminine, so we say *la mano.*)
- Some nouns that refer to people change the last letter to become masculine or feminine. A male nurse is *el enfermero,* and a female nurse is *la enfermera.* Similarly, nouns indicating national origin or ethnicity, such as *norteamericano,* end in either *-o* or *-a,* according to the gender of the person to whom they refer. Ethnicities are not capitalized.

    Soy Marcos. Soy enfermero. Soy argentino.
    La doctora García es cirujana. No es argentina, es mexicana.

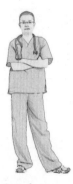 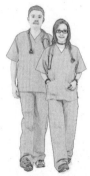 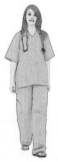 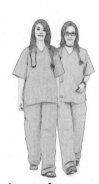

el enfermero   los enfermeros   la enfermera   las enfermeras

- The nouns for professions ending in *-iatra* and *-ista*, such as *el/la pediatra* and *el/la ortopedista*, can be either masculine or feminine. In these cases the definite articles indicate gender. A male pediatrician is *el pediatra*, while a female pediatrician is *la pediatra*, and the same is true for *el ortopedista* and *la ortopedista*.
- When speaking about a third person and using a title with the last name, the definite article is placed before the title, as in *El doctor Brito es chileno*. The definite article is not used when addressing someone, as in *Buenas tardes, doctor Brito*.
- Nouns ending in *-e*, such as *paciente* and *estudiante*, can be either masculine or feminine, depending on the gender of the person. A male student is *el estudiante*, while a female student is *la estudiante*. Words ending in *-ción*, such as *la infección*, are feminine. Most words ending in *-ma* or *-pa* are masculine and are of Greek origin: for example, *el mapa*, *el problema*, and *el sistema*.
- To make nouns plural in Spanish we add *-s* to nouns that end in vowels and *-es* to those ending in consonants. The articles and nouns must always agree in gender and number. The plural masculine article is *los*, and the plural feminine article is *las*.

Singular	*Plural*
el enfermero	los enfermeros
la enfermera	las enfermeras
el doctor	los doctores
la doctora	las doctoras
el hospital	los hospitales

HACIA PRECISIÓN

 1.7 Ejercicio _____

Change the nouns to agree with the gender of the person.

> The letter *ñ* is pronounced like the "ni" in the word "onion."

Modelo: El señor Nieves es secretario. / la señora Nieves
—El señor Nieves es secretario; la señora Nieves es secretaria.

A. El doctor Colón es neurólogo. / la doctora Palma
B. El doctor Aquino es odontólogo. / la doctora Losada
C. Ana es trabajadora social. / Tomás
D. El señor García es consejero. / la señora Marques
E. Leomara es farmacéutica. / Alfredo
F. El doctor Mena es psiquiatra. / la doctora Mariano
G. La doctora López es cardióloga. / el doctor López
H. La doctora Negrón es dentista. / el doctor José Peña Ortiz

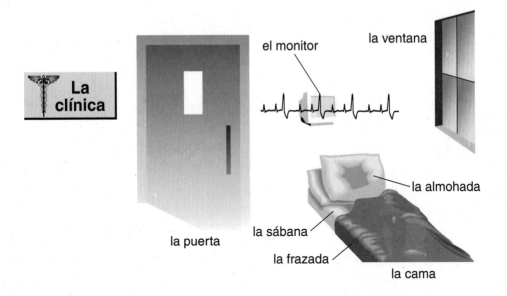

el monitor

la ventana

La clínica

la almohada

la puerta

la sábana

la frazada

la cama

 1.8 Ejercicio

Give the plural of the following nouns and definite articles.

Modelo: la trabajadora social / las trabajadoras sociales

A. la clínica   _____ _____

B. la puerta   _____ _____

C. el monitor   _____ _____

D. la cama   _____ _____

E. la sábana   _____ _____

F. la frazada   _____ _____

G. la almohada   _____ _____

H. el doctor   _____ _____

I. el hospital   _____ _____

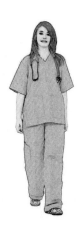
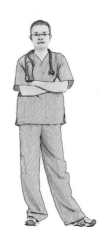

Somos enfermeros.

Estructura: Los sujetos y el verbo *ser* (*Subject Pronouns and the Verb* Ser)

- A sentence requires a subject and a verb. Subjects and verbs can be in the first, second, or third person. Speaking in the first person is to speak of oneself. Speaking in the second person is to ask about or tell about the person or persons whom you are addressing. Speaking in the third person is to ask or tell about someone else.

	Singular	*Plural*
First person	*yo* (I)	*nosotros* (we, masculine and mixed gender)
		nosotras (we, feminine)
Second person	*tú* (you, familiar)	*vosotros** (you, familiar)
	usted (you, formal)	*ustedes* (you, formal)
Third person	*él* (he)	*ellos* (they, masculine and mixed gender)
	ella (she)	*ellas* (they, feminine)

* Vosotros is used in Spain and not presented in this text. Latin Americans generally understand this form but use *ustedes* for the second person plural.

- In the second person, note that *tú* is normally used when addressing a child or someone with whom you are on a first-name basis. With adults, using *tú* where *usted* would be proper may offend. Ethnic groups from the Caribbean use the *tú* form with adults more readily than others, but one should use *usted* when in doubt. In the third person, note that *él* means "he" and *el* means "the."
- The plural masculine forms *nosotros* and *ellos* are used for a group of all males or a mixed group of males and females; the plural feminine forms *nosotras* and *ellas* are used with groups of all females.
- The verb *ser* means "to be." Use it to tell your name, occupation, characteristics, and national origin. As in English (I am, you are), the verb changes its form depending on its subject. Note that with the forms *soy* and *eres,* the pronoun is implied, but the form *es* can mean *you are, she is, he is,* or *it is* and may require a subject to clarify its meaning. The subject and verb may be reversed to form a question: *¿Es usted doctor?* Many grammars show a verb conjugation chart like this:

yo **soy**	I am	**Soy** Manuel.
tú **eres**	you are	**Eres** inteligente.
usted, él, ella **es**	you are; he, she is	**¿Es** usted la madre?
nosotros, nosotras **somos**	we are	Tú y yo **somos** mexicanas.
ustedes, ellos, ellas **son**	you (plural), they are	Ellos **son** cardiólogos.

HACIA PRECISIÓN

 1.9 Ejercicio

You work in an emergency room. In the spaces, indicate whether you would use *tú* or *usted* with the following people. Recall that *tú* is used when addressing a child or someone with whom you are on a first-name basis.

A. the Spanish-speaking nurse who usually works with you _____

B. your patient, age five _____

C. your new pediatric patient's mother _____

D. the new cardiologist from Guatemala, whom you've not met _____

E. a friend from Spanish class who meets you for lunch _____

F. your new patient, age forty-seven _____

1.10 Ejercicio

Subject pronouns can substitute for the name of a person and act as the subject of the verb. Identify the implied Spanish pronouns or subjects and add the appropriate form of the verb *ser,* as in the example. Note that the Spanish word *y* means "and," and is pronounced like "ee" in the English word "see."

Modelo: Juan   <u>él es</u>

A. el Sr. Romero	_____	F. la clase y yo	_____
B. Juan y yo	_____	G. los doctores	_____
C. Sergio y Ana	_____	H. el doctor y el enfermero	_____
D. las enfermeras	_____	I. la clínica	_____
E. la familia	_____	J. usted, usted y usted	_____

 ## Vocabulario: Las profesiones

Palabras de frecuente uso

el asociado médico,* la asociada médica	physician's assistant
el/la ayudante de enfermero	nurse's aide
el cardiólogo, la cardióloga	cardiologist
el cirujano, la cirujana	surgeon
el/la dentista	dentist
el odontólogo, la odontóloga	dentist
el/la dietista	dietitian
el doctor, la doctora	doctor
el médico, la médica	doctor
el enfermero, la enfermera	nurse
el/la estudiante de medicina	medical student
el farmacéutico, la farmacéutica	pharmacist

*The Spanish translation of "physician's assistant," *asociado médico,* was adopted by the American Academy of Physician Assistants in 1998 and reaffirmed in 2003. Due to the profession's uniqueness to the United States, the nurse practitioner does not have a concise counterpart in Spanish. Depending on state laws, you may say, *un enfermero con licencia para diagnosticar y tratar padecimientos y recetar medicamentos* (a nurse who has a license to diagnose and treat ailments and prescribe medications).

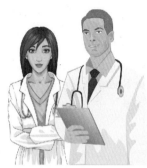

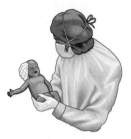

el obstetra

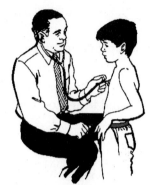

la doctora   el doctor

el pediatra

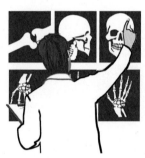

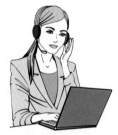

la secretaria

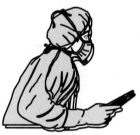

la radióloga

la cirujana

el ginecólogo,* la ginecóloga	gynecologist
el médico general, la médica general	general practitioner
el médico/la médica de cabecera	general practitioner
el médico internista, la médica internista	internist
el neurólogo, la neuróloga	neurologist
el/la obstetra	obstetrician
el/la ortopedista	orthopedist
el otorrinolaringólogo, la otorrinolaringóloga	ENT doctor
el/la pediatra	pediatrician
el psicólogo, la psicóloga	psychologist
el/la psiquiatra	psychiatrist
el radiólogo, la radióloga	radiologist
el/la recepcionista	receptionist
el secretario, la secretaria	secretary
el técnico de radiografía, la técnica de radiografía	x-ray technician

*The letter *g* is like a harsh, throaty English "h" when it precedes the vowels *e* and *i*. It is like the "g" in the English word "go" before the vowels *a, o,* and *u. Ginecólogo* contains an example of both. *J* is always pronounced like a throaty English "h," as in *cirujano.* Many words have accents that guide pronunciation.

el terapeuta físico, la terapeuta física	physical therapist
el terapeuta respiratorio, la terapeuta respiratoria	respiratory therapist
el trabajador social, la trabajadora social	social worker

Preguntas útiles

¿En qué trabaja usted?	What do you do for work?
¿Cuál es su especialidad?	What is your specialty?

Palabras para completar su léxico

el alergólogo, la alergóloga	allergist
el anestesiólogo, la anestesióloga	anesthesiologist
el audiólogo, la audióloga	audiologist
el comadrón, la comadrona	midwife
el consejero, la consejera	counselor
el dermatólogo, la dermatóloga	dermatologist
el endocrinólogo, la endocrinóloga	endocrinologist
el/la higienista dental	dental hygienist
el neumólogo, la neumóloga	pulmonologist
el/la nutricionista	nutritionist
el oftalmólogo, la oftalmóloga	ophthalmologist
el oncólogo, la oncóloga	oncologist
el partero, la partera	midwife
el podólogo, la podóloga	podiatrist
el reumatólogo, la reumatóloga	rheumatologist
el terapeuta, la terapeuta	therapist
el/la terapeuta del habla	speech therapist
el urólogo, la uróloga	urologist

HACIA PRECISIÓN

 1.11 Ejercicio_____

Words that look or sound similar in two languages and have the same meaning are called "close cognates." Those that look or sound similar and have different meanings are called "false cognates" and may lead to misunderstanding. You'll safely assume the meaning of the following close cognates. Listen to the instructor read the following patient chief concerns, and refer him or her to the appropriate discipline. Some have multiple correct responses.

Modelo:	Profesor:	Sufro de migrañas.
	Estudiantes:	Usted debe consultar con un neurólogo.

usted debe consultar
you should consult

A. Necesito una inyección.

B. Sufro de problemas cardíacos.

C. Sufro de diabetes.

D. Necesito una colecistectomía.

E. Sufro de cáncer de los pulmones.

F. Sufro de cataratas.

G. Necesito un rayo equis.

H. Necesito una dieta especial.

I. Sufro de problemas emocionales.

J. Sufro de artritis.

K. Tengo la clavícula fracturada.

L. Sufro de psoriasis.

M. Mi bebé tiene fiebre.

N. Me duele una muela.

- Spanish does not use the definite article *el* or *la* (the) or the indefinite article *un* or *una* (a, an) after the verb *ser* when stating a profession or nationality, unless the noun is modified.

Soy médico.	I am a doctor.
Ella es puertorriqueña.	She is Puerto Rican.
El Dr. Ortíz es un buen doctor.	Dr. Ortíz is a good doctor.

- The definite article is used with titles. *Ella es la doctora Meléndez.* Such titles as *doctor/doctora* and *señor/señora* are capitalized only when abbreviated (*Dr./Dra.* and *Sr./Sra.*).

HACIA FLUIDEZ

 1.12 Actividad _____

It is time for a soirée! Find the Spanish name for your current—or future—profession. Next, move around the classroom making introductions and asking questions to complete your knowledge.

> Modelo: —Buenas tardes. Soy Roberto. Soy enfermero.
> —Mucho gusto, Roberto. Soy Nancy.
> —Encantado. ¿En qué trabaja usted?
> —Soy médica.
> —¿Cuál es su especialidad?
> —Soy oftalmóloga.

Continue until you have spoken with everyone. When you have finished, take turns reporting your findings to the class. For example, *Ella es Nancy. Es oftalmóloga. Él es William. Es cirujano.* To make an introduction, say, *Clase, les presento a Nancy. Es oftalmóloga.*

1.13 Drama improvisado _____

Let's play our first game of "Categories." Form a circle, everybody holding one finger up. The first person makes eye contact with a person across the circle and states the name of a profession (*la uróloga,* for example). That person lowers his or her finger, makes eye contact with another, and states the name of a different profession. Continue until everyone has a profession (no duplicates), with the first person being last to receive one. Recall who said what to you and what you said to whom. Next, go through the list in that same order multiple times. Make eye contact with your receiver prior to speaking. This is a fun way to use Spanish without translating. Later, we shall work at speaking two or three lists simultaneously.

 1.14 Drama improvisado _____

Let's play our first game of "Party Quirks." The instructor will choose a host and then give five or six students a folded slip of paper on which a medical profession has been written. Next, the host stands in the front of the room preparing a party, talking aloud about the preparation in Spanish if possible (e.g., naming foods as they are set on an imaginary table). One of the chosen students knocks on an imaginary door. The host opens the door and welcomes the guest inside. Both exchange small talk while the student portrays the role of his or her assigned profession using gestures, questions, and statements, saying anything but the name of the profession. Perhaps portray part of an exam. At a lull in the conversation, another student knocks. At the end, the host must guess each student's profession: *Zahra es odontóloga; Marek es ortopedista,* and so on. Then the instructor may interview partygoers to demonstrate the forms of the verb *ser.* If one profession is assigned to more than one student, you'll be able to practice the plural forms as well (*Susan y Rashid son otorrinolaringólogos*).

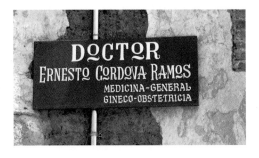

¿Cuáles son las tres especialidades del Dr. Ernesto Córdova Ramos?

Vocabulario: Los países y las identidades nacionales (*Countries and Ethnicities*)

Región	*País*	*Identidad nacional*
Europa		
	España	español/española
América del Norte		
	los Estados Unidos	estadounidense, norteamericano/a
	México	mexicano/a
El Caribe		
	Cuba	cubano/a
	la República Dominicana	dominicano/a
	Puerto Rico	puertorriqueño/a
América Central		
	Guatemala	guatemalteco/a
	Honduras	hondureño/a
	El Salvador	salvadoreño/a
	Nicaragua	nicaragüense
	Costa Rica	costarricense
	Panamá	panameño/a
América del Sur		
	Venezuela	venezolano/a
	Colombia	colombiano/a
	Ecuador	ecuatoriano/a
	Perú	peruano/a
	Bolivia	boliviano/a
	Paraguay	paraguayo/a
	Chile	chileno/a
	Uruguay	uruguayo/a
	Argentina	argentino/a

Preguntas útiles

¿De dónde es usted?	Where are you (formal) from?
¿De dónde eres?	Where are you (informal) from?

Expresiones útiles

Soy de Colombia.	I am from Colombia.
Soy colombiano/a.	I am Colombian.
La doctora es colombiana.	The doctor is Colombian.

> Some ethnic groups have popular words for their national identity. For example, Puerto Ricans may call themselves *boricuas* or *borinqueños/as*; Dominicans, *quisqueyanos/as*; and Costa Ricans, *ticos/as*. Puerto Rico is not a "country"; its people are full U.S. citizens. Immigrants to the United States may add the extension *americano/a* to their national origin when they wish to, as in *colombianoamericano*.

 ## Ask Your Patient's Name

«¿Cómo se llama usted?» *(What is your name?)*

Recall that *¿Cómo se llama usted?* means "What is your name?" Literally, it means "How do you call yourself?" The Spanish *ll* is pronounced like the English "y," although you'll notice that some groups give Spanish *ll* and *y* more of an English "j" or "zh" sound. The reflexive pronouns *se* and *te* are discussed in chapter 11. Here are some variations.

¿Cómo se llama usted?	What is your name?
¿Cómo te llamas?*	What is your name?
Me llamo Arturo.	My name is Arturo.
¿Cómo se llama el/la bebé?	What is the baby's name?
¿Cómo se llama el/la niño/a?	What is the child's name?
Él se llama Armando.	His name is Armando.
Ella se llama Roselín.	Her name is Roselín.

*This is the informal (*tú*) form, used with children and acquaintances.

HACIA FLUIDEZ

 1.15 Actividad _____

With so many new friends, it is time to update your contacts. Ask students who sit near you their name, profession, and national origin. Write the information for each and check your spelling.

Nombre: _____

Profesión: _____

Nacionalidad: _____

 1.16 Actividad _____

Role-play a case conference or morning rounds. Introduce yourselves to the rest of the class by name, occupation, and national origin.

Modelo: Estudiante: Hola. Me llamo Cristóbal. Soy dietista. Soy de los Estados Unidos.

Clase: Hola Cristóbal. Mucho gusto.

When you have finished, see who can introduce all of the people in the room. For example, *Ella es Nancy; es trabajadora social. Él es Bill; es cirujano. Es estadounidense.* If you forget someone's personal information, ask for it again.

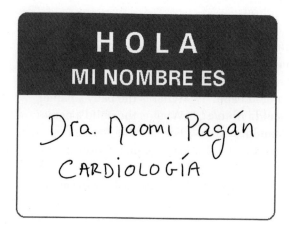

(1.17) Drama improvisado —————————————————

Play *"¿Cómo te llamas?"* Form a circle. The first student says his or her name, using *Me llamo* [*nombre*]. *Soy* [*profesión*]. While saying it, he or she makes a unique gesture (wave, bow, courtesy, bob, jump, etc.). Each student repeats the same sentences (using the first student's name, profession, and gesture). After going around the circle (quickly as you can!), the first student does it a second time, and the next student in line goes. Continue in this way until you know everyone's name. It is important to set a rhythm and follow it, to achieve a team dynamic.

 ## Describe People

 ## Vocabulario: Características personales

The verb *ser* is used to describe physical characteristics and personality traits. The following words are often used with *ser:*

rubio/a	blond, fair	**moreno/a***	brunette, dark
mayor, anciano/a	older, elderly	**joven**	young
grande	big	**pequeño/a**	small
alto/a	tall	**bajo/a**	short (height)
largo/a	long	**corto/a**	short (length)
mediano/a	medium	**gordo/a, obeso/a**	fat, obese
delgado/a	thin	**flaco/a**	skinny
bonito/a	pretty	**guapo/a**	handsome
feo/a	ugly	**bueno/a**	good
inteligente	intelligent	**simpático/a**	kind
amable	kind	**agradable**	pleasant
trabajador/a	hardworking	**muy****	very

*There is regional variation in the use of the word *moreno/a,* which is often used to refer to people with black hair in Spain and people in Spanish-speaking America with a rather dark complexion.

**Muy is an adverb and as such modifies an adjective. So say what you are thinking: *"Soy inteligente y muy guapo"*.

Preguntas útiles

¿Cómo es Marta?	What is Marta like?
¿Cómo está Marta?	How is Marta feeling?

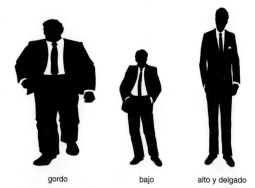

gordo   bajo   alto y delgado

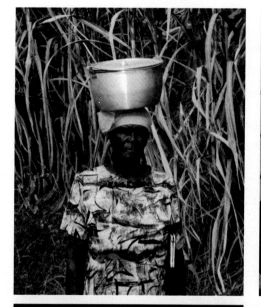

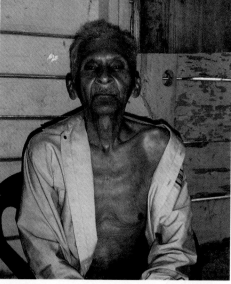

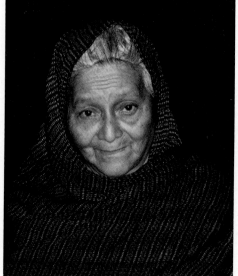

Above, left: Doña Gloria es dominicana y es morena. Su padre era de Haití.

Above, right: Don Samuel es rubio y anciano. Es muy delgado. Sus padres eran cubanos.

Left: Doña Otilia es de un pueblo de la región Mixe de Oaxaca, México. Es indígena y no habla español. Habla un dialecto precolombino.

Estructura: La concordancia de adjetivos, sustantivos y artículos indefinidos (*Agreement of Adjectives, Nouns, and Indefinite Articles*)

- Adjectives, like nouns, have gender (*género*) and number (*número*). Adjectives ending in -*o* change to -*a* to become feminine (e.g., *Jorge es alto; Miguelina es alta*). Adjectives ending in a vowel add -*s* to become plural and those ending in a consonant add -*es*.
- When an adjective modifies a noun, it must agree with that noun in gender and number. In Spanish a descriptive adjective normally *follows* the noun.

el ojo infectado	the infected eye
los ojos infectados	the infected eyes
la herida infectada	the infected wound
las heridas infectadas	the infected wounds
El enfermero es alto.	The (male) nurse is tall.
La doctora es delgada.	The (female) doctor is thin.

- Adjectives ending in -*e* modify both masculine and feminine nouns.

El niño es amable.	The boy is nice.
La niña es inteligente.	The girl is intelligent.

- The indefinite articles are *un, una, unos,* and *unas*. They correspond to "a," "an," and "some" in English and show both gender and number. The indefinite article is generally not used after forms of the verb *ser*, unless the object is modified. Verbs do not have gender, but the articles, nouns, and adjectives must agree in both gender and number. When referring to a mixed group of males and females, the male forms are used.

Marco es enfermero.	Marco is a nurse.
Marco es un enfermero nuevo.	Marco is a new nurse.
Ana es neuróloga.	Ana is a neurologist.
Ana es una neuróloga amable.	Ana is a kind neurologist.
Marco y Ana son altos.	Marco and Ana are tall.

HACIA PRECISIÓN

 1.18 Ejercicio_____

The instructor will ask for the opposite of each of the following words. For example, *¿Cuál es el opuesto de flaco?* Respond: *El opuesto de flaco es gordo.*

¿cuál? what?
opuesto opposite

A. alto   G. corto
B. delgado   H. joven
C. bajo   I. largo
D. pequeño   J. feo
E. anciano   K. gordo
F. grande   L. bonito

    1.19 Ejercicio

Recall that the indefinite article does not usually follow the verb *ser* unless an adjective is added. Agree with the descriptions of the following people. Remember to use the correct indefinite article when the noun is followed by an adjective.

Modelo: La profesora es simpática.
         Sí, es una profesora simpática.

A. La doctora es inteligente.   E. El médico es alto.
B. Los estudiantes son interesantes.   F. Los pacientes son delgados.
C. La enfermera es joven.   G. Los doctores son mayores.
D. El profesor es guapo.   H. El neurólogo es simpático.

    1.20 Ejercicio

To make a statement negative, place the word *no* before the verb. *Juan es alto* becomes *Juan no es alto.* When answering a question, you can use the word *no* twice. *¿Es alto Juan? No, Juan no es alto.* In this exercise, the first sentence tells you something about someone and the second sentence asks about his or her opposite. Notice that the gender also changes in each. Make the adjectives agree with their nouns.

Modelo: —Luis es alto. ¿Cómo es Guillermina?
         —Guillermina no es alta. Es baja.

A. Pedro es feo. ¿Cómo es Estrella?
B. Marta es gorda. ¿Cómo es Juan?
C. Miguel es alto. ¿Cómo es Rosa?
D. Ana es baja. ¿Cómo es Marco?
E. María es mayor. ¿Cómo es José?
F. Carlos es guapo. ¿Cómo es Ana?
G. Luis es delgado. ¿Cómo es Estrella?
H. Juana es joven. ¿Cómo es Timoteo?

HACIA FLUIDEZ

  1.21 Actividad _____

Look at the chart that follows and describe the following people. For example, *Cristina Rojas y Samuel Ortiz son enfermeros.* Then, ask questions of classmates: *¿Cómo es el doctor Andino? ¿Cuál es la especialidad de la doctora Droz?*

Nombre	Profesión	Nacionalidad	Características físicas
Cristina Rojas	enfermera	mexicana	joven, alta, delgada
Felipe Andino	cirujano	chileno	bajo, guapo, agradable
Carmen Machado	cirujana	mexicana	baja, simpática
Raquel Droz	obstetra	chilena	alta, delgada
Samuel Ortiz	enfermero	argentino	joven, alto, delgado

 1.22 Actividad 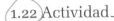_____

Describe the following people by drawing conclusions from the information presented in the chart. Note that while the titles *señor* and *señora* are used with the last name, the titles *don* and *doña,* which refer to seniors, are used with first names.

Nombre	Estatura (Height)	Peso (Weight)	Edad (Age)
Doña Afortunada	5 pies	200 libras	68 años
Don Amilcar	6 pies, 3 pulgadas	151 libras	72 años
Arturito	40 pulgadas	85 libras	5 años
Aurelina	44 pulgadas	42 libras	5 años

pie	foot
pulgada	inch
libra	pound

 ## Pronunciación de las vocales (*Pronunciation of Vowels*)

- For the most part, Spanish is pronounced as it is written. If you can spell it, you can say it. If you hear it spoken, you can write it. Imagine speaking by telephone to a Spanish-speaking receptionist. You leave one message for Guillermina Estelvina Rodríguez Asunción de Torres and another for Bill Jones. Then comes the obvious question, *¿Cómo se escribe Jones?* (How do you spell Jones?) The Spanish alphabet appears in appendix 1.

- Each vowel in Spanish has only one fundamental sound. Listen to and mimic native speakers, comparing your pronunciation to theirs. In class, practice exercises like *ma - me - mi - mo - mu* and *ta - te - ti - to - tu.*

Vowel	Like the English . . .		Examples from Spanish	
a	ah	mama	mano	mamograma
e	eh	way	vena	cerebro
i	ee	police	crisis	biopsia
o	oh	flow	droga	social
u	oo	rude	pulso	músculo

- Two vowels together are pronounced separately unless they form a diphthong. Practice the following: *pie* (pi-**E**), *idea* (i-**DE**-a), *fiebre* (fi-**E**-bre), *luego* (lu-**E**-go), *heroína* (e-ro-**I**-na), and *codeína* (co-de-**I**-na). When unstressed *i* or *u* falls next to another vowel in a syllable, it unites with that vowel to form a diphthong. The vowels still sound the same, but they are pronounced as one syllable. Examples are *aire, seis, oigo,* and *pausa.*
- In spoken Spanish, vowels create linkages across word boundaries. For example, *mucho gusto* sounds like a single word. *¿Es usted la madre?* may sound like *¿esustedlamadre?* Practice the linkages in *los hospitales* and *la clínica.*
- Fun-loving students might practice this well-known refrain of fresh children: *A, E, I, O, U, ¡más sabe el burro que tú!,* which means "A, E, I, O, U; a donkey knows more than you!" Courageous students might practice the following *trabalenguas,* or tongue-twisters.

Mi mamá me mima mucho. Mimo a mi mamá.
Como poco coco como, poco coco compro.
Corto caña, caña corto; corto caña, caña corto; corto caña, caña corto.
Poquito a poquito Paquito empaca poquitas copitas en pocos paquetes.
Si Pancha plancha con cuatro planchas, ¿con cuántas planchas plancha Pancha?

Exposición

Each chapter has a strong emphasis on interpersonal communication. The audio and video programs on the website will help with interpretive communication and demonstrate specific linguistic tasks that are pertinent to medical settings. The textbook and the website develop reading comprehension and writing skills.

Exposición is a feature that guides you into the presentational mode of communication, applying a specific new skill in each chapter.

CHAPTER 1 SKILL: INTRODUCING AND DESCRIBING YOURSELɪ AND OTHERS

For this presentation, imagine you have decided to practice Spanish and serve others on a medical mission. In preparation for the trip, team members introduce themselves by creating a profile on a social media website.

Listen to the sample profile on the audio program.

Write the following on a sheet of paper:

> your name
> your nationality and/or origin
> your profession
> some adjectives that describe your appearance and personality (look up adjectives that you want to use and do not find in the text)

Create complete sentences similar to those in the sample profile. Use the information you wrote down. Remember to use the first person singular of the verb *ser* to describe yourself. Use the Spanish that you know, to avoid translating from English to Spanish. Translation is a much more complex function.

Exchange your profile with a classmate. Write a summary of that person's description, using the third person singular form of the verb *ser*.

Your instructor may ask you to submit your description for feedback or may ask you to post it on your class website.

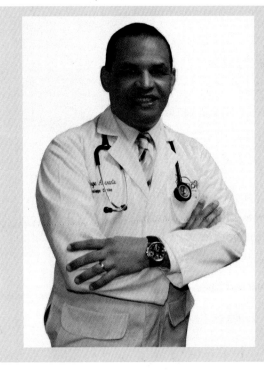

Hola. Soy el doctor Jorge Amarante. Me llamo Jorge. Soy dominicano, de San Francisco de Macorís. Soy nutriólogo clínico. Soy delgado y no muy alto. Soy simpático y muy trabajador. Mi página de Internet es www.elnutriologo.com.

El doctor Jorge Amarante

Take a break to visit the book's website!

The fifth edition has a more robust website. Take a few moments to review the ways in which the website can facilitate and consolidate your learning. You'll find an audio program, a video program, self-correcting electronic workbook activities, and downloadable forms including history-taking forms from the book. You can download audio files to your phone, computer, or personal digital player. Here are some of the protagonists you'll meet in the video.

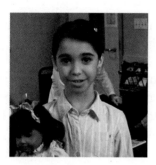

Mi nombre es Elsita. Mi papá se llama Francisco Flores, y mi mamá se llama Marisol García de Flores. Mi muñeca se llama Samantha. Ella está enferma. Le duelen los oídos. Necesita consultar con un otorrinolaringólogo.

Elsita Flores con su muñeca Samantha

Me llamo Francisco Flores. Soy casado. Mi esposa se llama Marisol García de Flores. Tenemos una hija. Ella se llama Elsita.

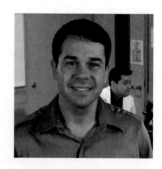

Francisco Flores

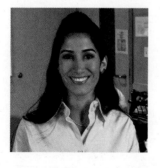

Soy Marisol García de Flores. Soy dominicana, de Santo Domingo. Mi padre tiene problema con la próstata, pero está bien, gracias a Dios. Vamos a consultar con un urólogo.

Marisol García de Flores

Soy el doctor Vargas. Soy de Puerto Rico. Soy médico generalista. No soy especialista. Trabajo con una variedad de problemas médicos.

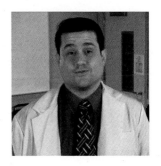

El doctor Vargas

Cultural Note: Spanish-speakers in the United States

¿Hablas español?

According to the United States Census Bureau data released in October 2015, less than 80 percent of persons over the age of five spoke only English at home. More than 38 million (13 percent of the U.S. population) spoke Spanish at home, making Spanish the second-most-spoken language in the United States. Chinese languages were the third-most-spoken languages, spoken by just 1 percent of the population. Of the Hispanic population, 36 percent were foreign born, and 74 percent of those over age five spoke Spanish at home. Los Angeles was the fifth largest Spanish-speaking city in the world. The Association of Spanish Language Academies predicts that the United States will be home to the world's largest Spanish-speaking population by 2050, and that within three or four generations 10 percent of the world population will understand Spanish. *Estás en América, ¡habla español!*

Soy latino

The term "Hispanic" was adopted during the Nixon administration to replace "Spanish-American." Some North Americans refer to people whose native language is Spanish as being "Spanish people." Actually, the word "Spanish" refers only to the people and culture of Spain. Non-indigenous persons who originate in other Spanish-speaking countries may be called Hispanic, Latino/a, or Spanish-speaking. No individual is typical. Whatever

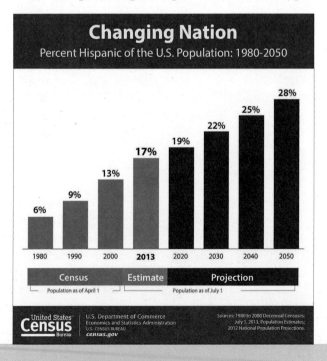

Changing Nation
Percent Hispanic of the U.S. Population: 1980-2050

1980: 6%
1990: 9%
2000: 13%
2013: 17%
2020: 19%
2030: 22%
2040: 25%
2050: 28%

Census — Population as of April 1
Estimate
Projection — Population as of July 1

United States Census Bureau
U.S. Department of Commerce
Economics and Statistics Administration
U.S. CENSUS BUREAU
census.gov

Sources: 1980 to 2000 Decennial Censuses;
July 1, 2013, Population Estimates;
2012 National Population Projections.

term a person prefers, it does not necessarily identify his or her place of birth, national origin, citizenship, languages spoken, racial blend, appearance, or cultural identity. Note that most Latinos living in the United States are United States citizens, although some are legal resident aliens, and a very small percentage are undocumented. Over two-thirds of Mexican Americans were born in the United States (some of them are descended from people who lived in parts of Mexico that were annexed by the United States). The Caribbean island of Puerto Rico became a United States territory after the Spanish-American War of 1898. Puerto Ricans were granted United States citizenship in 1917.

La colonización

The first Spanish explorers arrived in Mesoamerica before the Pilgrims boarded the *Mayflower*. The Italian admiral Christopher Columbus (Cristóbal Colón) received funding from Queen Isabella I of Castile (*Isabel la Católica*) and King Ferdinand II of Aragon and colonized Hispaniola (now the Dominican Republic and Haiti) in 1492. Juan Ponce de León landed on the shores of what is now Florida in 1513.

After his conquest of Cuba, Hernán Cortés entered Mexico in 1519. The megalopolis that is *la ciudad de México* today had been founded by the Mexica in 1325 as Tenochtitlan and Tlatelolco. For ninety years prior to the arrival of Cortés, ancient Mexico was dominated by descendants of the Mexica, sometimes referred to as the Aztec coalition, which demanded tributes and warriors from aboriginal peoples but did not achieve hegemony. This coalition, under the leadership of Cuauhtémoc (a cousin of emperor Moctezuma II) was defeated by Cortés at Tlatelolco in 1521. A monument there says, *El 13 de agosto de 1521, heroicamente defendido por Cuauhtémoc, cayó Tlatelolco en poder de Hernán Cortés. No fue triunfo ni derrota: fue el doloroso nacimiento del pueblo mestizo que es el México de hoy* ("On August 13, 1521, heroically defended by Cuauhtémoc, Tlatelolco fell under the rule of Hernán Cortés. It was neither a triumph nor a defeat: it was the painful birth of the Mestizo community that is today's Mexico").

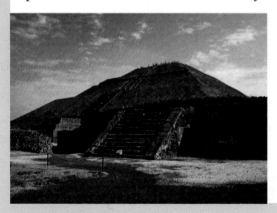

Teotihuacán was Mesoamerica's most celebrated capital between 300 and 100 BC. It was a huge metropolis with a dense, multiethnic population. Construction of these famous pyramids began there in the first century AD. The Spanish conquest took hold in 1521.

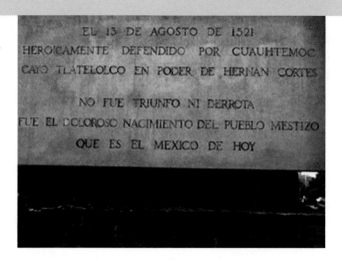

EL 13 DE AGOSTO DE 1521
HEROICAMENTE DEFENDIDO POR CUAUHTEMOC
CAYÓ TLATELOLCO EN PODER DE HERNAN CORTES

NO FUE TRIUNFO NI DERROTA
FUE EL DOLOROSO NACIMIENTO DEL PUEBLO MESTIZO
QUE ES EL MEXICO DE HOY

El sueño americano (The American Dream)

Spanish-speaking countries continue to be a large source of immigration to the United States. Although some people flee political oppression, many are loyal family members who seek education or the opportunity to work and send financial support to those who remain behind. The move to a foreign land (and sometimes the trip itself) constitutes great personal sacrifice. Spanish-speaking immigrants arrive in the United States every day. No longer concentrated in a few urban areas, they are very widely dispersed. Although most immigrant families assimilate by the third generation in the host culture, many still identify highly with their country of origin and strive to pass on their ethnic traditions and language to their children.

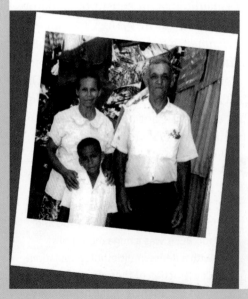

Consider the stress of leaving children and parents behind and working in a foreign place to support them economically.

Vocabulario del primer capítulo

Saludos y despedidas

Hola.	Hello.
Buenos días.	Good morning.
Buenas tardes.	Good afternoon.
Buenas noches.	Good evening; good night.
¿Cómo está usted?	How are you?
¿Cómo estás?	How are you?
Estoy bien, gracias.	I am fine, thank you.
Muy bien.	Very well.
Me alegro.	I'm glad.
¿Y usted?	And you?
Estoy mal.	I'm ill.
Lo siento.	I'm sorry.
De nada.	You're welcome.
Mucho gusto.	Pleased to meet you.
Encantado/a.	Pleased to meet you.
El gusto es mío.	The pleasure is mine.
Igual / Igualmente.	Same here.
Adiós.	Good-bye.
Hasta luego.	See you later.

Las profesiones

el/la asociado/a médico/a	physician's assistant
el/la ayudante de enfermero	nurse's aide
el/la cardiólogo/a	cardiologist
el/la cirujano/a	surgeon
el/la dentista	dentist
el/la odontólogo/a	dentist
el/la dietista	dietitian
el doctor, la doctora	doctor
el/la médico/a	doctor
el/la enfermero/a	nurse
el/la estudiante de medicina	medical student
el/la farmacéutico/a	pharmacist
el/la ginecólogo/a	gynecologist
el/la médico/a general	general practitioner
el/la médico/a de cabecera	general practitioner
el/la médico/a internista	internist
el/la neurólogo/a	neurologist
el/la obstetra	obstetrician
el/la ortopedista	orthopedist
el/la otorrinolaringólogo/a	ENT doctor
el/la pediatra	pediatrician
el/la psicólogo/a	psychologist
el/la psiquiatra	psychiatrist
el/la radiólogo/a	radiologist

el/la recepcionista	receptionist
el/la secretario/a	secretary
el/la técnico/a de radiografía	x-ray technician
el/la terapeuta físico/a	physical therapist
el/la terapeuta respiratorio/a	respiratory therapist
el/la trabajador/a social	social worker

Palabras para completar su léxico

el/la alergólogo/a	allergist
el/la anestesiólogo/a	anesthesiologist
el/la audiólogo/a	audiologist
el comadrón, la comadrona	midwife
el/la consejero/a	counselor
el/la dermatólogo/a	dermatologist
el/la endocrinólogo/a	endocrinologist
el/la higienista dental	dental hygienist
el/la neumólogo/a	pulmonologist
el/la nutricionista	nutritionist
el/la oftalmólogo/a	ophthalmologist
el/la oncólogo/a	oncologist
el/la partero/a	midwife
el/la podólogo/a	podiatrist
el/la reumatólogo/a	rheumatologist
el/la terapeuta	therapist
el/la terapeuta del habla	speech therapist
el/la urólogo/a	urologist

Las identidades nacionales

español/española	Spaniard, Spanish
estadounidense, norteamericano/a	American, North American
mexicano/a	Mexican
cubano/a	Cuban
dominicano/a	Dominican
puertorriqueño/a	Puerto Rican
guatemalteco/a	Guatemalan
hondureño/a	Honduran
salvadoreño/a	Salvadorian
nicaragüense	Nicaraguan
costarricense	Costa Rican
panameño/a	Panamanian
venezolano/a	Venezuelan
colombiano/a	Colombian
ecuatoriano/a	Ecuadorian
peruano/a	Peruvian
boliviano/a	Bolivian
paraguayo/a	Paraguayan
chileno/a	Chilean
uruguayo/a	Uruguayan
argentino/a	Argentinian

Características personales

rubio/a	blond, fair	**moreno/a**	brunette, dark
mayor, anciano/a	older, elderly	**joven**	young
grande	big	**pequeño/a**	small
alto/a	tall	**bajo/a**	short (height)
largo/a	long	**corto/a**	short (length)
mediano/a	medium	**gordo/a, obeso/a**	fat, obese
delgado/a	thin	**flaco/a**	skinny
bonito/a	pretty	**guapo/a**	handsome
feo/a	ugly	**bueno/a**	good
inteligente	intelligent	**simpático/a**	kind
amable	kind	**agradable**	pleasant
trabajador/a	hardworking	**muy**	very

Preguntas útiles

¿Cómo se llama usted?	What is your name?
¿De dónde es usted?	Where are you (formal) from?
¿De dónde eres?	Where are you (informal) from?
¿En qué trabaja usted?	What do you do for work?
¿Cuál es su especialidad?	What is your specialty?
¿Cómo es Marta?	What is Marta like?
¿Cómo está Marta?	How is Marta feeling?

Expresiones útiles

Soy el doctor Vargas.	I am doctor Vargas.
Soy la doctora González.	I am doctor González.
Me llamo Francisco Flores.	My name is Francisco Flores.
Soy de Puerto Rico.	I am from Puerto Rico.
Soy puertorriqueño.	I am Puerto Rican.
Le presento a la doctora García.	I introduce you to Doctor García.
Es cardióloga.	She is a cardiologist.

Chapter 2
«¿Cómo está usted?»

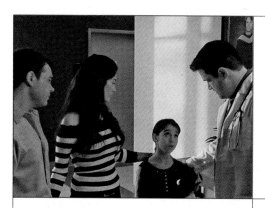

Communication Goals

Vocabulary

Structure

Cultural Note

Website   www.yalebooks.com/medicalspanish

Video   *Trama: ¿Cómo está usted? Demostración: La orientación*

Audio   *Los sentimientos; El dolor; ¿Dónde está?; Días de la semana;* Pronunciation of
   Stress and the Written Accent; *Ejercicio 2.22; Exposición*

Electronic Workbook

B y the end of this chapter you will be able to ask patients how they feel and to ask questions to clarify various states of feelings. You will learn how to ask and give information about the location of people and places. You will know the difference between the two verbs that mean "to be" (*ser* and *estar*) and when to use each. You will learn the days of the week in Spanish, begin to talk about weekly schedules, and test whether your patient is oriented to person, place, and time.

Ask How Your Patient Is Feeling

Diálogo

Dr. Vargas: Buenas tardes, don Francisco. Buenas tardes, doña Marisol. Hola, Elsita.
Sr. Flores: Buenas tardes, doctor.
Sra. Flores: ¿Cómo está usted?
Dr. Vargas: Yo estoy bien, gracias a Dios. Y ustedes, ¿cómo están?
Sr. Flores: Estamos un poco cansados, doctor. Elsita está enfermita.
Dr. Vargas: Lo siento. ¿Qué te pasa, Elsita?

Sometimes in fast-paced North American society we ask, "How are you?" without waiting for a response. In some cultures, such brevity may be interpreted as disinterest. The Latin American cultural norm is to wait for a response and to ask about family as well. (Family relationships are treated in chapter 5.)

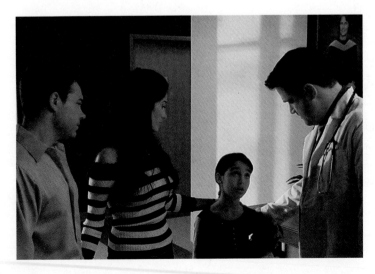

«¿Qué te pasa, Elsita?»

Vocabulario: Los sentimientos (*Feelings*)

bien	well, good	**mal**	not well, ill
feliz	happy	**triste**	sad
regular	okay	**así así**	so-so
enfermo/a	ill, sick	**cansado/a**	tired
mejor	better	**peor**	worse
igual	the same	**más o menos**	so-so
nervioso/a	nervous	**preocupado/a**	worried

Preguntas útiles

¿Cómo está usted?	How are you (formal)?
¿Cómo estás?	How are you (informal)?
¿Qué tal?	How are you (informal)?
¿Cómo está la familia?	How is your family?

Expresiones útiles

Estoy bien, gracias.	I am fine, thank you.
Gracias a Dios.	Thank God.
Me alegro.	I am glad to hear it.
No estoy bien.	I am not well.
Lo siento.	I am sorry.
Estoy en la lucha.	I am hanging in there ("in the battle").

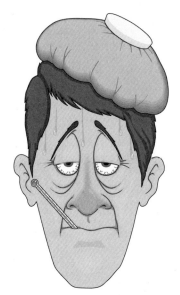

«Estoy mal».

Estructura: El verbo *estar* (*To Be*)

- The verb *estar,* like the verb *ser,* means "to be." *Ser* is used to express time, origin, ethnicity, profession, possession, and physical or personality traits: for example, *Soy la doctora Jiménez. Soy de Argentina. Estar* is used to express a state of being or condition, including how one feels and where someone or something is located. Thus *estar* is used to ask "How are you?" and "Where are you?"
- These are the forms of the verb *estar* in the present tense.

yo	**Estoy** cansado.
tú	**¿Estás** bien?
él, ella, usted	El paciente **está** mejor.
nosotros/nosotras	**Estamos** contentos.
ellos, ellas, ustedes	Los niños **están** enfermos.

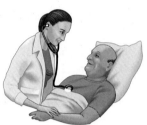

El paciente está mejor.
La doctora está contenta.

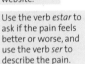

The pain scale is available for download from the website.

Use the verb *estar* to ask if the pain feels better or worse, and use the verb *ser* to describe the pain.

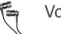 Vocabulario: El dolor (*Pain*)

¿Cómo está el dolor ahora?	How is the pain now?
¿Cómo es el dolor?	What is the pain like?
Señale el dibujo.	Point to the drawing.
Señale con el dedo.	Point with your finger.
No duele.	It doesn't hurt.
Duele un poco.	It hurts a little.
Es tolerable.	It is tolerable.
Duele mucho.	It hurts a lot.
Es intolerable.	It is not tolerable.
No aguanto el dolor.	I can't stand the pain.

¿Cómo está el dolor?
Señale el dibujo que corresponda.

0 1   2   3   4   5   6   7   8   9   10

No duele   Duele un poco   Tolerable   Duele mucho   Intolerable

HACIA PRECISIÓN

 2.1 Ejercicio _____ _____

Complete each sentence with the correct form of the verb *estar*. Then, if space and materials permit, do a graffiti exercise, in which you write additional complete sentences on the board, leaving a blank underline where the verb should go. Then switch places to finish each other's sentences prior to a group editing session to correct the final versions.

A. Mi mamá _____ enferma.

B. ¿_____ (tú) bien?

C. (Yo) _____ mucho mejor, gracias a Dios.

D. Mis pacientes _____ mejores.

E. Marisol y yo _____ preocupados por Elsita.

F. La clínica _____ en la Maple Street.

G. El odontólogo _____ en la clínica los lunes.

Tú is implied by the verb form, as are *yo* and *nosotros*.

HACIA FLUIDEZ

 2.2 Actividad _____

Circulate in the classroom asking each student how he or she feels. Give appropriate group feedback to each response. Recall that you can use *me alegro* and *lo siento*.

Modelo: Clase: Buenas tardes. ¿Cómo está usted?
         Estudiante 1:   Buenas tardes. No estoy bien. Estoy enfermo/a.
         Clase: ¿Está mejor, igual o peor?
         Estudiante 2:   Peor.
         Clase: Lo siento (pobre-c-i-i-i-t-o/a).

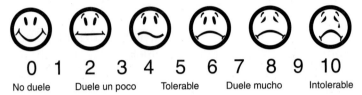

¿Cómo está el dolor?
Señale el dibujo que corresponda.

0 1 2 3 4 5 6 7 8 9 10

No duele   Duele un poco   Tolerable   Duele mucho   Intolerable

 2.3 Drama improvisado _____

Look at the illustration of a pain scale, *¿Cómo está el dolor?* Choose any number and think of how to express that level of pain by gestures and facial expressions. In a group in front of the classroom, each acts out his or her chosen intensity of pain. As a group, use these cues to line up according to intensity of pain from comfortable to agonizing. Then discuss your chosen ordering to see how you did. For example, ask *¿Cómo está el dolor?* and instruct *Señale el dibujo que corresponde* or *Señale con el dedo.*

 2.4 Drama improvisado_____

Play "Party Quirks," which you learned in chapter 1. Choose a party host and five partygoers to play. The instructor will give the five partygoers a folded note on which is written a feeling from the vocabulary list. The host prepares a party in front of the room. The chosen students take turns knocking on the door, entering the party, and exchanging small talk with each person while demonstrating the assigned feeling or emotion using gestures, questions, and statements. Say anything but the name of your assigned feeling. For example, student Paul receives *preocupado* and circulates with a worried expression, telling people *Mi madre está enferma; mi padre está enfermo.* At the end of play, with the help of the remaining students, the host must identify each person's affective state, for example, *Paul está preocupado,* and so on.

 ## Ask Where People and Places Are Located

As you learned, the verb *estar* is used to ask or say where a person, place, or thing is located. *¿Dónde está la clínica?* means "Where is the clinic?" Used in questions, interrogative words have written accents.

Vocabulario: «¿Dónde está?» (*Where is it?*)

a la derecha	on/to the right
a la izquierda	on/to the left
derecho	straight ahead
al final del pasillo	at the end of the hallway
en el primer piso / en la primera planta*	on the first floor

*In Spanish-speaking countries, the ground floor of a building is usually called *la planta baja,* and the next floor up is *el primer piso* or *la primera planta.* Here are the ordinal numbers from first to tenth: primero/a, segundo/a, tercero/a, cuarto/a, quinto/a, sexto/a, séptimo/a, octavo/a, noveno/a, décimo/a. You can see them on the illustration of an elevator sign on p. 42. Note that *primero* and *tercero* drop the final -*o* before a masculine singular noun. As adjectives, the ordinal numbers have gender, as in *la segunda puerta a la izquierda.*

Preguntas útiles

¿Dónde está el laboratorio?	Where is the laboratory?

Expresiones útiles

Está a la derecha, al final del pasillo.	It is on the right, at the end of the hallway.

HACIA PRECISIÓN

2.5 Ejercicio _____

Complete each sentence with the correct form of the verb *estar.*

> The Spanish *en* is used for the English "in," "at," and "on."

A. (Yo) _____ en casa.

B. ¿Dónde _____ usted?

C. ¿_____ (tú) en el baño?

D. Mis hijos y yo _____ en la cafetería.

E. El pediatra _____ en el consultorio hoy.

F. El doctor y la enfermera _____ en la clínica con un paciente.

G. La clínica ambulatoria _____ en el primer piso.

H. (Yo) _____ en la segunda planta.

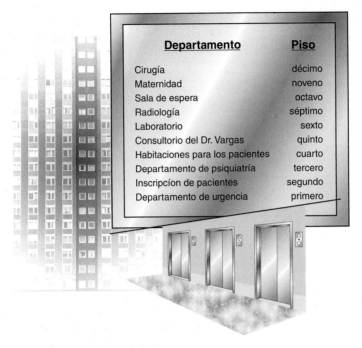

Departamento	Piso
Cirugía	décimo
Maternidad	noveno
Sala de espera	octavo
Radiología	séptimo
Laboratorio	sexto
Consultorio del Dr. Vargas	quinto
Habitaciones para los pacientes	cuarto
Departamento de psiquiatría	tercero
Inscripcíon de pacientes	segundo
Departamento de urgencia	primero

El departamento de psiquiatría está en el tercer piso.

HACIA FLUIDEZ

 2.6 Actividad _____

Look at the elevator sign and the vocabulary list *"¿Dónde está?,"* and in groups of two or three, ask and tell where various areas of the hospital are located.

 2.7 Actividad _____

Think about the hospital or clinic with which you are most familiar. Draw the building elevations and a floor plan. Next, in pairs or small groups take turns asking and giving directions to specific places that are located on the drawings.

 ## Estructura: Haciendo preguntas (*Forming Questions*)

- To form a question, place the subject pronoun after the verb.

¿Está usted contento?	Are you happy?
¿Está el doctor en la clínica?	Is the doctor at the clinic?

- You may form a question from a statement by changing intonation.

¿Usted está contento?	You are happy?
¿El doctor está en la clínica?	The doctor is in the clinic?

- The expressions *¿no?*, *¿verdad?*, or *¿no es verdad?* may be placed at the end of a statement to form a question.

Juan está enfermo, ¿no?	Juan is ill, isn't he?
Juan está mejor, ¿verdad?	Juan is better, right?
Juan está contento, ¿no es verdad?	Juan is happy, isn't that right?

 ## Vocabulario: Los días de la semana

el lunes	Monday
el martes	Tuesday
el miércoles	Wednesday
el jueves	Thursday
el viernes	Friday
el sábado	Saturday
el domingo	Sunday
el fin de semana	weekend
todos los días	every day
de lunes a viernes	from Monday to Friday
Hoy es lunes.	Today is Monday.
mañana	morning, tomorrow
el lunes que viene	next Monday
el próximo martes	next Tuesday

Preguntas útiles

¿Qué día es hoy?	What day is it today?
¿Dónde está usted los lunes?	Where are you on Mondays?

Notice that the days of the week do not start with a capital letter in Spanish. Notice, too, that the definite article is omitted with the days of the week when used after the verb *ser*. For example, *Hoy es lunes; mañana es martes.* When it is used, the definite article can differentiate between *this* Monday and *every* Monday. For example,

Estoy en el hospital *el lunes.*	I am at the hospital *this Monday.*
Estoy en el hospital *los lunes.*	I am at the hospital *on Mondays.*

HACIA FLUIDEZ

 2.8 Actividad _____

In pairs, ask and answer questions to practice the days of the week.

Modelo: Estudiante 1: Si hoy es lunes, ¿qué día es mañana?
           Estudiante 2: Si hoy es lunes, mañana es martes.

 2.9 Actividad _____

The past participles *abierto* (open) and *cerrado* (closed) are used as adjectives and therefore must agree in gender with the noun they modify. For example,

El laboratorio está abierto los martes.
La clínica está abierta los domingos.

Refer to the *Horario de servicios del Hospital de Cardiología* and ask a partner whether specific departments are open or closed on specific days. Remember that these questions are formed by placing the subject after the verb.

Hospital de cardiología
Horario de servicios

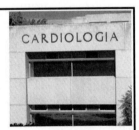

«Estamos abiertos en las horas más convenientes para usted.»

Departamento	Horas
Farmacia	De lunes a sábado. Cerrada los domingos.
Laboratorio	De lunes a viernes. Cerrado los fines de semana.
Depto. de cirugía	Los martes y jueves.
Clínica ambulatoria	Todos los días de 8 a 6.

Modelo: —¿Está abierta la farmacia los domingos?
          —No, la farmacia está cerrada los domingos.

 2.10 Actividad _____

Consult the *Horario del doctor.* Ask your partner where the doctor is on certain days, when he is at the clinic or hospital, and so on.

Horario del doctor	
lunes	la clínica
martes	el hospital
miércoles	la clínica
jueves	el hospital
viernes	el consultorio
sábado	libre
domingo	libre

Modelo: —¿Dónde está el doctor los lunes?
          —Los lunes el doctor está en la clínica.
          —¿Cuándo (*when*) está en el hospital el doctor?
          —El doctor está en el hospital los martes y los jueves.

 2.11 Actividad _____

Take turns telling about your schedule for various days of the week.

Modelo: Estoy en la clínica / en el hospital de lunes a viernes.
          Estoy en la clase los jueves.
          Estoy en casa los fines de semana.

 2.12 Drama improvisado _____

Play "Group Mind." Students stand in a circle and look down at the floor. One student says *lunes.* Other students, speaking one student at a time, advance the list in the order of days of the week. Do not follow the order in which you are standing or repeat the same sequence of students on successive trials. The turns are random and the order of the days is fixed. If two students speak at once, another student takes it back to *lunes* and a second trial commences. In cramped quarters, do this while seated in your places with heads down. The secret to a successful sequence is to slow the pace.

Estructura: *Ser* y *Estar* (*Choosing between* Ser *and* Estar)

- Recall the forms of *ser* and *estar* in the present tense.

Sujeto	Ser	Estar
yo	soy	estoy
tú	eres	estás
él, ella, usted	es	está
nosotros/as	somos	estamos
ellos, ellas, ustedes	son	están

- *Ser* is used when speaking of origins (birthplaces), professions, and nationalities. It is also used with adjectives that describe inherent characteristics, such as tall and intelligent, and to tell the day, date, and time. It does not tell the location of things and people, but it tells the location of an event.

Origin:	Soy de Colombia.
Nationality:	Soy norteamericano/a.
Profession:	Mi esposa es secretaria.
Characteristics:	Ella es alta y delgada.
Telling time:	Mañana es sábado.
Location of an event:	El examen es en el consultorio.

- *Estar* is used in connection with locations of things or people and with adjectives that describe states of being, such as emotions, feelings, and health, or conditions such as open, closed, broken, and swollen. Adjectives like *mejor* (better) and *cansado/a* (tired) describe conditions, so they are always used with *estar.*

Location:	Estoy en la clínica.
Emotions:	Gloria está deprimida.
Feelings:	¿Estás enfermo?
Conditions:	La clínica está abierta.

- Call it *Estar Wars,* but some adjectives take on different meanings, depending on whether they are used with *ser* or with *estar.* The use of *ser* implies enduring traits. The use of *estar* implies there has been a recent change. For example,

Ser	Estar
Ella es feliz.	**Ella está feliz.**
(*She is always happy.*)	(*She feels happy now.*)
Eres delgado.	**Estás delgado.**
(*You are thin.*)	(*You've lost weight.*)
Miguel es listo.	**Miguel está listo.**
(*Miguel is clever.*)	(*Miguel is ready.*)
María es bonita.	**María está bonita.**
(*María is beautiful.*)	(*María looks pretty today.*)

Although the words *loco* (crazy) and *borracho* (drunk) are slang and you would not use them in connection with a patient, imagine the difference in meanings when *ser* and *estar* are used!

HACIA PRECISIÓN

2.13 Ejercicio _____

Read the following story. Choose between *ser* and *estar* and supply the correct form of the verb in the spaces provided.

Buenos días. Me llamo Hilda Rodríguez Portocarrero. _____ enfermera en el hospital Nuestra Señora de la Altagracia. El hospital _____ grande y famoso. El hospital _____ en Lima, Perú. Trabajo con la doctora Kathi Collins. La doctora Collins _____ norteamericana. Ella _____ en el hospital todos los días, pero yo no. Los sábados yo _____ en la clínica y los domingos _____ en casa. Los domingos la clínica _____ cerrada. La doctora _____ alta y delgada. Yo _____ baja y no muy delgada. La doctora y yo _____ muy contentas.

2.14 Ejercicio _____

Here we identify the answer first and the question second. Like playing *Jeopardy,* complete the question that would have elicited each answer. Some will use *ser* and others will use *estar.*

A. Originalmente soy de Phoenix, Arizona.

—¿De dónde _____?

B. Estoy en el hospital de lunes a viernes.

—¿Cuándo _____ en el hospital?

C. Soy doctor de cabecera.

—¿Cuál _____ su profesión?

D. La enfermera es alta, morena y muy simpática.

—¿Cómo _____?

E. Estoy muy cansado.

—¿Cómo _____?

F. La pediatra es la doctora Marcelina Allende de Oviedo.

—¿Quién _____?

¿Quién?	Who?
¿Qué?	What?
¿Cómo?	How?
¿Dónde?	Where?
¿De dónde?	From where?

HACIA FLUIDEZ

 2.15 Actividad _____

Play a *Jeopardy*-like game using the personal descriptions from chapter 1. Use what you can observe as well as what you know about your classmates. One person tells something about a classmate, and the rest of the class tries to guess the person's identity by asking the question that would have elicited that information.

> Modelo: —Es una estudiante alta y rubia.
> —¿Cómo es Mary?
> —Es de Nueva York.
> —¿De dónde es Phyllis?
> —Es dentista.
> —¿Quién es Vladimir?

 2.16 Drama improvisado _____

Take turns in pairs sitting back-to-back in front of the classroom with imaginary phones in hand. You and your partner have never seen each other before and must share descriptions in order to connect when you meet at the airport (*el aeropuerto*). After greetings and introductions, one partner says, *Llego a las cuatro* (I arrive at four), and begins the exchange of self-descriptions. End with *Hasta las cuatro, entonces* (Until four o'clock, then).

Un chiste (*A Joke*)

Estudiante:	¿Cuál es correcto: Buenos Aires *está* en Brasil, o Buenos Aires *es* en Brasil?
Profesor:	Buenos Aires *está* en Brasil.
Estudiante:	No profesor, ¡Buenos Aires está en Argentina!

 ## Test a Patient's Orientation

Health care workers at times must assess whether a patient is oriented to person, place, and time. You can do this in Spanish with three questions you have already learned.

¿Cómo se llama usted?
¿Qué día es hoy?
¿Dónde estamos?

You'll learn to ask the date and the time in chapter 4. The question, *¿Dónde está usted?* does not always work well with patients who think concretely. Such patients tend to answer, *Estoy aquí* (I am here). *¿Dónde estamos?* or multiple choices may be more effective. For example, *¿Estamos en una casa, una escuela o una clínica?* Some exams test whether the patient knows the identity of the practitioner, as well, *¿Quién soy yo?*

HACIA FLUIDEZ

 2.17 Actividad _____

In small groups, demonstrate determining whether other group members are oriented to the three spheres of person, place, and time.

Vocabulario: Las especialidades

In chapter 1, we learned the names for various professions. Here are the names of corresponding specializations. You'll notice a pattern in the formation of most of the names for specialties and the adjective forms that indicate *what kind* of evaluation, procedure, or operation. They can be fun to say. The instructor will help you with the pronunciation of accents. A guide to pronouncing accents follows this section.

Profesión	*Especialidad*	*Adjetivo*
el/la alergólogo/a	la alergología	alergológico/a
el/la audiólogo/a	la audiología	audiológico/a
el/la cardiólogo/a	la cardiología	cardiológico/a
el/la dermatólogo/a	la dermatología	dermatológico/a
el/la endocrinólogo/a	la endocrinología	endocrinológico/a
el/la gastroenterólogo/a	la gastroenterología	gastroenterológico/a
el/la ginecólogo	la ginecología	ginecológico/a
el/la neurólogo/a	la neurología	neurológico/a
el/la obstetra	la obstetricia	obstétrico/a
el/la odontólogo/a	la odontología	odontológico/a
el/la oftalmólogo/a	la oftalmología	oftalmológico/a
el/la oncólogo/a	la oncología	oncológico/a
el/la ortopeda	la ortopedia	ortopédico/a
el/la otorrinolaringólogo/a	la otorrinolaringología	otorrinolaringológico/a
el/la pediatra	la pediatría	pediátrico/a

el/la psicólogo/a	la psicología	psicológico/a
el/la psiquiatra	la psiquiatría	psiquiátrico/a
el/la pulmonólogo/a	la pulmonología	pulmonológico/a
el/la radiólogo/a	la radiología	radiológico/a
el/la reumatólogo/a	la reumatología	reumatológico/a
el/la urólogo/a	la urología	urológico/a

The adjective forms are often used with the following nouns. Recall that adjectives must agree in gender and number with the nouns that they modify, for example, *el hospital psiquiátrico* and *la clínica psiquiátrica*. Words that end in *-ción* are always feminine.

Masculino	*Femenino*
el hospital	la clínica
el examen	la examinación
el procedimiento	la operación
el tratamiento	la evaluación

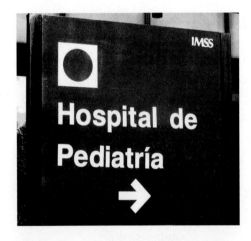

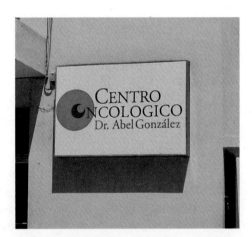

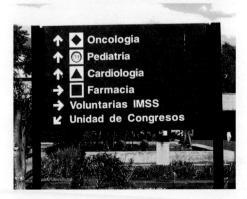

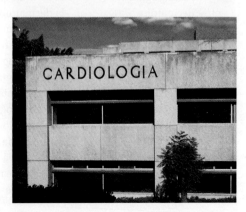

HACIA FLUIDEZ

 2.18 Actividad _____ _____

Ask where various professionals are, and answer using the adjective form for the profession, preceded by the noun *clínica* or *hospital,* as in the model.

Modelo: —¿Dónde está el oftalmólogo?
  —El oftalmólogo está en la clínica oftalmológica / el hospital oftalmológico.

 2.19 Actividad _____

Tell your partner what kind of evaluation or procedure he or she needs, where, and with whom, as in the example. The place can be a hospital or a clinic. To indicate the hospital or the clinic, you may use either the name for the specialty, as in *la clínica de psiquiatría,* or its adjective form, as in *la clínica psiquiátrica.*

Modelo: Sr. Ramos, una evaluación psiquiátrica
  —Sr. Ramos, usted necesita una evaluación psiquiátrica.
  —¿Dónde?
  —En el hospital psiquiátrico.
  —¿Con quién?   **¿Con quién?** With whom?
  —Con el psiquiatra.

A. Señora Camacho, una operación cardíaca
B. Doña Olga, un examen ginecológico
C. Señor Durán, un examen neurológico
D. Don Alfredo, un procedimiento urológico
E. Señora Quiñones, un tratamiento oftalmológico
F. Don Roberto, una evaluación psicológica

 2.20 Actividad _____

In pairs, make brief conversations based on the following ailments, whose names are close cognates with English. Say your chief complaint, and your partner will tell you what kind of evaluation or procedure you need and where to get it.

Modelo: prostatitis
  —Sufro de prostatitis (*I suffer from prostatitis*).
  —Necesita consultar con un urólogo. Hay un buen urólogo en la clínica de urología.

A. otitis   E. asma
B. glaucoma   F. ataques epilépticos
C. angina   G. dermatitis
D. cáncer   H. esquizofrenia

 2.21 Drama improvisado————————————————————

Play "*¿Quién es usted?*" A student leaves the room, and the class chooses a medical specialty from the vocabulary list, so that everyone knows it except the student who left. The student returns to the room and stands facing the instructor. The instructor asks questions, including *¿Quién es usted?* and *¿Cuál es su especialidad?* One or two students stand a distance behind the instructor, looking toward the student and miming appropriate responses. (If the instructor looks back at them, they must pretend they were not helping.) The student answers the questions based on clues from the mimes until the correct information is stated. Play several rounds.

Pronunciación del acento prosódico y el acento ortográfico (*Pronunciation of Stress and the Written Accent*)

The oral stress point or prosody of a word is sometimes indicated by an acute accent. For example, the word *está* is stressed on the last syllable, and the word *clínica* is stressed on the first syllable. In the absence of a written accent mark, there are two rules.

- In words that end with a vowel, the letter *n,* or the letter *s,* the oral stress is on the next-to-last syllable. Examples are *plaza, mano, pulso, hablan, examen,* and *epidermis.* The instructor will help you with the pronunciation of these words.
- In words ending with consonants other than *n* or *s,* the oral stress or accent is on the last syllable, as in *hospital, general,* and *regular.*
- Written accent marks are used when a word will otherwise break these two rules, as in *pulmón, útil,* and *sábado.* Written accent marks are also used when the spoken accent is before the penultimate syllable, as in *clínica, estómago,* and *odontólogo.* To know whether to use a written accent mark, you first must know how to pronounce the word properly.
- In summary, a written accent mark is required on the prosodic syllable when a word ending in a vowel, *n,* or *s* is stressed on the last syllable, when a word ending in any other consonant is stressed on any syllable but the last, and wherever two or more syllables remain after the syllable that receives the oral stress.

- There are other circumstances that require written accent marks. For example, when certain vowels are pronounced separately, as in *odontología*; and when two homonyms have different meanings, as in *mi* (my) and *mí* (to me). We'll point these out later, because if you can do the following exercises, you are off to a great start.

HACIA PRECISIÓN

  2.22 Ejercicio_____

With help from the instructor, practice saying the following words and tongue-twister.

amigo	diurética	colon	social
aspirina	farmacia	resucitación	gastritis
hablar	natural	ambulancia	antibiótico

Trabalengua: El otorrinolaringólogo está en el hospital de otorrinolaringología para una operación otorrinolaringológica.

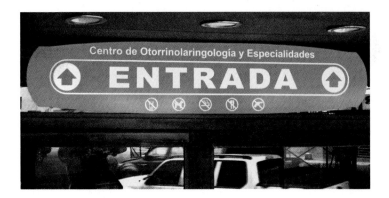

HACIA PRECISIÓN

 2.23 Ejercicio _____

Listen to your instructor say the following words. Then, write written accent marks where needed. Use a pencil, in order to make corrections when finished.

| A. facil | C. abril | E. perone | G. oncologo |
| B. dificil | D. cafe | F. sabado | H. final |

Exposición

CHAPTER 2 SKILL: PRESENTING INFORMATION

You are going to create a sign or graphic for a new clinic, based on information that you will hear about it and its specialties, tests and procedures, days of operation, doctors, and the floors on which specific services are located.

1. Listen to the announcement for the new clinic.

2. Take notes as you listen.

- Name of the clinic: _____

- Two specializations it offers: _____

- Specific doctors by name and profession: _____

- A type of service or procedure it offers: _____

- Its days of operation: _____

- The floors on which specific services are located: _____

3. Take the information from your notes and use it to create a sign or graphic to share electronically.

Cultural Note: Attitudes and Ourselves

Entre dos mundos (Between Two Worlds)

Exploring our attitudes toward groups that differ from our own is an essential step in learning a new language. There are two common outcomes when groups coexist in society. When *pluralism* prevails, groups retain and preserve their unique cultural characteristics, such as foods, language, and traditions. When there is *assimilation,* the norms, values, and practices of the majority culture are embraced. Although most Latinos assimilate by the third generation, some continue to go to their own neighborhood grocers and churches, watch television in Spanish, and fill out government forms in their native language. How do you feel about pluralism and assimilation?

A study by the Pew Research Center's Hispanic Trends Project revealed that Spanish-speakers learn English at a rate that is similar to that of immigrants who arrived a century ago. The first-generation immigrant retains native-speaker proficiency for his or her original language; bilingualism peaks in the second generation; and Spanish fades during the third generation.

Many consider it to be especially controversial to impose English on Spanish-language immigrants, and especially on people of Puerto Rican heritage, who are not considered immigrants. They are born United States citizens, serve in the United States military, and speak Spanish as their native tongue. These are among the arguments advanced by some Latinos for bilingual government services.

It may take five years or more for an immigrant to become proficient in English as a second language. Because of advances in communication and transportation, Spanish-speakers who immigrate to the United States today are more likely to maintain close ties to their native countries than

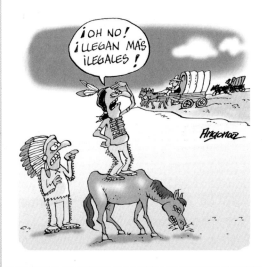

Cortesía del humorista
Pepe Angonoa

the immigrants of two generations ago. This makes them more likely to keep speaking their native language.

Caras vemos, corazones no sabemos
(We see faces, but we don't know hearts)

There seems to be a basic human tendency to "fill in the blanks" by assuming that we can perceive more about a person than what is apparent by appearance alone. Thus, we are prone to make generalizations based on skin tone, ethnicity, socioeconomic situation, and accent and English proficiency. The illogical aspects of such stereotypes are that they over-emphasize both the similarities between members of a group and the differences between groups. Stereotypes and over-generalized beliefs, when combined with judgment about what is favorable, constitute prejudice. It can be argued that most of us hold some prejudicial views. Discrimination, on the other hand, is the unfair *treatment* of another person based on prejudice. When we become aware of our beliefs, we can strive to keep them from causing us to treat others unfairly.

We can observe ourselves for signs of unhealthy attitudes. Complete the following sentences without sharing your answers.

1. My parents think that Spanish-speakers are . . .
2. I like Spanish-speakers who . . .
3. I am suspicious of Spanish-speakers who . . .
4. Latino men tend to be . . .
5. Latinas tend to be . . .
6. Immigrants generally . . .
7. Undocumented aliens usually . . .

Do your answers betray either positive or negative generalizations, or both? Even positive stereotypes (for example, that Latinos like to hug, respect doctors, and value family) tend to rob individuals of their individuality. How might your generalizations influence your treatment of others? Recall that in the diaspora there are Latinos who speak only Spanish, those who speak only English, and those who are bilingual and polyglot. Most are United States citizens, others are resident aliens, and a few are without documents. There are those whose skin tones resemble those of their white European ancestors, those who more resemble indigenous peoples, and those who have the physical characteristics of the African people who were enslaved and traded to the Spanish colonies. Some indigenous Indians from Latin America do not speak Spanish but have their own native languages. The Latino individual may face discrimination based on diverse prejudices involving race, ethnicity, language, customs, immigration, legal status, or socioeconomic situation.

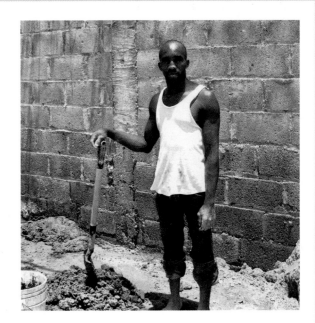

Discrimination based on skin tone is common to many cultures.

Vocabulario del capítulo dos

Los sentimientos

bien	well, good	**mal**	not well, ill
feliz	happy	**triste**	sad
regular	okay	**así así**	so-so
enfermo/a	ill, sick	**cansado/a**	tired
mejor	better	**peor**	worse
igual	the same	**más o menos**	so-so
nervioso/a	nervous	**preocupado/a**	worried

El dolor

¿Cómo está el dolor ahora?	How is the pain now?
¿Cómo es el dolor?	What is the pain like?
Señale el dibujo.	Point to the drawing.
Señale con el dedo.	Point with your finger.
No duele.	It doesn't hurt.
Duele un poco.	It hurts a little.
Es tolerable.	It is tolerable.
Duele mucho.	It hurts a lot.
Es intolerable.	It is not tolerable.
No aguanto el dolor.	I can't stand the pain.

«¿Dónde está?»

a la derecha	on/to the right
a la izquierda	on/to the left
derecho	straight ahead
al final del pasillo	at the end of the hallway
en el primer piso / en la primera planta	on the first floor

Los días de la semana

el lunes	Monday
el martes	Tuesday
el miércoles	Wednesday
el jueves	Thursday
el viernes	Friday
el sábado	Saturday
el domingo	Sunday
el fin de semana	weekend
todos los días	every day
de lunes a viernes	from Monday to Friday
Hoy es lunes.	Today is Monday.
mañana	morning, tomorrow
el lunes que viene	next Monday
el próximo martes	next Tuesday

Las especialidades

Profesión	Especialidad	Adjetivo
el/la alergólogo/a	la alergología	alergológico/a
el/la audiólogo/a	la audiología	audiológico/a
el/la cardiólogo/a	la cardiología	cardiológico/a
el/la dermatólogo/a	la dermatología	dermatológico/a
el/la endocrinólogo/a	la endocrinología	endocrinológico/a
el/la gastroenterólogo/a	la gastroenterología	gastroenterológico/a
el/la ginecólogo	la ginecología	ginecológico/a
el/la neurólogo/a	la neurología	neurológico/a
el/la obstetra	la obstetricia	obstétrico/a
el/la odontólogo/a	la odontología	odontológico/a
el/la oftalmólogo/a	la oftalmología	oftalmológico/a
el/la oncólogo/a	la oncología	oncológico/a
el/la ortopeda	la ortopedia	ortopédico/a
el/la otorrinolaringólogo/a	la otorrinolaringología	otorrinolaringológico/a
el/la pediatra	la pediatría	pediátrico/a
el/la psicólogo/a	la psicología	psicológico/a
el/la psiquiatra	la psiquiatría	psiquiátrico/a
el/la pulmonólogo/a	la pulmonología	pulmonológico/a
el/la radiólogo/a	la radiología	radiológico/a
el/la reumatólogo/a	la reumatología	reumatológico/a
el/la urólogo/a	la urología	urológico/a

Preguntas útiles

¿Cómo está usted?	How are you (formal)?
¿Cómo estás?	How are you (informal)?
¿Qué tal?	How are you (informal)?
¿Cómo está la familia?	How is your family?
¿Qué día es hoy?	What day is it today?
¿Dónde está el laboratorio?	Where is the laboratory?
¿Qué día es?	What day is it?
¿Dónde está usted los lunes?	Where are you on Mondays?

Expresiones útiles

Estoy bien, gracias.	I am fine, thank you.
Gracias a Dios.	Thank God.
Me alegro.	I am glad to hear it.
No estoy bien.	I am not well.
Lo siento.	I am sorry.
Estoy en la lucha.	I am hanging in there.
Está a la derecha, al final del pasillo.	It is on the right, at the end of the hallway.

Chapter 3
«¿Qué le pasa?»

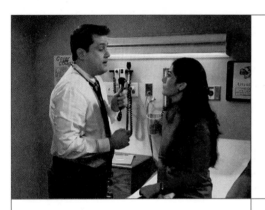

Communication Goals

Vocabulary

Structure

Cultural Note

Website   www.yalebooks.com/medicalspanish

Video   *Trama: ¿Qué le pasa?; Demostración: La comodidad*

Audio   *¿Qué tiene?; La gripe; Las partes del cuerpo; El dolor;* Pronunciation of *G, C, J,* and
   H; Exposición

Electronic Workbook

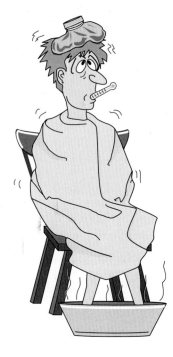

«Tengo gripe».

By the end of this chapter you will be able to ask patients what symptoms and how much pain they are experiencing. You will know the complaints associated with colds and flu season, and how to ask whether a patient feels hot, cold, hungry, thirsty, or sleepy. You will be familiar with the Spanish names for parts of the body and for injuries like cuts, burns, swelling, infections, and broken bones.

Discuss Colds and Influenza

Vocabulario: ¿Qué tiene? (*What is the matter?*)

¿Qué tiene?	What is the matter?
¿Qué tiene el niño/bebé?	What is the matter with the child/baby?
¿Qué le pasa?	What is happening (with you, with him/her)?
¿Qué síntomas tiene?	What symptoms do you have?
¿Qué problema tiene hoy?	What problem do you (does he/she) have today?
Estoy resfriado/a.	I have a cold.
Tengo gripe.	I have the flu.
No tengo nada.	There's nothing wrong with me.

¿Qué tiene? means literally, "What do you have?" and elicits a description of symptoms. If nothing is wrong, say, *No tengo nada.* The double negative is necessary in Spanish. After reviewing the verb *tener,* we shall learn a group of the most common complaints: cold and flu symptoms.

Estructura: El verbo *tener* (*To Have*)

- Recall that verbs change form depending on the subject or the doer.

yo	**Tengo** gripe.	I have the flu.
tú	¿Qué síntomas **tienes**?	What symptoms do you have?
él, ella, usted	**¿Tiene** usted fiebre?	Do you have a fever?
nosotros/as	Juan y yo **tenemos** diarrea.	Juan and I have diarrhea.
ellos, ellas, ustedes	Los niños **tienen** fiebre.	The children have fever.

- Symptoms following the verb *tener* may not require an article unless the symptom is modified by an adjective.

Tengo fatiga.	I am short of breath.
Tengo dolor de cabeza.	I have a headache.
Tengo una fiebre alta.	I have a high fever.
Tengo la nariz congestionada.	My nose is congested.

- Conditions that are participles used with the verb *estar* are used as adjectives. They change to agree in gender and number with the noun that they modify.

Estoy resfriado/a.	I have a cold.
¿Está usted estreñido/a?	Are you constipated?

HACIA PRECISIÓN

3.1 Ejercicio_____

To move into sentence-length discourse, think of a simple sentence as having three parts: a subject, a verb, and an ending that says something about the subject (the latter two are the *predicate*). Form sentences by choosing a subject from column **A**, supplying the correct form of the verb *tener* from column **B**, and finishing with an object or object phrase from column **C**. For example, *Juan tiene gripe.* Say these aloud in class. Your instructor may have you write sentences on the board and then conduct a group editing session. If you want to clarify words in column C, a vocabulary list follows this exercise.

A	B	C
Juan		fatiga.
Ana		gripe.
Yo	tengo	diarrea.
Tú	tienes	escalofríos.
La niña	tiene	dolor de cabeza.
Nosotros	tenemos	una gripe terrible.
Los pacientes	tienen	catarro y dolor de garganta.
Mi madre		una fiebre de cuarenta grados.

Vocabulario: El resfrío y la gripe (*Common Cold and Flu*)

la alergia	allergy
la influenza	influenza
el virus	virus
la gripe	flu, common cold
el resfrío, el resfriado	common cold
el catarro	mucus, common cold, congestion
la monga	common cold (Puerto Rico)
la gripa	common cold (Colombia)

El plural de *el virus* es *los virus*.

Los síntomas

la congestión nasal	stuffy nose
la nariz tapada	stuffy (blocked) nose
el goteo post-nasal	post-nasal drip
la flema verdosa	greenish sputum

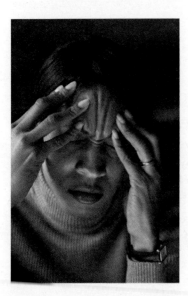

«Tengo un dolor de cabeza horrible. Me duele mucho la cabeza».

la fiebre	fever
la náusea	nausea
el vómito	vomit, vomiting
la tos	cough
el estornudo	sneeze
el mareo	dizziness
los escalofríos	chills
los sudores nocturnos	night sweats
la falta de aire	shortness of breath
la fatiga, la dificultad para respirar	shortness of breath
la diarrea	diarrhea
el estreñimiento	constipation
el malestar general	malaise

El dolor

el dolor de cabeza	headache
el dolor de cuerpo	body ache
el dolor de garganta	sore throat

Preguntas útiles

¿Tiene mareo?	Are you dizzy (lightheaded, faint)?
¿Está usted mareado/a?	Are you dizzy (lightheaded, faint)?
¿Tose mucho?	Do you cough a lot?
¿Es una tos seca?	Is it a dry cough?

Gripe, resfrío, resfriado, and *catarro* are interchangeable. An old adage says, *Gripe les da a los ricos; catarro a los pobres* (the rich get the flu; the poor get congestion). A similar refrain says, *Alergia les da a los ricos; raquiña a los pobres* (the rich get allergies; the poor get itching). Latinos may be prone to the belief that exposure to the cold, such as leaving a window open at night, may allow *frío* to enter the body, resulting in illness.

HACIA FLUIDEZ

3.2 Actividad _____

This activity sheet is available for download from the website.

Conduct medical research. Find out what symptoms classmates most typically have when they have a cold. Using the questionnaire, move about the classroom asking, *Cuando está resfriado/a, ¿qué síntomas tiene?* Report the results of your study to the class: *Los síntomas más comunes del resfriado son . . .* and, *William tiene dolor de garganta cuando está resfriado.*

Cuestionario de síntomas	
Síntoma	*Nombre de compañero/a*
Fiebre	
Catarro	
Goteo post-nasal	
Dolor de cabeza	
Congestión nasal	
Malestar general	
Una tos seca	
Falta de aire	

 3.3 Actividad

Take turns tastefully acting out the symptoms of colds and flu, while other students guess which you are miming. The interchange might go like this:

Clase:	¿Cómo estás, William?
Estudiante:	No muy bien. Estoy enfermo.
Clase:	¿Qué te pasa?
Estudiante:	(*Mime a symptom.*)
Clase:	¡Tienes _____!
Estudiante:	¡Sí! Tengo _____ (*or*) No, no tengo _____.

 3.4 Actividad

With a partner, observe the two pictures of Marina, who suffers from a common cold. Identify the symptoms that she currently demonstrates.

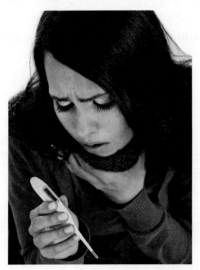 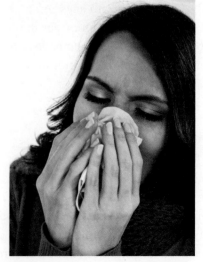

«Soy Marina y estoy mal. Tengo una gripe terrible».

3.5 Drama improvisado_____

Form a circle if space permits. In the alternative, choose an order for taking turns from your seats. As you did in *Ejercicio 3.1,* think of sentences as having a beginning (subject), a middle (conjugated verb), and an ending (a symptom or condition, for example). Going in order around the circle, up and down aisles or rows, or in groups of three, make sentences spontaneously.

Modelo:	Student 1:	Mis padres
	Student 2:	tienen
	Student 3:	una fiebre alta.
	All:	Mis padres tienen una fiebre alta.

This collaboration requires listening as well as speaking, as the second person must supply the correct form of the verb, and the third person must state a condition or symptom that is associated with the subject. Set a rhythm for the sentences by tapping your thighs or desks, and consider accelerating gradually. After each sentence, the class percussively repeats the sentence without breaking rhythm, and the pattern continues.

Lectura: El resfriado común

Follow the text as the instructor or a classmate reads about the common cold. Then answer the questions that follow. You will be able to guess the meaning of some of the new verbs. Less obvious verbs include *durar* (to last), *tomar* (to take), *fumar* (to smoke), *bajar* (to lower), *aliviar* (to relieve), and *descansar* (to rest).

Un virus causa el resfriado. Hay casi doscientos (200) virus que causan el resfriado. Los síntomas incluyen catarro, dolor de garganta, tos, dolor de cabeza y malestares. El resfriado dura de una hasta dos semanas. Los niños normalmente tienen resfriado hasta seis veces al año. Los adultos usualmente tienen dos o tres resfriados al año.

de … hasta	from … to
remedios caseros	home remedies
jugo	juice
limón	lemon
jengibre	ginger
canela	cinnamon
debe	you should

Existen varios remedios caseros para el resfriado. Por ejemplo, debe tomar muchos líquidos como el agua o jugo para aliviar la congestión de la nariz. La sopa de pollo o una infusión (un té) de limón, jengibre y canela son muy buenos para aliviar el frío del cuerpo. Debe usar un vaporizador en la casa. No debe fumar cigarrillos. La aspirina, el ibuprofeno y el acetaminofén bajan la fiebre y alivian los dolores. Los niños con fiebre no deben tomar aspirina. Es muy importante descansar.

Los antibióticos no curan el resfriado, pero el resfriado a veces causa una infección bacteriana como la bronquitis, la sinusitis o la pulmonía. Los antibióticos son para curar las infecciones bacterianas. Debe consultar con un médico o visitar a una clínica si tiene síntomas de una infección bacteriana como una fiebre alta, fiebre con escalofríos, fiebre persistente, dolor en el pecho cuando tose o esputo amarillo verdoso o de un color oscuro.

amarillo verdoso yellow-greenish
oscuro dark

HACIA FLUIDEZ

 3.6 Actividad _____

With a partner, take turns asking and responding to these reading comprehension questions.

A. ¿Qué causa los resfriados?
B. ¿Cuánto tiempo dura un resfriado?
C. ¿Curan el resfriado los antibióticos?
D. ¿Cuáles son los síntomas de las infecciones bacterianas?
E. ¿Cuáles son los remedios que alivian la congestión nasal?
F. ¿Cuáles son los remedios que bajan la fiebre y alivian los dolores?
G. ¿Qué debo hacer si tengo una fiebre persistente?

 3.7 Actividad _____

You are a doctor who is treating a patient who is suffering from a common cold. Your partner is your patient, who believes that he or she needs an antibiotic. Educate your patient and negotiate the treatment.

 ## Ask Whether a Patient Feels Comfortable

Vocabulario: La comodidad (*Comfort*)

- *Tener* is also used to express hunger, thirst, sensations of heat and cold, and sleepiness. These expressions are translated for meaning, not word for word.

  ¿Tiene usted **hambre**?   Are you hungry?

- Drive states such as hunger and thirst are used as nouns and do not change form to agree with the gender of the person.

  Miguel tiene **sueño**.   María tiene **sueño**.

- Here are some idiomatic expressions using *tener* to practice in the exercises that follow.

Tengo **hambre**.	I am hungry.
¿Tiene **sed**?	Are you thirsty?
No tengo **calor**.	I don't feel like it is hot.
Los niños tienen **frío**.	The children feel like it is cold.
¿Tiene **sueño**?	Are you sleepy?
¿Tiene **prisa**?	Are you in a hurry?
¿Tiene **miedo** el niño?	Is the child afraid?
Usted tiene **razón**.	You are right.

- Recall that the verb *estar* is used with the adjectives *cansado/a* (tired) and *contento/a* (happy). *El niño está caliente* means the child has a fever (is hot to the touch). *El niño tiene calor* refers to the child's subjective experience of feeling that the day or the room is hot.

HACIA PRECISIÓN

 3.8 Ejercicio_____

To aid your memorization, associate the following cues with one or more of the *tener* idioms, as in the examples. *Buenísimo/a* means "exceptionally good."

Modelo: el café   El café es buenísimo cuando tengo sueño.
        las frutas Las frutas son buenísimas cuando tengo hambre.

A. una cama
B. un carro deportivo (*a sports car*)
C. una frazada
D. un osito de peluche (*a stuffed bear*)
E. una hamburguesa
F. un ventilador (*a fan*)
G. un vaso de agua (*a glass of water*)
H. una discusión (*an argument*)

HACIA FLUIDEZ

 3.9 Actividad _____

If classroom space allows, divide large areas of the blackboard into the categories *hambre, sed, frío, calor,* and so on. In the appropriate areas, write whatever words or phrases in Spanish that you already know and associate with these feelings. This "semantic graffiti" helps create memory cues that are not English.

Modelo: *Hambre*   *Calor*
           Quiero Taco Bell.   enero en Argentina
           arroz con pollo   la playa

 3.10 Actividad_____

The instructor will hand out index cards, each with one of the *tener* idioms on it. Take turns miming the idiom on your card. Ask, *¿Qué tengo?* The rest of the class will report, *¡Tienes _____!* Watch out—perhaps the instructor will add a few trick cards, like *Tengo dolor de cabeza* or *Tengo catarro.*

This activity sheet is available for download from the website.

 3.11 Drama improvisado

Circulate in the classroom with the following *cuestionario* and ask classmates whether they are hungry, thirsty, and so forth. After gathering your data, report your findings to the rest of the class. For example, *Susan tiene frío cuando está en el hospital y yo no.*

Circunstancia	*Nombre de compañero/a: sí o no*
Tener razón siempre	
Tener frío cuando está en el hospital	
Tener miedo de las inyecciones	
Tener prisa por la mañana	
Tener sueño a las ocho (8:00) de la noche	
Tener hambre a medianoche (*midnight*)	
Tener calor cuando está en la clase	

 3.12 Drama improvisado_____

Play another game of "Party Quirks." Choose a host. The instructor gives five students a note on which is written a state of discomfort. The host goes to the front of the room and prepares a party. The five students take turns knocking on the door, entering the party, and exchanging small talk with the host while demonstrating the assigned state using gestures, questions, and statements. The name of the assigned state is taboo. For example, student Emily receives *hambre,* and asks, for example, *¿Tienes una hamburguesa?* At the end of play, with the help of the class, the host must guess each person's state of comfort, for example, *Emily tiene hambre,* and so on.

Vocabulario: Las partes del cuerpo (*Parts of the Body*)

This section requires some memorization. Practice the following anatomical words during the next week while you are bathing, drying yourself, dressing, and so on. Name it as you dry it, so that kinesthesia cues memory as well. If you make index cards for studying, write the names in Spanish only. If needed, add a sketch of the body part. This will help you avoid depending on English cues. Share with the class other techniques for memorization. Rote memory is a slow and tedious process. It is more helpful to elaborate on the new vocabulary by making drawings, sentences, and other associations. You'll find some helpful flashcards on the companion website.

La cabeza (*Head*)

el cráneo	cranium
el cabello, el pelo	hair

La cara (*Face*)

la frente	forehead
el ojo	eye
el pómulo, la mejilla	cheekbone, cheek
la nariz	nose
el seno frontal/paranasal	frontal/nasal sinus
la oreja	ear (outer)
el oído	ear (inner)
la mandíbula	jaw
la barbilla	chin
la garganta	throat

el cabello
la frente
el ojo
la oreja
la nariz
la boca
la garganta

La cabeza

A *seno* is a cavity, hence the word's use for a sinus and a mammary gland. The adjectives differentiating nasal sinuses include *frontal, etmoidal, maxilar,* and *esfenoidal.*

La boca (*Mouth*)

el labio	lip
la lengua	tongue
el diente	tooth
la muela	molar
la encía	gum

Las partes del cuerpo (*Parts of the Body*)

el pecho, el tórax	chest
el pecho, el seno	breast, mammary gland
el brazo	arm
la mano	hand
el dedo	finger
la uña	fingernail
el abdomen	abdomen
la barriga, la panza (*popular*)	abdomen
el ombligo	navel
el recto, el ano	rectum, anus
el pene	penis
el escroto	scrotum
la vagina	vagina
el gluteo	buttock
la nalga, el pompis (*popular*)	buttock
la pierna	leg
el muslo	thigh
el pie	foot
el talón	heel
el dedo del pie	toe
la uña del dedo del pie	toenail

Note that although *la nalga* (Caribbean) and *el pompis* (Mexico, Central America) are not clinical terms, they are readily understood and their use is not likely to be offensive.

Las articulaciones (*Joints*)

la articulación, la coyuntura	joint
el cuello	neck
la espalda	back
la espina dorsal	spine
la vértebra	vertebra
el hombro	shoulder

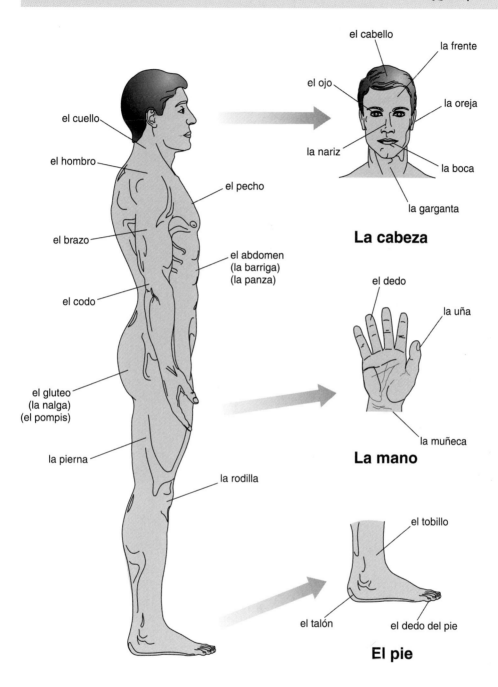

el cabello
la frente
el ojo
la oreja
la nariz
la boca
la garganta

La cabeza

el cuello
el hombro
el pecho
el brazo
el abdomen
(la barriga)
(la panza)
el codo

el dedo
la uña
la muñeca

La mano

el gluteo
(la nalga)
(el pompis)
la pierna
la rodilla

el tobillo
el talón
el dedo del pie

El pie

el codo	elbow
la muñeca, el radio	wrist
el nudillo	knuckle
la cadera	hip
la rodilla	knee
el tobillo	ankle

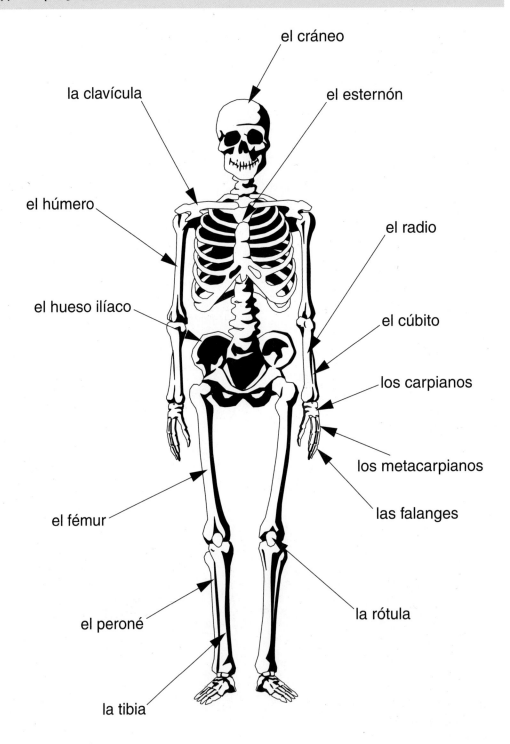

el cráneo

la clavícula

el esternón

el húmero

el radio

el hueso ilíaco

el cúbito

los carpianos

los metacarpianos

las falanges

el fémur

el peroné

la rótula

la tibia

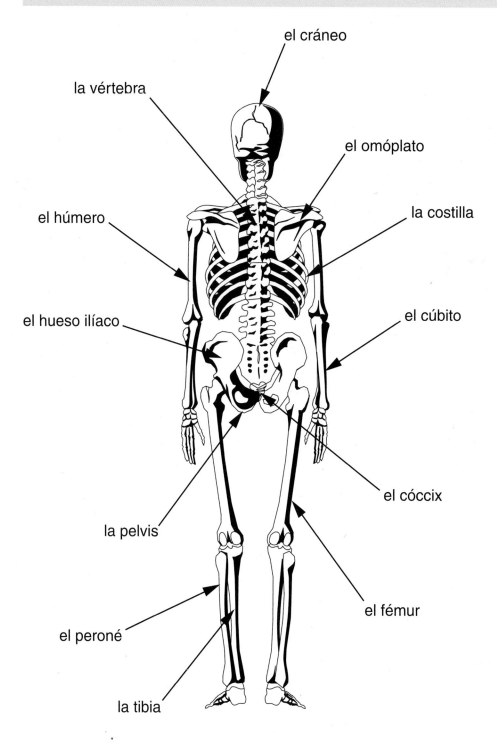

el cráneo

la vértebra

el omóplato

la costilla

el húmero

el hueso ilíaco

el cúbito

el cóccix

la pelvis

el fémur

el peroné

la tibia

Los huesos (*Bones*)

la clavícula	clavicle
el omóplato	scapula
el esternón	sternum
la costilla	rib
el húmero	humerus
el radio	radius
el cúbito	ulna
el carpo	carpus
el metacarpo	metacarpus
carpiano/a	carpal
la falange	phalange
el sacro	sacrum
el íleon	ilium
la pelvis	pelvis
el cóccix	coccyx
el fémur	femur
la patela, la rótula	kneecap
la tibia	tibia
el peroné	fibula
el tarso	tarsus
el metatarso	metatarsus

Los músculos (*Muscles*)

el bíceps braquial/femoral	biceps
el cuádriceps	quadriceps
deltoides	deltoid
dorsal	dorsal
esternocleidomastoideo	sternocleideomastoid
gemelo	gastrocnemius
glúteo mayor	gluteus maximus
masetero	masseter
pectoral mayor	pectoralis major
el recto abdominal	rectus abdominis
el recto femoral	rectus femoris
el sartorio	sartorius
el serrato	serratus
tibial anterior	tibialis anterior
el trapecio	trapezius
el tríceps braquial/femoral	triceps

The names of many muscles are adjectives. Because they modify the implied masculine noun *músculo,* they are used in the masculine form. Those that are nouns are written with a definite article. Note that to avoid the risk of overwhelming you

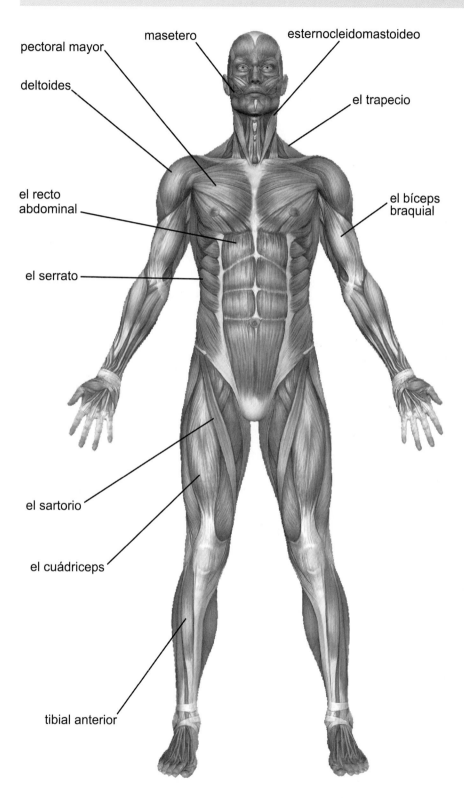

pectoral mayor

deltoides

el recto
abdominal

el serrato

el sartorio

el cuádriceps

tibial anterior

masetero

esternocleidomastoideo

el trapecio

el bíceps
braquial

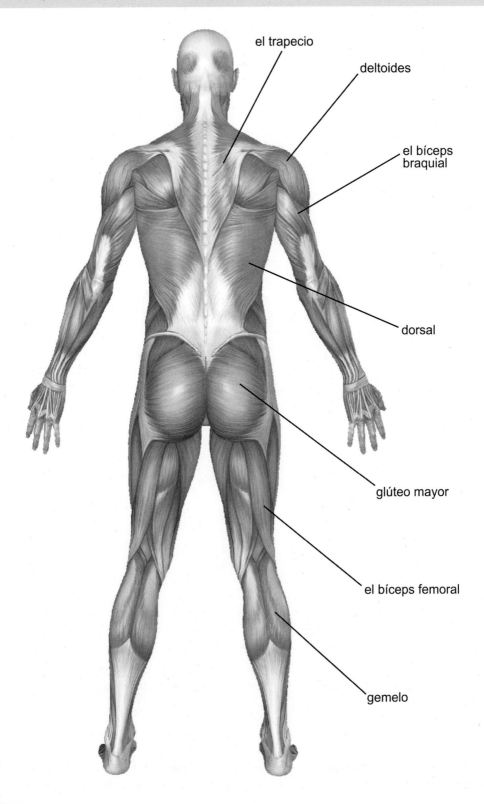

el trapecio

deltoides

el bíceps braquial

dorsal

glúteo mayor

el bíceps femoral

gemelo

with the Spanish names for organs, too, we present these in chapter 10, where you'll practice them in the context of surgical history and surgery. If you need them now, you can find them there.

HACIA FLUIDEZ

 3.13 Actividad _____

Choose a leader to drill the class by calling out body parts. In response, repeat the word and move or point to the part on your own body.

 3.14 Actividad _____

Your instructor will bring a Mr. Potato Head or a disassembled Halloween skeleton to the class and distribute the components to you and your classmates. Answer the instructor's questions, such as *¿Quién tiene la oreja?* and take turns naming the parts you picked as you put them on the model. As you do, feel free to elaborate with any related information that comes to mind. For example, *Es la oreja, no es el oído*, or *Aquí está la nariz. La nariz está congestionada.*

 3.15 Actividad _____

Students take turns as "police artist," drawing a face on the blackboard according to a description by other class members. Guidance may include, for example, *tiene la nariz grande; las orejas son pequeñas y no tiene dientes.* Later, describe the various sketches while pointing to each aspect.

 3.16 Actividad _____

Play "*Simón dice*" (like the game "Simon Says"). Stand while one class member chooses a part of the body and says, *Simón dice mueva la cabeza* or *No mueva las caderas.* Obey his or her commands. Sometimes he or she will give commands that don't begin with *Simón dice.* In those cases, anyone who obeys that command is out of the game and must sit down. The last person standing wins!

 3.17 Drama improvisado _____

Play "Categories." Form a circle. Everyone raises a finger. The first student points to another student anywhere in the circle and says a part of the body. The student who was signaled then points to another student, says another part of the body, and lowers his or her finger. Continue in this way until everyone has a word. The last word must go to the student who initiated the list. Next, repeat the list from the first student to the last, making eye contact before giving the word (you must remember who said what to you and what you said to whom). After several repetitions, a different student goes first and the group makes a new list, for example, bones, joints, or muscles. When finished, try doing both of the lists at the same time. (As the first list progresses, the student who started the second list will start again. Eye contact is essential.)

 ## Discuss Pain

 ### Estructura: El verbo *doler* (*To Hurt, Ache*)

- In chapter 2 you learned that "pain" in Spanish is *el dolor.*

Tengo dolor de cabeza.	I have a headache.
¿Tiene dolor?	Do you have pain?
¿Dónde está el dolor?	Where is the pain?
Enséñame dónde duele.	Show me where it hurts.

- The verb *doler* means "to ache, to hurt." The third person (*duele* or *duelen*) is used because a part (or parts) of the body *does* the hurting. *Me duele la cabeza* is literally "The head hurts me," and translated for meaning, "My head hurts." Spanish-speakers use the indirect article *me* to indicate who feels the hurt, and avoid redundancy by saying *la cabeza.*
- The indirect objects—*me, te, le, nos,* or *les*—are placed before the verb and represent the person who is in pain. *Le* represents "you," "him," and "her."

Me duele el cuerpo.	My body hurts.
¿Le duele la garganta?	Does your throat hurt?
¿Qué le duele?	What hurts you (him, her)?
¿Qué le duele a Roberto?	What hurts Roberto?

- When the subject (what hurts) is plural, the verb must also be plural.

Me duele el ojo izquierdo.	My left eye hurts.
Me duelen los ojos.	My eyes hurt.
A ella le duelen los oídos.	Her (inner) ears hurt.

HACIA FLUIDEZ

   3.18 Actividad _____ _____

This is a guessing game. One student thinks of a body part that is hurting, and classmates guess. Whenever you say the name of a body part, point to that part of yourself while saying the word to reinforce the meaning.

Modelo: —¿Le duele la cabeza?
         —No, no me duele la cabeza.

Take turns guessing until the student says, *¡Sí, eso es!* (Yes, that is it!). Then start over with a new student.

   3.19 Drama improvisado _____

This is an elimination game. Because it is so much like play, we shall use the informal article *te*. The instructor makes duplicate index cards or slips of paper with the Spanish name (or a drawing) of a body part written on each and distributes them to all students. (In the case of an odd number of students, the instructor plays, too). Circulate and identify the student who has the same pain as you, asking, for example, *¿Te duele el hombro?* If the other student has been assigned this body part, he or she dramatically says, *¡Sí, el hombro me duele mucho!* and both take their seats.

   Vocabulario: El dolor (*Pain*)

¿Cómo está el dolor?	How is the pain?
¿Le duele mucho?	Does it hurt a lot?
Me duele muchísimo.	It hurts a great deal.
. . . **mucho**	. . . a lot
. . . **un poco**	. . . a little
. . . **un poquito**	. . . a tiny bit
Está peor.	It's worse.
Está igual.	It's the same.
Está regular.	It's so-so.
Está mejor.	It's better.
¿Cuál es el brazo que le duele?	Which is the arm that hurts?
Es el brazo izquierdo/derecho.	It is the left/right arm.
Señale con el dedo.	Point with your finger.
¿Cómo es el dolor?	What is the pain like?

¿Es un dolor sordo?	Is it a dull ache?
. . . **agudo/punzante**	. . . sharp
. . . **quemante/ardiente**	. . . burning
. . . **pesado**	. . . crushing
. . . **un dolor que corre**	. . . a radiating pain

The verb *estar* refers to the state of the pain (*El dolor* **está** *igual*), and the verb *ser* is used to describe the pain (**Es** *un dolor pesado*). "Right" and "left" are adjectives and must agree in gender with the noun they modify (*Me duele la pierna derecha y el brazo izquierdo*). Use definite articles and not the possessive adjectives with parts of the body (*Me duele* **el** *brazo*).

 ## Diagnose Injuries

Vocabulario: Las heridas (*Injuries*)

Las heridas

el golpe	bump, blow
la laceración	laceration
el corte, la cortada, el tajo	cut
la cortadura	bad cut
la quemadura	burn
la herida de bala, el balazo*	gunshot wound
la puñalada	stab wound
la infección	infection

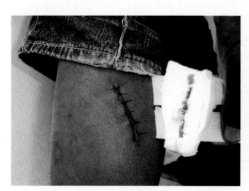 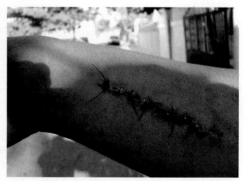

La pierna de Digo está cortada. ¿Qué tiene Lucas?

*In this context, the suffix -*azo* added to a noun generally implies an injury caused by that object. For example, getting hit by a bullet is *un balazo;* by a board, *un tablazo;* by a book, *un librazo;* by a chair, *un sillazo;* by an elbow, *un codazo;* and walking out into the tropical sun, *un solazo.*

la hinchazón	swelling
la torcedura, el esguince	sprain
la luxación, la dislocación	dislocation (of a bone)
los politraumatismos	multiple injuries

Tipos de fracturas

la fractura abierta (compuesta)	open (compound) fracture
la fractura conminuta	comminuted fracture
la fractura espiral	spiral fracture
la fractura oblicua	transverse fracture
la fractura simple	simple fracture

Expresiones útiles

Apalíquese una crema antibiótica.	Apply an antibiotic cream.
Apalíquese hielo.	Apply ice.
Usted necesita puntos.	You need stitches.
Usted necesita un yeso.	You need a cast.
Necesita una venda.	You need (he, she, it needs) a bandage.

Estructura: El participio pasado (*The Past Participle*)

- The preceding vocabulary for injuries are nouns and are often used with *tener.*

Usted tiene una infección.	You have an infection.
Tengo un golpe en la cabeza.	I have a bump on my head.

- In addition, as you saw earlier in the chapter, you may use a past participle as an adjective that modifies the injured part of the body. To form the past participle, add *-ado* to the stems of verbs that end in *-ar,* and *-ido* to the stems of verbs that end in *-er* or *-ir.* For example, the verb *fracturar* (to fracture) changes to *fracturado* (and *fracturada*) and *torcer* (to twist, sprain) changes to *torcido/a* (twisted, sprained). Note that *romper* is irregular in the past participle, and less clinical sounding than *quebrar,* but is commonly used. Here is a mnemonic device: if you can pinch an inch, it must be *hinchado*!

cortar	to cut	→	**cortado/a**	cut
quemar	to burn	→	**quemado/a**	burned
hinchar	to swell	→	**hinchado/a**	swollen
torcer	to sprain	→	**torcido/a**	sprained
infectar	to infect	→	**infectado/a**	infected

inflamar	to inflame	→	**inflamado/a**	inflamed
quebrar	to break	→	**quebrado/a**	broken
fracturar	to fracture	→	**fracturado/a**	fractured
romper	to break	→	**roto/a**	broken

- When the past participle is used as an adjective, it must follow the noun and agree with it in gender and number.

el brazo quebrado	the broken arm
la pierna quebrada	the broken leg
los ojos infectados	the infected eyes

- The past participle can be used with the verb *estar* as well as with the verb *tener.*

| **El brazo está fracturado.** | The arm is fractured. |
| **José tiene el brazo fracturado.** | José has a fractured arm. |

HACIA PRECISIÓN

 3.20 Ejercicio _____

Tell the patient that the body part is sprained but not broken.

Modelo: la muñeca
      —La muñeca no está quebrada, gracias a Dios; está torcida.

A. la rodilla   E. el dedo
B. los tobillos   F. la espalda
C. el cuello   G. el tobillo izquierdo
D. las muñecas   H. el radio derecho

 3.21 Ejercicio _____

Give some more good news. Say that the indicated part of the body is swollen but not infected.

Modelo: el dedo
      —El dedo está hinchado, pero no está infectado.

A. la encía   E. el dedo del pie
B. los labios   F. el codo izquierdo
C. la rodilla   G. la lengua
D. los tobillos   H. el ojo derecho

HACIA FLUIDEZ

 3.22 Actividad _____ _____

With a partner, read the x-ray images that are on the next page. Then identify the diagnosis of a broken bone as if to a patient. Recall that gender and number must agree when you use a past participle as an adjective. Vary your sentences by using the verb *tener,* as in *Usted tiene el brazo quebrado* and the verb *estar,* as in *Su brazo está quebrado.*

 3.23 Actividad _____ _____

Speak Spanish continuously—and test your memory—during this activity. The first student says, *Miguel tuvo* (had) *un accidente automovilístico, el pobrecito. Tiene el brazo quebrado.* The class repeats the report from the beginning. The next student adds yet another medical complaint, for example, *También tiene los tobillos hinchados.* The class repeats the entire report from the beginning **también** also before the next student adds to the list of injuries, and so on.

 3.24 Drama improvisado _____ _____

When you have finished *Actividad* 3.23, act out (or overact) a conversation with Miguel's parent or sibling in which you let him or her know what injuries Miguel sustained in the accident. The family member, repeating each portion of news, reacts with hyperbolic disbelief or anxiety, while you are a calming influence. Words of disbelief and words of assurance include

¡Dios mío, el pobrecito!	My God, the poor fellow!
¡No puede ser!	It can't be!
¡No lo puedo creer!	I can't believe it!
No se preocupe.	Don't worry.
Todo va a estar bien.	Everything is going to be all right.
Haremos todo lo posible.	We will do everything we can.

 3.25 Drama improvisado _____ _____

Play "*Enfermero con tres cabezas.*" Three students stand arm-in-arm and give a shift report to the class as if they were one person. Taking turns, each student tells only one word of the report at a time. For example, *El-paciente-* **la habitación** room *en-la-habitación-tres-tiene-el-brazo-infectado* and so on. Keep track of the agreement of nouns and adjectives. Do not plan ahead. You'll have to pay

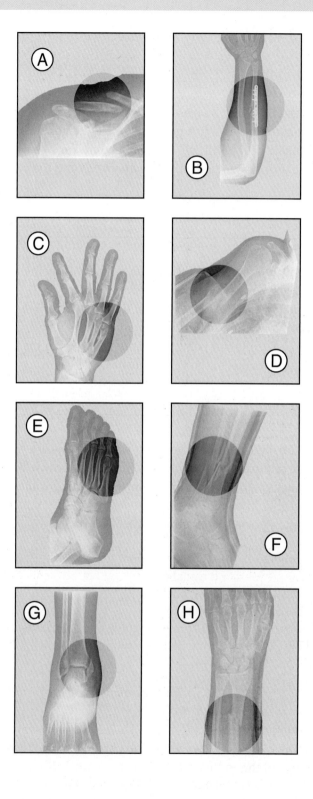

attention to articles so that you match the body part and the injury in gender and number. The results may be hilarious.

 3.26 Reciclaje ————————————————————————

Reciclaje activities near the end of each chapter help you to consolidate earlier skills. With a partner, demonstrate for the class an interview that starts with shared greetings. Resist the temptation to start with the chief complaint. Focus instead on introducing yourself by name and profession, on the patient's names, national origin, feeling state, and comfort (if he or she feels well, feels cold or thirsty, and so on). Then establish the chief complaint.

 3.27 Reciclaje ————————————————————————

Play a variation of "Categories" to review the vocabulary from chapters 1, 2, and 3. The instructor addresses a student and says, *Di* (say) *cinco partes del cuerpo.* That student lists five parts of the body. After each item, the class counts, *uno, dos, tres, cuatro, cinco: cinco partes del cuerpo.* Other categories may include, for example, *profesiones, especialidades, etnicidades* (ethnicities), *días de la semana, síntomas de la gripe, partes de la cabeza, huesos, músculos,* and *heridas.*

 3.28 Reciclaje ————————————————————————

Recall that in chapter 2 we learned to ask about pain. We asked, *¿Estás mejor, igual o peor?* Add this new information to what you know. Ask a partner about his or her pain, and prepare a skit you can perform for the class. Begin with *¿Qué le duele?* and then work towards a more specific description, as in the example. You may also want to use the pain scale from chapter 2, which appears following this exercise.

Modelo: —¿Qué le duele?
—Me duele la mano.
—¿Cuál es la mano que le duele?
—Me duele la mano izquierda.
—¿Cómo está el dolor? ¿Está peor, igual o mejor?
—Está un poco mejor, gracias.
—¿Cómo es el dolor?
—Es un dolor sordo.

As a variation, conduct an interview of this type with a patient who responds only *sí* or *no.*

¿Cómo está el dolor?
Señale el dibujo que corresponda.

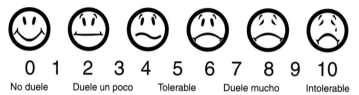

0 1	2 3	4 5	6 7	8 9	10
No duele	Duele un poco	Tolerable	Duele mucho	Intolerable	

Pronunciación de *G, C, J* y *H* (*Pronunciation of* G, C, J, *and* H)

- The letter *g* is pronounced like a harsh, throaty English "h" when it precedes the vowels *e* and *i*. It is a fricative sound, which means that to produce it, air passes through a slightly constricted airway. Examples are *general, género,* and *ginecología.* It is pronounced as the English "g" in "go" before consonants and the vowels *a, o,* and *u.* Examples are *gracias, gripe, garganta, gordo,* and *gusto.* To preserve this "g" sound before the vowels *e* and *i,* the letter *u* is inserted in the written word, as in *guerra* (war), *guitarra,* and the family name *Rodríguez.*
- The letter *c* is pronounced like the English "c" in "cent" when it precedes the vowels *e* and *i.* (In some parts of Spain this is pronounced like the English "th.") Examples are *cerebro* and *cirugía.* It is pronounced like the English "k" or the "c" in "coin" before the vowels *a, o,* and *u,* and before consonants. Examples are *cansado, catarro, cortar, codo, Cuba, clínica,* and *recto.*
- *J* is pronounced like a throaty English "h," as in *ojo, oreja,* and *jueves.* Spanish *h* is always silent, as in *herida, hambre,* and *hospital.* Note that the *g* is soft in the Spanish word for surgery, *cirugía,* because it is followed by *i.* To preserve the soft sound, the word for surgeon is written with a *j* (*cirujano*) as a spelling accommodation.

Exposición

 CHAPTER 3 SKILL: SUMMARIZING AND PRESENTING INFORMATION

You are going to invent a patient and the details of his or her ailment in order to prepare a case study to share with the class.

1. Listen to the audio for the chapter 3 *Exposición*. Take notes as a health professional describes what is wrong.

    Nombre: _____

    Nombre del doctor de cabecera: _____

    Parte del cuerpo: _____

    Problema: _____

    Tipo de dolor: _____

    ¿Cómo está el dolor? _____

    ¿Con qué especialidad debe consultar? _____

2. Now, using this case as a model, think of a different patient and a different ailment, and create a new case study. Include similar information to what you heard in the patient's description.

3. Share your case study with the rest of the class in a mock case conference.

Cultural Note: Expressions for Every Day

La lengua, aunque no tiene huesos, los quiebra
(Although the tongue has no bones, it breaks them)

You will become comfortable with the medical interview as a nonnative speaker of Spanish. Listen carefully to other Spanish conversations to

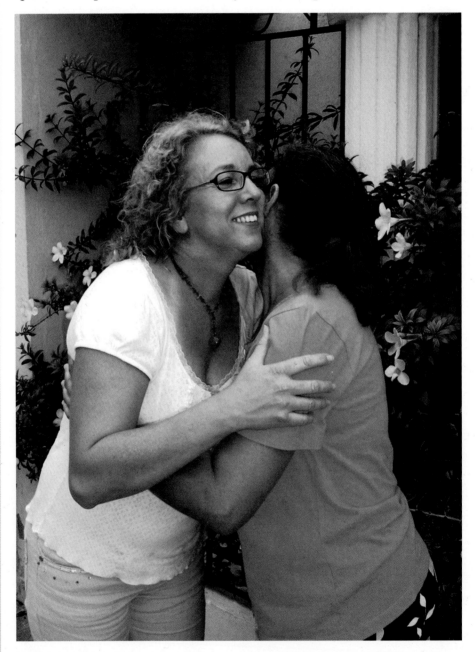

«¡Mucho gusto!»

become familiar with natural daily expressions and cultural styles of communication. In faster-paced urban and industrial areas of the world some people have traded good manners for efficiency. But in general, Spanish speakers strive to make social interactions warm, friendly, and courteous.

El tener respeto is a quality of the self in which one always expresses deference to the other person in an interpersonal exchange. It constitutes a cultural norm that accords value to the other person. Failure to do so is *una falta de respeto.* Many polite expressions are part of everyday life. For example, when you enter a room, it is customary to greet each person individually, which may involve shaking hands with everyone. You might say, *Hola, ¿cómo está usted?* You'll notice that Latinos normally wait for a response after asking the question. Personal relationships are friendly. Kisses and hugs (*besos y abrazos*) are common. Sometimes Latino children do not make eye contact with an adult, having been taught that to do so would be disrespectful.

You may also notice that Latinos who have not fully assimilated into North American culture may have closer personal space tolerances. They may unconsciously judge the North American to be aloof for maintaining greater interpersonal distance. North Americans sometimes avoid eye contact when uncomfortable with physical closeness and unconsciously back off.

You'll recall the Spanish equivalents of some common courtesies:

por favor	please
muchas gracias	many thanks
de nada	you're welcome
mucho gusto / encantado/a	pleased to meet you
Al contrario, el gusto es mío.	To the contrary, the pleasure is mine.
un placer	a pleasure / you're welcome

After introducing oneself or being introduced to another person, it would be proper to say, *Encantado* (or *Encantada*), which is like "enchanted" and means "Pleased to meet you." You can also say, *Mucho gusto,* to which the other person might respond, *El gusto es mío. Igual* or the adverb *Igualmente* is used for "Same here." In a professional context you might say, *A sus órdenes* (At your service) or *Para servirle* (In order to serve you).

When leaving a room, one customarily asks permission. *Con su permiso* means "With your permission." (The term *perdón* is reserved for asking forgiveness after bumping, interrupting, or otherwise offending, while *permiso* is used before the interruption.) "I am going to return soon" is *Voy a volver pronto,* or *Vuelvo ahora.*

Vocabulario del capítulo tres

¿Qué tiene?

¿Qué tiene?	What is the matter?
¿Qué tiene el niño/bebé?	What is the matter with the child/baby?
¿Qué le pasa?	What is happening (with you, him, or her)?
¿Qué síntomas tiene?	What symptoms do you have?
¿Qué problema tiene hoy?	What problem do you have today?
Estoy resfriado/a.	I have a cold.
Tengo gripe.	I have the flu.
No tengo nada.	There's nothing wrong with me.

El resfrío y la gripe

la alergia	allergy
la influenza	influenza
el virus	virus
la gripe	flu, common cold
el resfrío, el resfriado	common cold
el catarro	mucus, common cold, congestion
la monga	common cold (Puerto Rico)
la gripa	common cold (Colombia)

Los síntomas

la congestión nasal	stuffy nose
la nariz tapada	stuffy (blocked) nose
el goteo post-nasal	post-nasal drip
la flema verdosa	greenish sputum
la fiebre	fever
la náusea	nausea
el vómito	vomit, vomiting
la tos	cough
el estornudo	sneeze
el mareo	dizziness
los escalofríos	chills
los sudores nocturnos	night sweats
la falta de aire	shortness of breath
la fatiga, la dificultad para respirar	shortness of breath
la diarrea	diarrhea
el estreñimiento	constipation
el malestar general	malaise

La comodidad

el dolor de cabeza	headache
el dolor en el cuerpo	body ache

el dolor de garganta	sore throat
el hambre	hunger
el sed	thirst
el calor	heat
el frío	cold
el sueño	sleepiness
la prisa	rush
el miedo	fear
la razón	correctness

La cabeza

el cráneo	cranium
el cabello, el pelo	hair
la frente	forehead
el ojo	eye
el pómulo, la mejilla	cheekbone, cheek
la nariz	nose
el seno frontal/paranasal	frontal/paranasal sinus
la oreja	ear (outer)
el oído	ear (inner)
la mandíbula	jaw
la barbilla	chin
el labio	lip
la lengua	tongue
el diente	tooth
la muela	molar
la encía	gum

Las partes del cuerpo

la garganta	throat
el pecho, el tórax	chest
el pecho, el seno	breast, mammary gland
el brazo	arm
la mano	hand
el dedo	finger
la uña	fingernail
el abdomen	abdomen
la barriga, la panza (*popular*)	abdomen
el ombligo	navel
el recto, el ano	rectum, anus
el pene	penis
el escroto	scrotum
la vagina	vagina
el gluteo	buttock

la nalga, el pompis (*popular*)	buttock
la pierna	leg
el muslo	thigh
el pie	foot
el talón	heel
el dedo del pie	toe
la uña del dedo del pie	toenail

Las articulaciones

la articulación, la coyuntura	joint
el cuello	neck
la espalda	back
la espina dorsal	spine
la vértebra	vertebra
el hombro	shoulder
el codo	elbow
la muñeca, el radio	wrist
el nudillo	knuckle
la cadera	hip
la rodilla	knee
el tobillo	ankle

Los huesos

la clavícula	clavicle
el omóplato	scapula
el esternón	sternum
la costilla	rib
el húmero	humerus
el radio	radius
el cúbito	ulna
el carpo	carpus
el metacarpo	metacarpus
carpiano/a	carpal
la falange	phalange
el sacro	sacrum
el íleon	ilium
la pelvis	pelvis
el cóccix	coccyx
el fémur	femur
la patela, la rótula	kneecap
la tibia	tibia
el peroné	fibula
el tarso	tarsus
el metatarso	metatarsus

Los músculos

el bíceps braquial/femoral	biceps
el cuádriceps	quadriceps
deltoides	deltoid
dorsal	dorsal
esternocleidomastoideo	sternocleideomastoid
gemelo	gastrocnemius
glúteo mayor	gluteus maximus
masetero	masseter
pectoral mayor	pectoralis major
el recto abdominal	rectus abdominis
el recto femoral	rectus femoris
el sartorio	sartorius
el serrato	serratus
tibial anterior	tibialis anterior
el trapecio	trapezius
el tríceps braquial/femoral	triceps

El dolor

¿Cómo está el dolor?	How is the pain?
¿Le duele mucho?	Does it hurt a lot?
Me duele muchísimo.	It hurts a great deal.
. . . mucho	. . . a lot
. . . un poco	. . . a little
. . . un poquito	. . . a tiny bit
Está peor.	It's worse.
Está igual.	It's the same.
Está regular.	It's so-so.
Está mejor.	It's better.
¿Cuál es el brazo que le duele?	Which is the arm that hurts?
Es el brazo izquierdo/derecho.	It is the left/right arm.
Señale con el dedo.	Point with your finger.
¿Cómo es el dolor?	What is the pain like?
¿Es un dolor sordo?	Is it a dull ache?
. . . agudo/punzante	. . . sharp
. . . quemante/ardiente	. . . burning
. . . pesado	. . . crushing
. . . un dolor que corre	. . . a radiating pain

Las heridas

el golpe	bump, blow
la laceración	laceration
el corte, la cortada, el tajo	cut
la cortadura	bad cut

la quemadura	burn
la herida de bala, el balazo	gunshot wound
la puñalada	stab wound
la infección	infection
la hinchazón	swelling
la torcedura, el esguince	sprain
la luxación, la dislocación	dislocation (of a bone)
los politraumatismos	multiple injuries

Tipos de fracturas

la fractura abierta (compuesta)	open (compound) fracture
la fractura conminuta	comminuted fracture
la fractura espiral	spiral fracture
la fractura oblicua	transverse fracture
la fractura simple	simple fracture

Preguntas útiles

¿Tiene mareo?	Are you dizzy (lightheaded, faint)?
¿Está usted mareado/a?	Are you dizzy (lightheaded, faint)?
¿Tose mucho?	Do you cough a lot?
¿Es una tos seca?	Is it a dry cough?

Expresiones útiles

Aplíquese una crema antibiótica.	Apply an antibiotic cream.
Aplíquese hielo.	Apply ice.
Usted necesita puntos.	You need stitches.
Usted necesita un yeso.	You need a cast.
Necesita una venda.	You need (he, she, it needs) a bandage.

Chapter 4
El recepcionista

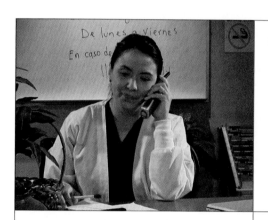

Communication Goals

Tell a Patient His or Her Vital
  Signs   98
Take a Telephone Message   102
Make Dates for Future
  Appointments   107
Ask and Tell Age   109
Conduct a Registration or Admissions
  Interview   112

Vocabulary

Numbers from Zero to 1,000   98
The Month, the Date, and the
  Time   107
Personal Information   112

Structure

Possession   104
Forming Questions   105

Cultural Note

What's in a Name? 117

Website   www.yalebooks.com/medicalspanish
  Video   *Trama: La recepcionista; Demostración: Los números de teléfono*
  Audio   *Los meses del año;* Telling Time; *Los datos personales;* Pronunciation of *Ñ, R, RR,
    LL,* and *Y; Exposición*
  Electronic Workbook

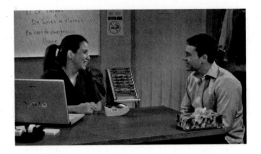

By the end of this chapter you will know the vocabulary that is used when receiving patients for admission at a medical office or hospital. You will be able to count to a thousand, report vital signs, and take telephone numbers. You will be able to negotiate with patients the dates and times of follow-up appointments. You'll be able to ask the patient's name, address, date of birth, and insurance and other information critical to the admissions process. In the cultural note, you will learn why Latinos may use two last names.

 ## Tell a Patient His or Her Vital Signs

Vocabulario: Los números del cero al 1.000

Practice saying aloud the numbers from zero to ten. Build rhythm and fluency.

0	cero	4	cuatro	8	ocho
1	uno	5	cinco	9	nueve
2	dos	6	seis	10	diez
3	tres	7	siete		

Notice the words for eleven through fifteen and the multiples of ten. The rest of the numbers to ninety-nine will be intuitive.

11	once	21	veintiuno	31	treinta y uno
12	doce	22	veintidós	32	treinta y dos
13	trece	23	veintitrés	33	treinta y tres
14	catorce	24	veinticuatro	34	treinta y cuatro
15	quince	25	veinticinco	35	treinta y cinco
16	dieciséis	26	veintiséis	36	treinta y seis
17	diecisiete	27	veintisiete	37	treinta y siete
18	dieciocho	28	veintiocho	38	treinta y ocho
19	diecinueve	29	veintinueve	39	treinta y nueve
20	veinte	30	treinta	40	cuarenta

Notice the patterns. Zero to thirty are spelled as one word. After thirty, such numbers are spelled as three words. *Sesenta* has an *s* like *seis*. *Setenta* has a *t* like *siete*. Whether one word or three, native pronunciation usually involves linking the words as if they were one. (Recall how fast you counted when playing hide-and-seek as a child.) Notice the spelling of *quinientos*, *setecientos*, and *novecientos*.

50	cincuenta	190	ciento noventa
51	cincuenta y uno	199	ciento noventa y nueve
52	cincuenta y dos	200	doscientos
60	sesenta	225	doscientos veinticinco
70	setenta	300	trescientos
80	ochenta	351	trescientos cincuenta y uno
90	noventa	400	cuatrocientos
100	cien	500	quinientos
101	ciento uno	600	seiscientos
102	ciento dos	700	setecientos
130	ciento treinta	800	ochocientos
135	ciento treinta y cinco	900	novecientos
150	ciento cincuenta	1.000	mil

HACIA PRECISIÓN

 4.1 Ejercicio_____

Take turns with a fellow student asking the following questions. *¿Cuántos?* and *¿Cuántas?* mean "How many?" and must agree in gender and number with the nouns they precede.

Modelo: piernas
            —¿Cuántas piernas tienes?

A. costillas   D. orejas
B. dedos   E. dedos de los pies
C. vértebras   F. hermanos (*siblings*)

las vértebras
7 verticales
12 dorsales
5 lumbares

(*This exercise continues on page 100.*)

Now as a larger group, ask how many of the following there are. *Hay* means "there is" and "there are." Ad lib additional questions.

Modelo: días en la semana
—¿Cuántos días hay en una semana?

G. escritorios (*desks*) en la clase
H. solteros (*singles*) en la clase
I. libros (*books*) en la clase
J. personas con sangre del tipo O
K. sillas (*chairs*)

L. ventanas (*windows*) en la clase
M. vegetarianos en la clase
N. estudiantes de enfermería en la clase
O. personas que cumplen años en mayo
P. personas que usan lentes (*glasses*)

4.2 Ejercicio ___Answers on p.437___

Ask your partner what your body temperature is, starting over and taking turns for each of the following readings. The decimal point is expressed *punto,* as in *noventa y ocho punto ocho grados* (98.8 degrees). (This may frighten a patient who normally uses the metric system, in which 37 degrees is normal and 40 is a high fever!)

Modelo: 98.0   —¿Cuál es mi temperatura?
—Su temperatura está en noventa y ocho grados.

A. 98
B. 100.8
C. 97.4
D. 103

E. 104.2
F. 98.9
G. 101.2
H. 100.3

If you wish, you can add comments, for example,

Su temperatura está bien, no tiene fiebre.
Tiene fiebre.

4.3 Ejercicio _____ *Answers on p. 438*

✓ Likewise, ask about blood pressure. The word "over" is *sobre*, as in *ciento veinte sobre ochenta* (120/80). *Tensión arterial* may also be expressed *presión arterial* or *presión sanguinea.*

Modelo: (120/80) —¿Cuál es mi tensión arterial?
                         —Su tensión arterial está en ciento veinte sobre ochenta.

A. 110/68   E. 122/84
B. 166/110   F. 118/92
C. 134/80   G. 106/74
D. 128/70   H. 120/80

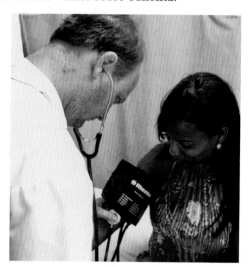

If you wish, you can add comments, for example,

Su tensión es normal, gracias a Dios.
Su tensión está alta / está baja.

«Su tensión arterial está en ciento veinte sobre ochenta. Es normal».

HACIA FLUIDEZ

4.4 Actividad _____

Using the vital signs record that follows, talk with a partner about the following patients. The following questions may help start your conversation.

A. ¿Quién tiene la presión alta?
B. ¿Quién tiene taquicardia?
C. ¿Quién tiene la presión baja?
D. ¿Quién tiene fiebre?
E. ¿Quiénes no tienen fiebre?
F. ¿Quién tiene los signos normales?

Paciente	Tensión arterial	Pulso	Temperatura
Sr. Bosch	128/78	90	103.8
Sr. García	160/110	160	98.9
Sra. Álvarez	90/55	84	98.7
Sra. Allende	120/70	68	97.9

4.5 Actividad ————————————————————————————

This will be more fun than tedious. Enjoy playing "*¿Cuántos dulces hay?*" The instructor will bring a small glass jar of candies such as M&Ms to class for counting. Pass it around, record names and guesses as to how many candies are in the jar, and then count the candies aloud to determine the winner.

 4.6 Drama improvisado ————————————————————————

Standing in a circle or staying in your places, your group identifies the numbers in a pattern or a sequence. Choose to go in order or to contribute numbers at will. The first person says a number. The second person says a number that may lead to the identification of a pattern. The third person says a number that firmly establishes the pattern, and subsequent students follow it. For example, the sequence can be odd numbers, multiples of any number, doubling numbers, or even the Fibonacci sequence!

 ## Take a Telephone Message

Los números telefónicos (*Telephone Numbers*)

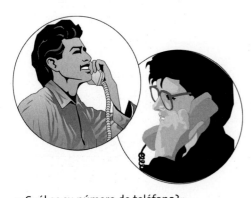

«¿Cuál es su número de teléfono?»

Telephone numbers may be expressed orally using individual numbers. However, where ten-digit numbers are used, the groups of three (such as area code) are often organized as a single number followed by a two-digit number. The groups of four are expressed as two, two-digit numbers. For example, (860) 977-4987 is said 8-60-9-77-49-87, or *ocho sesenta, nueve setenta y siete, cuarenta y nueve, ochenta y siete*. Zeros can change things. The number (203) 679-7000 is *dos cero tres, seis setenta y nueve, siete mil*, and the number (212) 305-7001 is *dos doce, tres cero cinco, setenta, cero uno*. When a double number, such as 77 appears, you may hear *doble siete* or *par de sietes* (pair of sevens). You'll need extra practice to differentiate sixes and sevens (66, 67, 76, 77), as they will sound similar until you have heard them a lot. Here is some additional vocabulary.

En este momento no está.	He/She is not here right now.
¿Quiere dejar un mensaje?	Do you want to leave a message?
¿Quién llama?	Who is calling?
¿Cuál es su número de teléfono?	What is your telephone number?
Mi número de teléfono es . . .	My telephone number is . . .

HACIA FLUIDEZ

 4.7 Actividad _____

Write down telephone numbers as your instructor dictates them. Then the instructor will write them on the board so that you can check your work. Next, students take turns telling work or other important phone numbers. See how many classmates comprehend the numbers that you give in Spanish. If you can telephone native-speaker friends via Skype, FaceTime or Messenger for everyone to hear, then make calls and see if you can comprehend native speakers telling phone numbers.

 4.8 Actividad _____

The instructor will pass out index cards with telephone numbers written on them. Each card will have an exact double. Circulate in the classroom exchanging telephone numbers until you have paired with the student who has the same phone number as you. Speak only Spanish, and don't show your card.

 4.9 Actividad _____

In pairs, prepare a telephone conversation that you can demonstrate for the class. You are the receptionist. Your partner calls to leave a telephone messages for a practitioner in the office, but he or she isn't there.

 4.10 Drama improvisado_____

Play "Answering Machine." Take turns being the answering machine at a clinic or hospital. Without planning or preparation, speak as fluently as you can, making up all information on the spot. Continue until you laugh aloud or have a breakdown, and another student takes a turn. In the case of a breakdown, the class will support you! Be spontaneous.

Modelo: "Gracias por llamar a la clínica Rosario, donde su salud es nuestra
prioridad. Para inglés, presione dos; para el departamento de pediatría, presione tres; para la pediatra Patricia Penélope Pérez Piña,
presione cuatro; para otorrinolaringología, presione cinco."

Estructura: Posesión

- English employs *'s* to indicate possession, as in "the doctor's office." To indicate possession in Spanish you can use the formula [*de* + noun], as in *el consultorio del doctor* (the doctor's office).

la casa de Juana	Juana's house
la casa de los padres de Juana	Juana's parents' house
el departamento de psiquiatría	the psychiatry department

- Spanish also uses possessive adjectives. Because *su* has a surplus of meanings,
it is best used where the context clarifies the reference. For example: *Mi doctora es la Dra. Suárez. Su clínica está en el centro de la ciudad.*

mi, mis	my
tu, tus	your (informal)
su, sus	your (formal), his, her, its, their
nuestro/a/os/as	our

- Possessive adjectives, like all adjectives, must agree in gender and number
with the nouns that they modify.

Mi casa es su casa.	My house is your house.
Mis padres están vivos.	My parents are alive.
Nuestro hospital es bueno.	Our hospital is good.
Nuestras ideas son buenas.	Our ideas are good.

HACIA PRECISIÓN

 4.11 Ejercicio _____

Read the following phrases aloud, saying the appropriate possessive adjective where indicated.

Modelo: la casa de Miguelito   __su__ casa

A. las sábanas de Elsa   _____ sábanas

B. la cama de usted   _____ cama

C. las frazadas de nosotros   _____ frazadas

D. los hijos de José y Rosa   _____ hijos

E. la silla de la doctora   _____ silla

F. el consultorio de la doctora López _____ consultorio

G. el estetoscopio mío   _____ estetoscopio

Estructura: Haciendo preguntas (*Forming Questions*)

- Changing the pitch from low to high when speaking can turn a statement into a question. Read the following statement while raising the pitch at the end: *Su cita es a las cuatro.* Intonation turns it into *¿Su cita es a las cuatro?* When questions are written, two question marks signal the event. Placing the subject after the verb also makes the question more obvious. *¿Es su cita a las cuatro?*
- You learned in chapter 2 that another way to ask a question is to make a statement followed by a marker such as *¿no?, ¿verdad?,* or *¿cierto?* For example, *Su cita es a las cuatro, ¿no?*
- To solicit more than a yes-or-no answer, use an interrogative word. These have an accent mark when used in a written question.

¿dónde?	where?	**¿adónde?**	to where?
¿de dónde?	from where?	**¿cómo?**	how?
¿cuándo?	when?	**¿quién/quiénes?**	who?
¿cuál/cuáles?	what? which?	**¿qué?**	what?
¿cuánto/a?	how much?	**¿cuántos/as?**	how many?
¿a qué hora?	at what time?		

- Note the difference between *¿por qué?* and *porque.* One asks and the other answers.

  —¿Por qué estudias español?
  —Estudio español porque quiero hablar con mis pacientes.

- Consider the following more complete questions.

  ¿De dónde es usted?   ¿Dónde están sus padres?
  ¿Cómo está usted?   ¿Cuándo es su cita?
  ¿Quién es su doctor?   ¿Cuál es el tobillo hinchado?
  ¿Qué le duele?   ¿Cuántos años tiene?
  ¿Qué hora es?   ¿A qué hora es su cita?

- *¿Qué?* and *¿Cuál?* are not always interchangeable. Before the verb *ser, ¿cuál?* means "what," as in *¿Cuál es su número de teléfono?* In many cases, *¿qué?* requests a definition or an explanation, and *¿cuál?* asks for a choice. For example,

  ¿Qué es la pulmonía?   What is pneumonia?
  ¿Qué le duele?   What hurts you?
  ¿Cuál es el hombro que le duele?   Which is the shoulder that hurts you?
  ¿Cuál es su número de teléfono?   What is your telephone number?

HACIA FLUIDEZ

 4.12 Actividad _____

Speak with other students. Practice several ways to ask for students' and their doctors' and dentists' names (circumlocution helps build flexibility).

  ¿Quién es su doctor?
  ¿Cómo se llama su odontólogo?
  ¿Tiene alergólogo? ¿Cuál es su nombre?

 4.13 Drama improvisado _____

Play an "answer-and-question" game show. Two teams write questions and answers that would be familiar to everyone. One team challenges the other with a *respuesta,* or answer, and the other team states the question that would have elicited that answer. The instructor moderates and keeps score. Here are some examples

Respuesta	*Pregunta*
Hoy es lunes.	¿Qué día es?
Me llamo Rafael.	¿Cómo te llamas?
Es un doctor para el corazón.	¿Qué es un cardiólogo?
Guadalajara está en México.	¿Dónde está Guadalajara?
Es una inflamación del pulmón.	¿Qué es la pulmonía?

Make Dates for Future Appointments

Vocabulario: El mes, la fecha y la hora (*The Month, the Date, and the Time*)

Los meses del año (*The Months of the Year*)

enero	January	**julio**	July
febrero	February	**agosto**	August
marzo	March	**septiembre**	September
abril	April	**octubre**	October
mayo	May	**noviembre**	November
junio	June	**diciembre**	December

1900	**mil novecientos**	**1960**	**mil novecientos sesenta**
2000	**dos mil**	**2018**	**dos mil dieciocho**

La fecha (*The Date*)

When writing the date, it is best to write out the name of the month. Using numbers can be confusing, because Spanish-speakers normally write the day before the month. Hence, October 5, 2018, is written 5-10-2018 in Spanish-speaking countries, while in the U.S. it is written 10-5-2018. In countries that use roman numerals for the month, this date would be 5-X-18. In the United States, writing the date 10-5-2020 might be understood by a Spanish speaker as either October 5, 2020, or May 10, 2020, depending on the individual's degree of acculturation. So, for clarity, write *el 5 de octubre de 2020* or *5 octubre 2020*. (Months of the year are not written with an initial capital letter unless they begin a sentence.) The first day of the month has special treatment: *Hoy es el primero de mayo.*

¿Qué día es?	What day is it?
Hoy es jueves.	Today is Thursday.
¿Cuál es la fecha de hoy?	What is today's date?
Hoy es el cinco de febrero.	Today is February 5.
¿Cuál es su fecha de nacimiento?	What is your date of birth?

La hora (*Telling Time*)

Notice that *y* is used for the first thirty minutes after the hour, while *menos* is used for the twenty-nine minutes that precede the following hour. With the worldwide proliferation of digital watches, some Spanish speakers now use digital time. For example, 10:45 in digital time is *Son las diez, cuarenta y cinco;* however, the traditional analog method is still common.

¿Qué hora es?	What time is it?
Es la una.	It is 1:00.
Son las dos.	It is 2:00.
Son las tres.	It is 3:00.
Son las tres y cinco.	It is 3:05.
Son las seis y media.	It is 6:30.
Son las siete y cuarto (y quince).	It is 7:15.
Son las diez menos cinco.	It is 9:55.
Es mediodía / Es medianoche.	It is midday / It is midnight.
Son las diez de la mañana.	It is 10:00 in the morning.
a las cuatro de la tarde	at 4:00 in the afternoon
a las diez de la noche	at 10:00 at night

> *Es la una* is singular, while *Son las dos* and all higher numbers are plural. *Cuarto* means "quarter."

HACIA PRECISIÓN

 4.14 Ejercicio _____

Look at the clock faces below and say the times, first as analog, and then as digital.

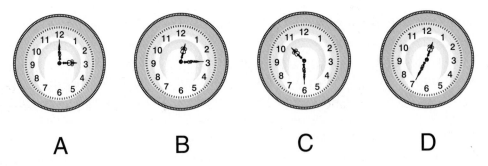

A   B   C   D

4.15 Ejercicio _____

Say the following times, translating from the English digital form to traditional analog Spanish. Afterwards, say them in Spanish digital time.

A. 10:45 a.m.   C. 8:30 p.m.   E. 3:56 p.m.   G. 1:00 p.m.
B. 6:15 a.m.   D. 11:55 p.m.   F. 6:05 p.m.   H. 5:29 a.m.

4.16 Ejercicio _____

To say, "You have an appointment with the doctor at 10:15," use *Usted tiene una cita con el doctor a las diez y cuarto.* Tell a partner about the following appointments in Spanish. When you have finished, switch roles.

A. You have an appointment with the dentist on Thursday, December 14 at 3:30 in the afternoon.
B. You have an appointment at the clinic on Tuesday, January 22 at 10:15 in the morning.
C. You have an appointment with Doctor Contreras Medina on Friday, February 28 at 6:45 in the evening.
D. Your mother has an appointment with the neurologist, Dr. Solano, on Wednesday, May 30 at 1:00 in the afternoon.

Ask and Tell Age

La edad (*Age*)

Use the verb *tener* to express age. The literal translation of *Tengo cincuenta años* is "I have fifty years," but its meaning in Spanish is clear. Never forget the importance of pronunciation. *Año* (pronounced "anyo") means "year," and *ano* you know from chapter 3!

¿Cuántos años tiene?	How old are you?
Tengo treinta años.	I am 30 years old.
¿En qué año estamos?	What year is this?
¿En qué año nació usted?	In what year were you born?
Nací en el año 2000.	I was born in the year 2000.

Nació and *nací* are from the past tense of the verb *nacer.*

HACIA FLUIDEZ

 4.17 Actividad _____

Refer to the chart below and ask and answer questions about it with a partner. For example:

¿Cuántos años tiene don Samuel? ¿Cuál es su fecha de nacimiento?

Nombre	Fecha de nacimiento
don Samuel	el 3 de octubre de 1955
Sara	el 14 de marzo de 1983
doña Olga	el 2 de mayo de 1941
Elsita	el 5 de febrero de 2017
el Sr. Arroyo	el primero de junio de 1968

 4.18 Actividad _____

Ask fellow students their age: *¿Cuántos años tiene usted?* Answer: *Tengo ____ años.* (It's all right to stretch—or shrink—the truth!) Can you find a student who is the same age as you? Ask fellow students their date of birth: *¿Cuál es su fecha de nacimiento?* Can you find a student who has the same birthday or birth month as you?

 4.19 Actividad _____

Play "Time Aerobics." Space permitting, the instructor or a student volunteer stands with his or her back to the class, positions his or her arms like the hands of a clock (big hand, little hand), and chants the time represented. Students, who are standing as well, copy the position and repeat the time. Here is a fun option: have someone beatbox and the class will create a rap hit. The instructor or a student chants the time in rap genre, and students repeat. When making rap games, use four to the bar and fit in the syllables. Tap the four-to-the-bar rhythm on your thighs. In the example, the downbeat is bold and dashes and plain text denote the offbeat.

Modelos: **Son**—**las**—**cinco** y **me**-dia.
Es—**la**—**una** de la **tar**-de.
Son—**las**—**tres** menos **quin**-ce.

4.20 Actividad _____

The instructor will use a cardboard clock with movable hands or a plastic "Will be back at . . ." clock from an office supplies store as a prop in the classroom. Students use it to practice asking and telling the time.

 4.21 Actividad _____

Look at the doctor's appointment book. With your partner, role-play the part of the receptionist, calling the patients to remind them about their appointments. When you have finished, switch roles. Recall that *Son las dos* means "It is two o'clock" and *a las dos* means "at two o'clock."

MARTA DURÁN LÓPEZ, MD

LUNES, 2 DE JULIO

1:00   Sr. Julio Ortiz

1:15   Sra. Acevedo

1:30   Anita Negrón

1:45   José Durán

2:00   Sra. Elsa Morel

MARTES, 3 DE JULIO

10:00   Srta. Paola Castro

10:15   Sra. Ana Dejesús

10:30   Sr. Pedro García

10:45   Alberto Gómez

4.22 Drama improvisado

Play "Group Mind." Students stand in a circle and look down at the floor. One student says *enero*. Speaking one student at a time, the group will state all of the months of the year. Do not follow the order in which you are standing or repeat the same sequence of students on successive trials. The turns are random and the order of the months is fixed. If two students speak at once, another student takes it back to *enero* and a new trial commences. In cramped quarters, do this while seated in your places with heads down. The secret of the group mind is to slow the pace.

 ## Conduct a Registration or Admissions Interview

 ### Vocabulario: Los datos personales

¿Cuál es su . . . ?	What is your . . . ?
nombre	name
apellido	last name
fecha de nacimiento	date of birth
número de Seguro Social	Social Security number
número de teléfono	telephone number
dirección	address
estado civil*	marital status
soltero/a	single
casado/a	married
separado/a	separated
divorciado/a	divorced
viudo/a	widower/widow
¿Dónde vive usted?	Where do you live?
¿Qué . . . ?	What . . . ?
calle	street
número	number
ciudad/pueblo	city/town
¿Tiene usted plan/seguro médico?	Do you have health insurance?

*In addition to *¿Cuál es su estado civil?* you can ask, *¿Está usted soltero/a?* or *¿Está usted casado/a?* Asking *¿Tiene pareja?* ("Do you have a partner?") removes the marriage implication. Note that *¿Es usted señorita?* may imply a question about virginity.

¿Cuál es el número de su póliza?

el Medicare

el Medicaid

la asistencia pública

¿Tiene la tarjeta?

¿A quién llamamos en caso de emergencia?

¿Tiene usted la custodia legal?

¿Es usted el tutor / la tutora legal?

Favor de firmar el permiso para el tratamiento.

What is your policy number?

Medicare

Medicaid

public assistance

Do you have the card?

Whom do we call in case of emergency?

Do you have legal custody?

Are you the legal guardian?

Please sign the consent to treatment form.

Medicaid es un plan médico público en los Estados Unidos para las personas que son pobres y tienen hijos o que son discapacitadas (*disabled*). Medicare es un plan médico público para las personas que tienen sesenta y cinco años o más o que son discapacitadas. Medicare Parte A cubre (*covers*) internamientos y cirugías (*hospitalizations and surgeries*), atención en centros de rehabilitación y asilos de ancianos, hospicio y servicios de asistencia médica a domicilio (*home health care*). Medicare Parte B cubre visitas médicas, pruebas de laboratorio y servicios y equipos médicos como camas de hospital, oxígeno y monitores de glucosa en la sangre que son necesarios para el diagnóstico o el tratamiento de una enfermedad o condición. También cubre equipos médicos duraderos como sillas de ruedas y andadores (*wheelchairs and walkers*) que son necesarios para tratar una enfermedad o condición. Parte B cubre salud mental y servicios para prevenir enfermedades (la vacuna para la gripe, por ejemplo) o detectar enfermedades. El paciente paga hasta 20 por ciento de los servicios de Parte B. La Parte D cubre medicamentos recetados.

HACIA FLUIDEZ

 4.23 Áctividad _____

Work with a partner to admit each other to the services of the Clínica Abreu using the form that appears here.

This *Formulario de inscripción* may be downloaded from the website.

A

Clínica Abreu
Formulario de inscripción del paciente

Nombre y apellidos: _____

Idioma: _____

Dirección: _____

Teléfono: _____

Fecha de nacimiento: _____

Número de seguro social: _____

Estado civil: _____

Plan médico: _____

Contacto de emergencia:

Nombre y apellidos: _____

Teléfono: _____

 4.24 Drama improvisado _____

Review the advertisement that follows. Take turns acting out telephone calls between a patient and the receptionist at the dental office of *la doctora* Dolores de Repente. Identify the service that you need, and work to set up an appointment and another for six months later. Create—or your instructor will randomly assign to other students—specific challenging scenarios. For example, you are experiencing a lot of pain, and the doctor's office is very busy; or the doctor's office does not seem to be very busy until you reveal that you do not have insurance.

Dra. Dolores D. Repente
servicios dentales para toda la familia

Limpiezas	**Extracciones**
Exámenes	**Implantes**
Dentaduras	**Coronas**
—completas y parciales	—de oro y de porcelana

Para más información llame al 809-356-8090.
Abierto de lunes a jueves desde las 9 hasta las 4.

Hablamos español e inglés.
La primera consulta es gratis.
Aceptamos la mayoría de los planes dentales.

 4.25 Reciclaje _____

In chapter 2 you learned how to determine whether a patient was oriented as to person, place, and time. Now you have expanded your repertoire to be able to ask about the date and about the names of towns and cities as well. Work with a partner to role-play for the class an interview to elicit whether a patient is oriented to the three spheres of person (name of patient and of interviewer); place (building, city, and state); and time (the day, month, and year).

 4.26 Reciclaje _____

Integrate what you have learned in the first four chapters. Set up a small clinic in the front of the classroom. Volunteer to play the parts of patient, patient family member, receptionist, and practitioner. The receptionist registers the patient, the practitioner enters the room, and introductions are made. Work out a situation in which the patient's diagnosis will be a sprained joint or a fractured bone, and schedule a follow-up visit with an orthopedist.

Pronunciación de Ñ, R, RR, LL y Y

- The Spanish alphabet (*el alfabeto* or *el abecedario*) has twenty-seven letters (see appendix 1). The letter that appears in Spanish but not in English is the letter *ñ*, although some grammars include *rr* in the alphabet.
- The letter *ñ* (called *eñe*) is pronounced like the "ni" in "onion" or the "ny" in "canyon." Some examples are: *uña, señor, doña, año, sueño,* and *niño.*
- The letter *r* is pronounced by tapping the palate softly with the tip of the tongue, almost as in the English "tt" in "butter" or the "dd" in "ladder." When *rr*

appears, it is trilled. Listen to good models and copy them. Say "brr," but with your tongue instead of your lips. Practice saying *pero* (but) and *perro* (dog). Do not be discouraged. There are regions where a dialect calls for a more throaty sound. Those who can, however, may trill the letter *r* when it starts a word. Hearing the Spanish *r* pronounced like an English retroflex "r" can be irritating to a native speaker. Practice saying *diarrea, catarro, carrera, roto, regular,* and *rótula.* Don't forget *otorrinolaringólogo*! Then try these tongue-twisters (*trabalenguas*):

> *Perro raro, pero perro al fin* (An odd dog, but a dog after all).
> *Qué rápido corren los carros del ferrocarril* (How fast the rail cars run).

- The letters *ll* when together are pronounced like English "y." The letter *y* (*ye*) is pronounced likewise, except when it stands alone in the word *y*, which is pronounced like Spanish *i*. Some examples are: *llamar, llegar, rodilla, yo, mayo,* and *yodo.* Caribbean Americans often give an English "j" sound to both "y" and "ll." In some countries it can sound like the English "g" in "genre."

Exposición

CHAPTER 4 SKILL: TAKING NOTES AND COMPLETING FORMS

You are going to listen to a practitioner ask specific questions needed for registering a patient, and to the patient's response to the questions. You will take notes and then prepare an intake or registration interview form based on the information that you hear in the audio file.

1. Listen to the interview and take note of the information that is being requested.
2. Use the information from your notes to create an intake or registration form.
3. Listen again and fill in the form with the information that the patient provided.
4. The instructor may choose to give you written feedback. Use the feedback to perfect your form and then share it with the class.

Cultural Note: What's in a Name?

This cultural note is in Spanish. You can do it! Take time to notice that many of the words are close cognates: words that sound like or look like their counterparts in English. Note which of the following words are close cognates and which are not.

normalmente	normally	**común**	common
costumbre	custom	**complicado/a**	complicated
comprender	to understand	**intentar**	to try
ayudar	to help	**proceso**	process
solicitar	apply for	**expediente**	file
clarificar	clarify	**manera**	manner
paterno/a	paternal	**materno/a**	maternal
primero/a	first	**segundo/a**	second
sencillo/a	simple	**seguir**	follow

Llamar al pan pan y al vino vino
(Call the bread, bread and the wine, wine)

Donde se habla español normalmente se usan dos apellidos, aunque es menos común en Argentina. Esta costumbre es un poco complicada para las personas que no comprenden el uso de dos apellidos e intentan ayudar al paciente con el proceso de solicitar un acta de nacimiento o para personas que buscan un expediente médico en la computadora.

apellido	last name
buscar	to seek
padre	father
madre	mother
hijo	son
abuelos	grandparents
casarse	to marry
seguir	to follow
por supuesto	of course

Vamos a clarificar. Cuando se usa un solo apellido es el apellido del padre (el apellido paterno). Cuando se usa dos apellidos, el primer apellido del padre va primero y el primer apellido de la madre va segundo. De esa manera Pedro Ortiz Pagán es hijo del señor Ortiz y la señora Pagán. Ya comprendemos por qué Pedro se llama Pedro Ortiz Pagán. También Pedro puede usar una forma un poco más sencilla y llamarse Pedro Ortiz.

Vamos a seguir con los nombres de la familia de Pedro Ortíz Pagán. Sus padres se llaman Luis Ortiz Moncado y María Pagán López. Los padres de Luis Ortiz Moncado (los abuelos paternos de Pedro) son el señor Ortiz y la señora Moncado. Los padres de María Pagán López (los abuelos maternos de Pedro) son el señor Pagán y la señora López.

Cuando una mujer se casa, usa su nombre completo de soltera o usa el apellido de su esposo como segundo apellido. Si Elsa Negrón García se casa con Pedro Ortíz Pagán, Elsa puede llamarse Elsa Negrón García o Elsa Negrón de Ortiz. Si Elsa vive en los Estados Unidos y decide seguir la cultura norteamericana, ella se llama Elsa Ortiz.

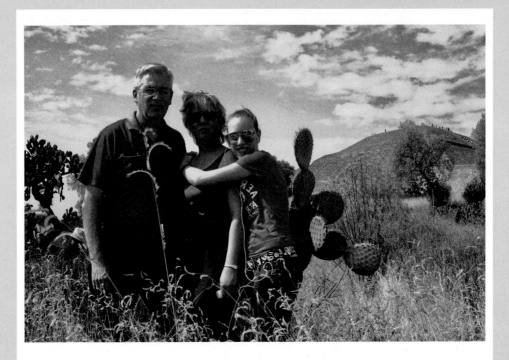

(de izquierda a derecha) Robert Chase, Clarisa Medina de Chase y Elsa Chase Medina

Ahora vamos a suponer que Pedro Ortiz Pagán y su esposa Elsa Negrón de Ortiz tienen dos hijos, Juan y Ana. Entonces los hijos se llaman Juan Ortiz Negrón y Ana Ortiz Negrón. Ahora, si Juan Ortiz Negrón se casa con Marta Ortiz García, ¿cómo se llamará su hijo Juancito? Juan Ortiz Ortiz, por supuesto. Finalmente, es común tener un segundo nombre (*middle name*) también. Si el segundo nombre de Juan Ortiz Ortiz es Oscar, él se llama Juan Oscar Ortiz Ortiz.

Vocabulario del capítulo cuatro

Los números del cero al 1.000

cero	0
uno	1
dos	2
tres	3
cuatro	4
cinco	5
seis	6
siete	7
ocho	8
nueve	9
diez	10
once	11
doce	12
trece	13
catorce	14
quince	15
dieciséis	16
diecisiete	17
dieciocho	18
diecinueve	19
veinte	20
veintiuno	21
treinta	30
treinta y uno	31
cuarenta	40
cincuenta	50
sesenta	60
setenta	70
ochenta	80
noventa	90
cien	100
ciento uno	101
ciento dos	102
ciento diez	110
doscientos	200
trescientos	300
cuatrocientos	400
quinientos	500
seiscientos	600
setecientos	700
ochocientos	800

novecientos	900
mil	1.000

El mes, la fecha y la hora

enero	January
febrero	February
marzo	March
abril	April
mayo	May
junio	June
julio	July
agosto	August
septiembre	September
octubre	October
noviembre	November
diciembre	December
1900	**mil novecientos**
1960	**mil novecientos sesenta**
2000	**dos mil**
2018	**dos mil dieciocho**

¿Qué día es?	What day is it?
Hoy es jueves.	Today is Thursday.
¿Cuál es la fecha de hoy?	What is today's date?
Hoy es el cinco de febrero.	Today is February 5.
¿Cuál es su fecha de nacimiento?	What is your date of birth?

¿Qué hora es?	What time is it?
Es la una.	It is 1:00.
Son las dos.	It is 2:00.
Son las tres.	It is 3:00.
Son las tres y cinco.	It is 3:05.
Son las seis y media.	It is 6:30.
Son las siete y cuarto (y quince).	It is 7:15.
Son las diez menos cinco.	It is 9:55.
Es mediodía / Es medianoche.	It is midday / It is midnight.
Son las diez de la mañana.	It is 10:00 in the morning.
a las cuatro de la tarde	at 4:00 in the afternoon
a las diez de la noche	at 10:00 at night

Es la una is singular, while *Son las dos* and all higher numbers are plural. *Cuarto* means "quarter."

Los datos personales

¿Cuál es su . . . ?	What is your . . . ?
nombre	name
apellido	last name

fecha de nacimiento	date of birth
número de Seguro Social	Social Security number
número de teléfono	telephone number
dirección	address
estado civil	marital status
soltero/a	single
casado/a	married
separado/a	separated
divorciado/a	divorced
viudo/a	widower/widow
¿Dónde vive usted?	Where do you live?
¿Qué . . . ?	What . . . ?
calle	street
número	number
ciudad/pueblo	city/town
¿Tiene usted plan/seguro médico?	Do you have health insurance?
¿Cuál es el número de su póliza?	What is your policy number?
el Medicare	Medicare
el Medicaid	Medicaid
la asistencia pública	public assistance
¿Tiene la tarjeta?	Do you have the card?
¿A quién llamamos en caso de emergencia?	Whom do we call in case of emergency?
¿Tiene usted la custodia legal?	Do you have legal custody?
¿Es usted el tutor / la tutora legal?	Are you the legal guardian?
Favor de firmar el permiso para el tratamiento.	Please sign the consent to treatment form.

Haciendo preguntas

¿dónde?	where?	¿adónde?	to where?
¿de dónde?	from where?	¿cómo?	how?
¿cuándo?	when?	¿quién/quiénes?	who?
¿cuál/cuáles?	what? which?	¿qué?	what?
¿cuánto/a?	how much?	¿cuántos/as?	how many?
¿a qué hora?	at what time?		

Chapter 5
La familia

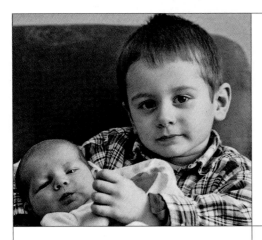

Communication Goals

Vocabulary

Structure

Cultural Note

Website   www.yalebooks.com/medicalspanish

  Video   *Trama: La historia clínica familiar; Demostración: ¿Cuáles idiomas habla?*

  Audio   *Los familiares; Ejercicio 5.10; Las enfermedades hereditarias;* Pronunciation of

    B and *V; Exposición*

  Electronic Workbook

B y the end of this chapter you will be able to name the various members of a family and to ask about basic family medical history. In the process you will greatly expand your repertoire of words that narrate action.

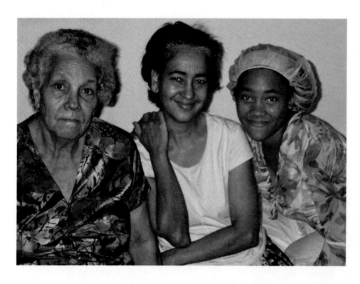

Hay tres generaciones: abuela, hija y nieta.

Ask about Family Constellation

Vocabulario: Los familiares (*Family Members*)

Palabras de frecuente uso

el padre, papá	father	**la madre, mamá**	mother
el esposo, el marido	husband	**la esposa, mujer**	wife
el hijo	son	**la hija**	daughter
el hermano	brother	**la hermana**	sister
el abuelo	grandfather	**la abuela**	grandmother
el nieto	grandson	**la nieta**	granddaughter
el tío	uncle	**la tía**	aunt
el sobrino	nephew	**la sobrina**	niece
el primo	male cousin	**la prima**	female cousin
el padrino	godfather	**la madrina**	godmother

Hijos means sons, but as a plural word it can refer to sons and daughters. *Hijas* refers only to daughters. In the same way, *padres* refers to parents, but *padre* only to father; and *hermanos* can refer to brothers and sisters or to brothers only.

—¿Tiene hijos? Do you have children?
—Sí, tengo dos hijos: un hijo y una hija. Yes, I have two: a son and a daughter.

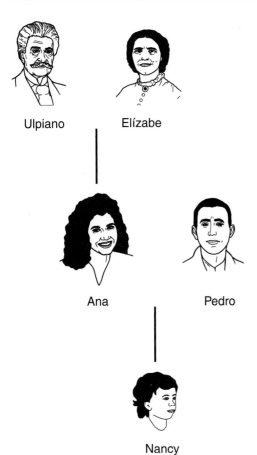

La familia de Ana. ¿Quiénes son? Por ejemplo,
Ana es la madre de Nancy.

Hola. Soy Ana. Soy hija única de mi papá y mamá. No tengo hermanos.   **único/a** only
Estoy casada. Mi esposo se llama Pedro. Tenemos una hija. Ella se llama
Nancy y tiene cinco años de edad. Aquí está un diagrama de mi familia.

Vocabulario: Más familiares (*More Family Members*)

Para completar su léxico

el tío abuelo	great-uncle	**la tía abuela**	great-aunt
el/la bisabuelo/a	great-grandparent	**el/la bisnieto/a**	great-grandchild
el suegro	father-in-law	**la suegra**	mother-in-law
el yerno	son-in-law	**la nuera**	daughter-in-law
el cuñado	brother-in-law	**la cuñada**	sister-in-law
el padrastro	stepfather	**la madrastra**	stepmother
el hijastro	stepson	**la hijastra**	stepdaughter
el hermanastro	stepbrother	**la hermanastra**	stepsister
el hermano de padre	half-brother	**la hermana de padre**	half-sister

el hermano de madre	half-brother	la hermana de madre	half-sister
el ahijado	godson	la ahijada	goddaughter
hijo de crianza	foster child	como familia	just like family

- To establish whether a caretaker who brings a child for medical care is the child's parent, ask *¿Es su hijo/a?* or *¿Es usted el padre / la madre del niño / de la niña?*
- A Spanish-speaker with two siblings may say *Tengo dos hermanos* or *Somos tres hermanos.* The latter is a cultural norm that more explicitly includes the speaker.
- The adjectives *paterno/a* and *materno/a* following a noun clarify whether the family member is related by father or by mother.

HACIA PRECISIÓN

 5.1 Ejercicio _____

Quiz a classmate by asking for the following family relationships, as in the example. Make up some additional questions on your own.

Modelo: el padre de mi abuela
—¿Quién es el padre de mi abuela?
—El padre de su abuela es su bisabuelo.

A. la esposa de mi hermano
B. el hijo de mi hijo
C. el hijo de mi padrastro
D. la hermana de mi madre

E. el hijo de mi tía
F. la hermana de mi primo
G. la madre de mi esposa
H. el hijo de mi esposa y su ex marido

 5.2 Ejercicio _____

Fill in the following blanks with the names of family relationships based on the diagram of Arturo Martínez Mendoza's family.

Hola. Me llamo Arturo. Mi _____ se llama Juan Martínez. Él tiene

una _____ que se llama Carmen y es mi _____. También

tiene un _____ que se llama Pedro y es mi _____. Soy el

_____ de mi tía Carmen y mi tío Pedro. Tío Pedro tiene dos hijos.

Ellos son mis _____. El padre de mi padre es mi _____ Ja-

vier Martínez. La esposa de mi abuelo es mi _____.

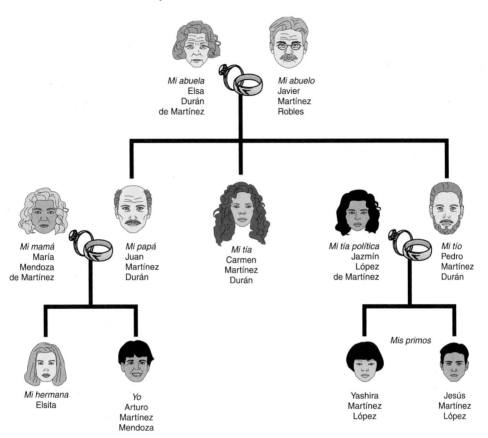

Mi Familia
por Arturo Martínez Mendoza

Mi abuela
Elsa
Durán
de Martínez

Mi abuelo
Javier
Martínez
Robles

Mi mamá
María
Mendoza
de Martínez

Mi papá
Juan
Martínez
Durán

Mi tía
Carmen
Martínez
Durán

Mi tía política
Jazmín
López
de Martínez

Mi tío
Pedro
Martínez
Durán

Mis primos

Mi hermana
Elsita

Yo
Arturo
Martínez
Mendoza

Yashira
Martínez
López

Jesús
Martínez
López

HACIA FLUIDEZ

 5.3 Actividad _____

Refer to the diagram *Mi familia, por Arturo Martínez Mendoza* and with a partner make as many questions and statements as you can about the family relationships. Ask, for example, *¿Tiene hermanos Yashira?* or *¿Quién es doña Elsa?* Recall that the titles *señor* and *señora* are used with last names, and the titles *don* and *doña* are used with first names.

 5.4 Actividad _____

Circulate in the classroom and ask classmates whether they have children, siblings, nieces and nephews, godparents, and so on, and their names and ages. Take notes, and report your findings to the class.

5.5 Actividad

As a variation of *Ejercicio* 5.1, the instructor will give each student an index card. Each card will have a perfect match. For example, if one card says *el hijo de mi tío,* its match says *primo.* Students circulate and find their match. If there are an odd number of students, the instructor plays, too.

 5.6 Actividad

Take turns showing the class a picture of your family or of an imaginary or fictitious family (the Simpsons, for example). Identify and describe family members. If your instructor gives you advance notice, e-mail or bring these on thumb drives for projection in the classroom. Break into spontaneous conversation where possible. For example:

> Modelo: —¿Quién es? ¿Es su hija?
> —Sí, es mi hija menor (*youngest*).
> —¿Cómo se llama y cuántos años tiene?
> —Se llama Susan y tiene diez años.

 5.7 Drama improvisado

Play "Tangled Web." Five or six students form a circle around one student. A student from the circle declares his or her family relationship to the student in the middle, for example, *Soy tu madre,* and the student in the middle declares his or her consequential relationship to that student: *Eres mi madre, soy tu hijo/a.* The next student then does the same with the student in the middle and with each student who has gone before. When you feel ready, suppose someone in the group divorced (*Soy tu ex esposo*) and married a person with children. Continue until you can no longer keep track of your tangled web!

 5.8 Drama improvisado

"*Velorio*" is a fun if not macabre variation of "Tangled Web." Create a "wake," in which one student lies comfortably on a few chairs, while his son or daughter sits alongside. The child has never met his family. Students approach one by one to pay their respects, and tell the child their relationship to the deceased. Then the child and family member announce their relationship to each other.

> Modelo: —Él fue (*was*) mi hermano favorito.
> —Usted es mi tío.
> —Sí, soy tu tío y eres mi sobrino.

Estructura: Los verbos regulares terminados con -ar, -er e -ir (*Regular Verbs Ending in* -ar, -er, *and* -ir)

- So far you have learned three verbs: *ser, estar,* and *tener.* Each morphs, or changes its form, according to its person. These three verbs are considered irregular, because their forms are idiosyncratic; that is, their forms don't follow a pattern that is repeatable with other verbs.
- Fortunately there are regular verbs that share common morphology. These are divided into three groups, based on their infinitive endings: *-ar, -er,* and *-ir.* Each group has a consistent set of forms.
- This is the morphology of the regular verb *hablar* (to talk or to speak):

yo	**Hablo** inglés y un poquito de español.
tú	¿**Hablas** inglés?
él, ella, usted	Mi mamá no **habla** inglés.
nosotros/as	En casa, **hablamos** español.
ellos, ellas, ustedes	Mis hijos **hablan** inglés, pero soy bilingüe.

- Regular verbs that end in *-er* have a consistent morphology. Here is the regular verb *comer* (to eat):

yo	En un restaurante italiano **como** espaguetis.
tú	¿**Comes** tacos al pastor?
él, ella, usted	Usted **come** muchas frutas.
nosotros/as	Mi esposa y yo **comemos** a las seis.
ellos, ellas, ustedes	Ellas **comen** en la cafetería.

- Regular verbs that end in *-ir* also have a consistent morphology. These differ from those that end in *-er* only in the first person plural (*nosotros/as*). Here is the regular verb *vivir* (to live):

yo	**Vivo** en una casa grande.
tú	¿Dónde **vives**?
él, ella, usted	Ella **vive** con mi madre.
nosotros/as	**Vivimos** en un departamento (*apartment*).
ellos, ellas, ustedes	¿**Viven** ustedes en Florida?

- People who learn Spanish as a primary language or via immersion do not necessarily recognize the designations "regular" and "irregular." These terms are shorthand to help second-language learners; for them, hearing that a particular verb is "regular" will signal its morphology.

Vocabulario: Algunos verbos regulares (*Some Regular Verbs*)

Verbos terminados en -*ar*

ayudar	to help
caminar	to walk
cocinar	to cook
comprar	to buy
cuidar	to care for
enseñar	to teach, show
estudiar	to study
examinar	to examine
llamar	to call
llegar	to arrive
necesitar	to need
practicar	to practice
preguntar	to ask a question
recetar	to prescribe
tomar	to take, drink
trabajar	to work
usar	to use
visitar	to visit

Verbos terminados en -*er*

aprender	to learn
beber	to drink
comer	to eat
leer	to read

Verbos terminados en -*ir*

abrir	to open
escribir	to write
sufrir de	to suffer from
vivir	to live

HACIA PRECISIÓN

 5.9 Ejercicio_____ _____

Identify the phrase or object in parenthesis that is more likely to appear with each verb.

    A. llegar (a las seis, por tres horas)
    B. recetar (una hamburguesa, medicina para el colesterol)
    C. caminar (en el parque, en la ambulancia)
    D. leer (las instrucciones, los pacientes)
    E. comprar (el doctor, el medicamento)
    F. escribir (el radio, una receta)
    G. cocinar (vegetales, las sábanas)
    H. sufrir de (una enfermera, una enfermedad)
    I. cuidar (a un paciente, a un estado civil)
    J. necesitar (una receta, la diabetes)
    K. comer (un elíxir, una ensalada)
    L. vivir (por cien años, la otorrinolaringóloga)

 5.10 Ejercicio _____

Read this paragraph aloud with the correct forms of the verbs.

Me llamo Shawn. _____ (ser) enfermero y _____ (trabajar) en la clínica de lunes a viernes. No _____ (vivir) lejos de la clínica y _____ (caminar) a la clínica todos los días. La clínica _____ (abrir) a las ocho de la mañana. La doctora Valerio _____ (trabajar) en la clínica también. Ella y yo _____ (cuidar) a nuestros pacientes. La doctora _____ (examinar) a los pacientes y _____ (recetar) los medicamentos. Yo _____ (enseñar) a los pacientes cómo tomar sus medicamentos. Los pacientes _____ (comprar) sus medicamentos en la farmacia y _____ (visitar) la clínica cuando están enfermos o _____ (necesitar) más medicamentos.

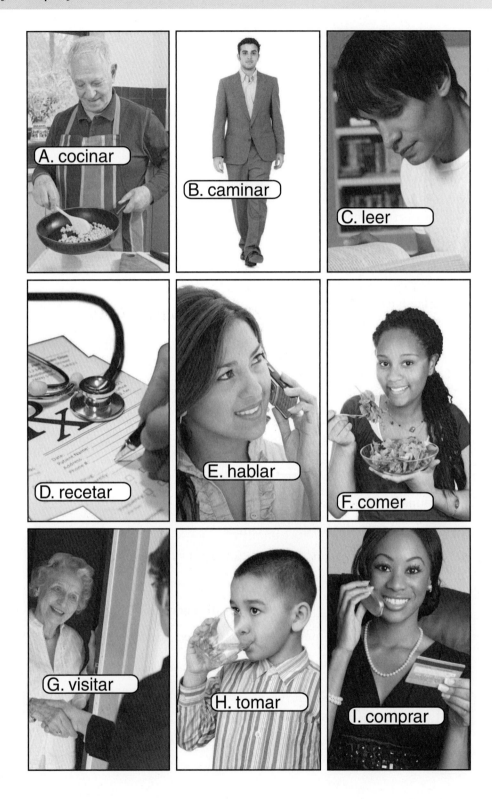

A. cocinar

B. caminar

C. leer

D. recetar

E. hablar

F. comer

G. visitar

H. tomar

I. comprar

5.11 Ejercicio

Complete the following sentences based on the photo collage.

A. Mi abuelo _____ vegetales para la familia.

B. Juan Miguel _____ al hospital para trabajar todos los días.

C. Usted _____ libros en inglés y español.

D. Los doctores _____ los medicamentos.

E. Marisol y su hermana _____ por teléfono todos los sábados.

F. Yo _____ mucha ensalada porque tiene fibra y muchas vitaminas.

G. Una enfermera _____ a mi abuela en su casa una vez a la semana.

H. Luisito _____ un vaso de agua porque tiene mucha sed.

I. Miguelina _____ libros por Internet con su tarjeta de crédito.

 5.12 Ejercicio

Work with a partner to ask and respond to the following questions. Although you would normally use the formal *usted* form with an adult patient, you'll practice the informal *tú* here with your classmate.

Modelo: sufrir de
—¿Sufres de migrañas?
—No, no sufro de migrañas, gracias a Dios.

A. caminar   ¿Caminas a la clase?
B. llegar   ¿A qué hora llegas a la clase?
C. tomar   ¿Tomas antiácidos por la noche?
D. trabajar   ¿Qué días de la semana trabajas?
E. abrir   ¿Abres la ventanas de tu casa en la noche?
F. practicar   ¿Con quién practicas el español?
G. leer   ¿Lees el libro de español por la noche?
H. beber   ¿Bebes bebidas alcohólicas todos los días?
I. estudiar   ¿Cuántas horas estudias los fines de semana?
J. sufrir de   ¿Sufres de alergias?

HACIA FLUIDEZ

 5.13 Actividad _____

Circulate in the classroom asking classmates which languages (*idiomas*) they speak and which are spoken by members of their family. We shall practice the informal register (*tú*) because we are talking among classmates. Identify bilingual and polyglot (multilingual) individuals and report your findings. (In Spanish, names of languages do not begin with a capital letter.)

Modelo: —¿Qué idiomas hablas?
—Hablo inglés.
—¿Qué idiomas hablan tus familiares?
—Mis abuelos hablan polaco.

español	Spanish	**inglés**	English
francés	French	**italiano**	Italian
alemán	German	**portugués**	Portuguese
chino	Chinese	**japonés**	Japanese
árabe	Arabic	**polaco**	Polish

 5.14 Actividad_____

This activity sheet is available for download from the website.

Conduct the following survey (*¡solo español, por favor!*) with five of your classmates. Write their names in the spaces according to how often they eat at various places. Then discuss your results with the class. Key: *a veces* (occasionally), *a menudo* (frequently), and *siempre* (always).

Comer . . .	A veces	A menudo	Siempre
. . . en casa			
. . . en la cafetería			
. . . en un restaurante			
. . . en casa de los padres			
. . . en el trabajo (*at work*)			

5.15 Drama improvisado————————————————————

Play "Three-headed Person." Space permitting, form a circle. Otherwise choose a pattern for taking turns while seated in the classroom, such as up and down rows. Recall that a sentence usually has a subject, a verb, and an ending. The first person states a subject (for example, *yo, usted, Juan, mis padres, la uróloga*). The next person supplies the verb, conjugated according to the subject. The third person provides an ending. Then the class repeats the whole sentence in loud and percussive tones.

> Modelo: —el doctor
> —examina
> —al paciente
> —El doctor examina al paciente.

   5.16 Drama improvisado————————————————————

Play "Party Quirks." Choose a host to throw a party, and ask the host to leave the room for a moment. The class will give five or six students a verb phrase, including a verb and an object, or a sentence ending (for example, *recetar un medicamento* or *llamar al odontólogo*). Next, the host returns and stands in the front of the room preparing a party, perhaps describing the space and preparations. One of the students knocks on an imaginary door (gesture knocking while tapping a foot on the floor for the sound). The host opens the door and welcomes the guest inside. Both exchange greetings and small talk. Then the student portrays the meaning of the verb phrase, using gestures, questions, and statements, and saying anything but the verb. For example, the student with *llamar al odontólogo* might use an imaginary cell phone to chat with the dentist's office complaining about a toothache and requesting an appointment. At a lull in the conversation, another student knocks. At the end, the host must guess each student's phrase.

   ## Estructura: La *a* personal (*The Personal a*)

- When a person receives the action of the verb directly, a preposition called the personal *a* is placed after the verb.

  > Visito **a** mi mamá todos los días.
  > La enfermera cuida **a** sus pacientes muy bien.
  > Sara llama a Susana todos los días.

- The preposition *a* and the masculine definite article *el* form the contraction *al* (*a* + *el* = *al*).

  > Llamo **al** doctor cuando estoy enfermo.

- The personal *a* is not needed when a person is not the direct object of the verb.

  Practico español en la comunidad.
  Necesito aspirina para el dolor de cabeza.

HACIA PRECISIÓN

 5.17 Ejercicio _____

Choose which of these sentences require the inclusion of the personal *a* and which do not, and write it in the provided spaces as needed.

A. Aprendo ___ español rápidamente.

B. Enseño inglés ___ mis padres.

C. Mi esposa y yo hablamos ___ español en casa.

D. Cuido ___ mis padres en la casa.

E. Visito ___ mi mamá todas las semanas.

F. Llamo ___ mi hermana por teléfono los domingos.

G. Mi hermano come ___ una hamburguesa al mediodía.

H. Mi tío bebe ___ tres tazas de café por la mañana.

 ## Take Family Medical History

 ## Vocabulario: Las enfermedades hereditarias

el alcoholismo	alcoholism
el asma*	asthma
el cáncer	cancer
la depresión	depression
la diabetes	diabetes
la distrofia muscular	muscular dystrophy

*Asma, like agua, is a feminine word that uses the masculine article el and a feminine adjective, for example, el asma crónica.

la enfermedad de Alzheimer	Alzheimer's disease
la enfermedad de Huntington	Huntington's disease
la hemofilia	hemophilia
la hipertensión	hypertension
los problemas cardíacos	cardiac problems
los problemas emocionales	emotional problems
el síndrome de Down	Down syndrome
la tensión alta	high blood pressure

Vivo and *muerto* are adjectives meaning "alive" and "dead," and therefore have gender and number. The definite article (*el, la*) is not used after *hay*, as in, *¿Hay asma en la familia?* To say that someone *had* an illness while implying a particular time, use the past tense *tuvo,* which we'll present in chapter 9.

The question *¿Ha tenido asma?* uses the present perfect tense. The helping verb *haber* combines with the present participle of the verb *tener* to ask if you, he, or she has had any particular illness, in this case asthma. You will learn more about this tense in chapter 10

Expresiones útiles

Su padre tiene la tensión alta.	Your father has high blood pressure.
Mi madre tuvo cáncer.	My mother had cancer.
Mi padre murió.	My father died.
Mi padre está muerto.	My father is dead.

Preguntas útiles

¿Están vivos sus padres?	Are your parents alive?
¿Qué enfermedades tenían?	What illnesses did they have?
¿De qué murió su madre?	From what did your mother die?
¿Hay asma en la familia?	Is there asthma in the family?
En su familia ¿alguien ha tenido asma?	Has anyone in your family had asthma?
¿Qué enfermedades hay en su familia?	What illnesses are there in your family?

HACIA FLUIDEZ

 5.18 Actividad _____

Form small groups and ask each other whether various relatives are living, as in the example. Ask about the cause of death, which may prompt you to refer to the glossary that appears at the end of the book. (Recall that the adjectives must agree in gender and number.)

> Modelo: —¿Está vivo su abuelo?
> —Sí, mi abuelo está vivo (or) No, mi abuelo murió.
> —(*if negative*) ¿De qué murió?
> —Mi abuelo murió de un infarto cardíaco.

 5.19 Actividad

In the same small groups, ask about several aspects of medical history, using the preceding vocabulary.

> Modelo: —¿Hay asma en su familia?
> —No, no hay asma (or) Sí, mi madre tiene (tuvo) asma.

Take Pediatric Family History

Historia médica de los padres biológicos

Recall some options for talking about family medical history.

> ¿Hay hipertensión en la familia?
> ¿Quién tuvo hipertensión?
> En la familia ¿alguien ha tenido problemas renales?
> Entre los dos padres biológicos ¿ha tenido alguien un retraso mental?
> Tengo diabetes. Mi padre tuvo diabetes también.
> Tuve un ataque al corazón.

 5.20 Actividad

This form is available for download from the website.

You are a pediatrician and your partner is a parent with a new baby. Using the form that has been provided, practice taking family medical history. Find out which family member had the illness or condition and take notes to share your results with the class. Use *ha tenido* to talk about an illness or condition that the person **has had** at some unspecified time in the past. Use *tuvo* to talk about an illness or condition that she or he **had,** when speaking in the context of a specific time or when speaking of a deceased person.

☐ Diabetes

☐ Hipertensión

☐ Fumador/a*

☐ Alergia

☐ Asma

☐ Epilepsia, convulsiones

☐ Malformación genética/congénita

☐ Problema renal

☐ Problema con huesos/articulaciones

☐ Cáncer

☐ Enfermedad de músculo/nervio

☐ Ataque al corazón antes de los sesenta años

☐ Accidente cerebrovascular

☐ Problema gastroenterológico

☐ Retraso mental

☐ Hemoglobinopatía

☐ (a) anemia drepanocítica

☐ (b) talasemia

☐ (c) hemoglobinopatía C ☐ S-C

☐ Sordera

☐ Hipercolesterolemia

☐ Problema urinario

☐ Otro†

†Favor de explicar:

_____

_____

_____

*In the case of *fumador/a* (smoker), use the verb *fumar* or the verb *ser. ¿Fuma usted? ¿Es usted fumador/a?*

Estructura: Los complementos directos (*Direct Object Pronouns*)

- The direct object pronoun represents the person or thing that directly receives the action of the verb. It can be used to replace the direct object noun. It sounds natural and reflects economy of language. These are the direct object pronouns.

me	¿Me necesitas?	Do you need me?
te	Te necesito.	I need you.
lo/la	Lo/la visito.	I visit you/him/her/it.
nos	Ellos nos esperan.	They are waiting for us.
los/las	Los cuido.	I take care of them.

- Direct object pronouns must agree in gender and number with the object noun they replace or refer to. They are used when the object noun has been mentioned or is understood. For example, here the object noun is mentioned in the question and replaced by the direct object in the answer.

—¿Usa usted insulina?

—¿Necesita el inhalador?

—Sí, *la* uso dos veces al día.

—No, no *lo* necesito.

—¿Tiene los supositorios? —No, no *los* tengo.
—¿Tomas café? —Sí, pero no *lo* tomo por la tarde.
—¿Cuándo visitas a tu mamá? —*La* visito los domingos.

HACIA FLUIDEZ

 5.21 Actividad_____

Notice the efficiency of the direct object pronoun. Take turns asking members of the class about what they drink. Use the direct object pronoun (*lo/la* or *los/las*) to answer the questions.

 Modelo: —¿Tomas café?
     —Sí, lo tomo por la mañana.
     —¿Tomas cerveza (*beer*)?
     —Sí. La tomo los viernes en la tarde.

 A. el té   E. las bebidas alcohólicas
 B. el vino (*wine*) F. el jugo de naranja (*orange juice*)
 C. el agua (*f*)   G. el jugo de ciruela (*prune juice*)
 D. la leche   H. el té de manzanilla (*chamomile tea*)

 5.22 Actividad_____

Ask a partner the following questions. Use the direct object pronoun when answering. The symbols (*m*) and (*f*) are provided to indicate the gender of the direct object noun. You'll know whether they are singular or plural.

 Modelo: —¿Toma aspirina (*f*) todos los días?
     —Sí, la tomo (*or*) No, no la tomo.

 A. ¿Toma antibióticos (*m*) cuando tiene resfriado?
 B. ¿Usa insulina (*f*) para la diabetes?
 C. ¿Usa el inhalador (*m*) cuando tiene fatiga?
 D. ¿Usa lentes (*m*) para leer?
 E. ¿Visita a sus hermanos (*m*) en Puerto Rico?
 F. ¿Necesita medicamento (*m*) para el dolor?
 G. ¿Bebe bebidas alcohólicas (*f*)?
 H. ¿Ayuda a sus padres (*m*) en la casa?

5.23 Actividad

Improvise skits in which a practitioner interviews a patient to determine his or her family medical history, personal history, current conditions, and habits with regard to alcohol, tobacco, and other substances. If desired, assign unusual roles, such as a hypochondriac or a "heart attack waiting to happen."

 5.24 Drama improvisado

Play the game show "Competitive Hypochondriac." Choose a panel of students. Each contestant tells of his or her aches, pains, injuries, and personal and family medical history. The object of the game is to amplify your own complaints while minimizing those of your opponents. A host should keep score, assigning points based on the amount of hyperbole.

 5.25 Reciclaje

Here's a description of *tío* Alfredo: *Tío Alfredo es rubio. Es alto y delgado. Trabaja como profesor y siempre llega tarde a la escuela. Él cuida a mi tía.* Describe *tía Mercedes*.

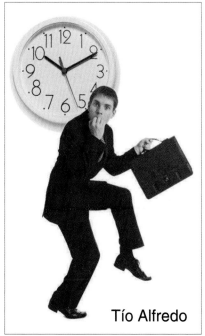

Tío Alfredo

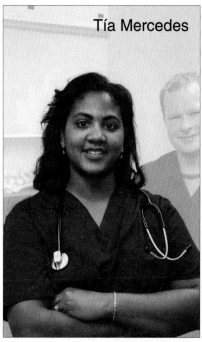

Tía Mercedes

5.26 Reciclaje _____

Take a blank sheet of paper and pretend it is a photo of a member of your family (or bring your own family photo). Use adjectives from chapter 1 as well as your new verbs to describe family members and to say something else about each. Note that in the list that follows, we have replaced *gordo/a* with *con sobrepeso* (overweight). It is used with the verb *estar,* because it is a state or condition.

rubio/a	moreno/a	anciano/a	joven
alto/a	bajo/a	delgado/a	mediano/a
con sobrepeso/a	bonito/a	guapo/a	bueno/a
inteligente	simpático/a	amable	agradable

 Reciclaje 5.27 _____

Recycle the names for injuries from chapter 3 and use them with the names for family relationships. You are an emergency room nurse. Role-play a skit in which you call the home of a patient who was in an accident. You wish to speak with a parent, however the imaginary phone gets passed from student to student. Each plays the role of a family member other than a parent and asks about the situation.

 ## Pronunciación de *B* y *V*

- The letters *b* and *v* are pronounced very similarly, both spoken a little more softly than the English "b," and neither quite like the English "v." Prior to 2010 in many geographical regions, their names in Spanish were *be* and *ve*. Because the letters and their names sounded alike, Spanish-speakers would request clarification by asking, ¿«*V*» *de vaca, o* «*b*» *de burro?* or ¿«*V*» *corta o* «*b*» *larga?* To help with this, in 2010 the *Real Academia Española* confirmed that the letter *v* should be called *uve,* and the letter *w* should be called *doble uve.* The complete Spanish alphabet appears in appendix 1.

vaca COW

- Practice the following words, and then tackle a pair of *trabalenguas.*

biopsia	fiebre	aborto
varicela	viruela	vivir

Veinte viudas con venas varicosas viven en una vivienda vieja.
¿Qué bebe el bebé? El bebé bebe leche buena de un biberón blanco.

Exposición

   CHAPTER 5 SKILL: DESCRIBING PEOPLE IN GREATER DETAIL

You are going to make a presentation about your family. It can be true to life or you can make up an imaginary family, whichever you prefer.

1. Listen as a person describes two family members. Notice the information she provides about each person and use the chart to take note of the information that is included.

	Descripción de la primera persona	Descripción de la segunda persona
nombre/relación		
edad		
profesión		
estado donde vive		
descripción		
historia médica		
padecimientos actuales		

2. Look at the chart and decide what kind of information you will include about each family member, real or imaginary, that you describe.
3. Write your description. Be sure that you include at least two family members.
4. Present your description to the class. You may choose to project on the classroom screen a photograph or other visual of the family members.
5. As you listen to your classmates' presentations, ask follow-up questions about their family members.

Cultural Note: *La familia*

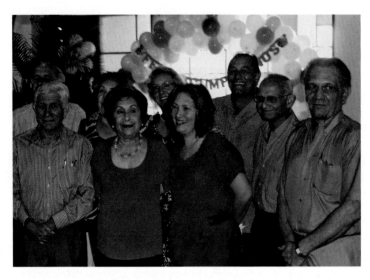

Un grupo de hermanos celebra un cumpleaños.

Often the Latino family is an extended family. Speaking of *mi familia,* Spanish-speakers may have in mind aunts, uncles, and cousins as well as brothers, sisters, and in-laws. This is no surprise to health care workers who have had the responsibility of limiting the number of visitors at a patient's bedside. In some countries, a family member must stay with a hospitalized patient for the purpose of delivering food, providing personal care, and making trips to a local pharmacy to purchase medications.

A *padrino* (godfather) or *madrina* (godmother) has almost equal standing with a parent, having promised to raise the child in the event the parents cannot. The child is expected to respect a godparent as a parent, although godparents count primarily as a support to the parents, or *compadres.* A hospital security guard outside the intensive care unit of a North American hospital once told a family member that visits were restricted to "immediate family only," to which the visitor replied, "I am his godfather."

Although children are highly valued and well cared for, they are not always the center of attention at family gatherings. In times past, an old saying dictated that *los muchachos hablan cuando las gallinas orinan* ("children talk when chickens urinate," comparable in meaning to "children should be seen and not heard").

Donde comen dos, comen tres

Family boundaries are flexible. Even a neighbor can be considered part of the family. A close friend might be called *primo, hermano* or *compadre.*

People say of these relationships, *somos como familia,* or "we're just like family."

The Latino family is a strong, primary support network for its members. Immigrants to the United States who are separated from family and homeland generally suffer a profound sense of loss. Many who emigrate leave their family reluctantly to work abroad and send money to support those who remain. Most leave children behind in the care of other relatives, and some choose to take or send children on perilous journeys to save them from recruitment by violent gangs.

Some Spanish speakers say, *Tengo tres hermanos*; others say, *Somos cuatro hermanos.* The latter demonstrates a cultural view that includes oneself in the count, unlike the concept of sibling rivalry. This is an example of the relation between worldview and language.

When working with a Latino family, a helper must assess the degree to which the family has retained, for its members, its highly influential cultural value. Family boundaries may be vague. Policies regarding confidentiality of a patient vis-à-vis the family may be misunderstood. What the broad family system believes about the nature of the distress itself will be a powerful factor in the patient's view of the problem being treated. The worth of the family to the individual and of the individual to the family must never be underestimated.

Vocabulario del capítulo cinco

Los familiares

el padre, papá	father	**la madre, mamá**	mother
el esposo, el marido	husband	**la esposa, mujer**	wife
el hijo	son	**la hija**	daughter
el hermano	brother	**la hermana**	sister
el abuelo	grandfather	**la abuela**	grandmother
el nieto	grandson	**la nieta**	granddaughter
el tío	uncle	**la tía**	aunt
el sobrino	nephew	**la sobrina**	niece
el primo	male cousin	**la prima**	female cousin
el padrino	godfather	**la madrina**	godmother

Más familiares

el tío abuelo	great-uncle	**la tía abuela**	great-aunt
el/la bisabuelo/a	great-grandparent	**el/la bisnieto/a**	great-grandchild
el suegro	father-in-law	**la suegra**	mother-in-law
el yerno	son-in-law	**la nuera**	daughter-in-law
el cuñado	brother-in-law	**la cuñada**	sister-in-law
el padrastro	stepfather	**la madrastra**	stepmother
el hijastro	stepson	**la hijastra**	stepdaughter
el hermanastro	stepbrother	**la hermanastra**	stepsister
el hermano de padre	half-brother	**la hermana de padre**	half-sister
el hermano de madre	half-brother	**la hermana de madre**	half-sister
el ahijado	godson	**la ahijada**	goddaughter
hijo de crianza	foster child	**como familia**	just like family

Algunos verbos regulares

ayudar	to help	**llegar**	to arrive
caminar	to walk	**necesitar**	to need
cocinar	to cook	**practicar**	to practice
comprar	to buy	**preguntar**	to ask a question
cuidar	to care for	**recetar**	to prescribe
enseñar	to teach, show	**tomar**	to take, drink
estudiar	to study	**trabajar**	to work
examinar	to examine	**usar**	to use
llamar	to call	**visitar**	to visit
aprender	to learn	**comer**	to eat
beber	to drink	**leer**	to read

abrir	to open	**sufrir de**	to suffer from
escribir	to write	**vivir**	to live

Algunos idiomas

español	Spanish	**inglés**	English
francés	French	**italiano**	Italian
alemán	German	**portugués**	Portuguese
chino	Chinese	**japonés**	Japanese
árabe	Arabic	**polaco**	Polish

Las enfermedades hereditarias

el alcoholismo	alcoholism
el asma	asthma
el cáncer	cancer
la depresión	depression
la diabetes	diabetes
la distrofia muscular	muscular dystrophy
la enfermedad de Alzheimer	Alzheimer's disease
la enfermedad de Huntington	Huntington's disease
la hemofilia	hemophilia
la hipertensión	hypertension
los problemas cardíacos	cardiac problems
los problemas emocionales	emotional problems
el síndrome de Down	Down syndrome
la tensión alta	high blood pressure

Enfermedades adicionales

el accidente cerebrovascular	cerebrovascular accident
la anemia drepanocítica	sickle cell anemia
el ataque al corazón	heart attack
la enfermedad de músculo/nervio	illness of muscles/nerves
la hemoglobinopatía	hemoglobinopathy
la malformación genética/congénita	genetic/congenital deformity
el problema con huesos/articulaciones	bone/joint problems
el retraso mental	mental retardation
la sordera	deafness
la talasemia	thalassemia

Historia médica de los padres biológicos

fumador/a	smoker
problema gastroenterológico	GI problem
alergia	allergy
epilepsia, convulsiones	epilepsy, convulsions
hemoglobinopatía	hemoglobinopathy

problema renal	kidney problem
problema con huesos/articulaciones	bone/joint problem
hipercolesterolemia	hypercholesterolemia
problema urinario	urinary problem
enfermedad de músculo/nervio	muscle/nerve disease

Expresiones útiles

Su padre tiene la tensión alta.	Your father has high blood pressure.
Mi madre tuvo cáncer.	My mother had cancer.
Mi padre murió.	My father died.
Mi padre está muerto.	My father is dead.

Preguntas útiles

¿Están vivos sus padres?	Are your parents alive?
¿Qué enfermedades tenían?	What illnesses did they have?
¿De qué murió su madre?	From what did your mother die?
¿Hay asma en la familia?	Is there asthma in the family?
En su familia ¿alguien ha tenido asma?	Has anyone in your family had asthma?
¿Qué enfermedades hay en su familia?	What illnesses are there in your family?

Chapter 6
La farmacia

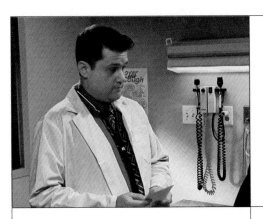

Communication Goals

Vocabulary

Structure

Cultural Note

Website   www.yalebooks.com/medicalspanish
   Video   *Trama: ¿Qué medicamentos toma?; Demostración: Cómo usar el inhalador*
   Audio   *Formas de medicamentos; Algunas clases de medicamentos; Las reacciones
      alérgicas; El asma; Exposición*
   Electronic Workbook

B y the end of this chapter you will be able to write and explain basic instructions for taking medicines. You will be able to ask about drug allergies and educate patients about side effects and allergic reactions. You will know how to make polite and direct commands and to use these when educating patients about medication regimens, the management of asthma, and the use of pill organizers.

From here on, many headings are in Spanish without translation. Instructions for most exercises and activities will appear in Spanish, although directions for *Drama improvisado* are English in many cases. This list of key words and phrases will get you started. The verbs are used as formal commands, which you'll learn in this chapter.

agregue	add
colabore	collaborate
complete	complete
conteste	answer
dé	give
escoja	choose
escriba	write
hable con compañeros	talk with classmates
haga oraciones completas	make complete sentences
identifique	identify
observe, vea	observe, see
pregunte	ask
use	use

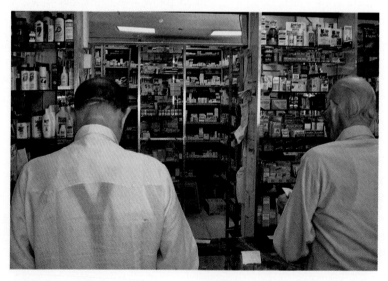

La farmacia está abierta.

Give Medication Instructions

In some areas, the pharmacist is the most accessible health care provider. In developing countries, many Spanish-speaking people will consult a pharmacist prior to going to see a doctor. The pharmacist may dispense a medication that would be controlled elsewhere. Some countries are trying to end this practice because of the emergence of treatment-resistant infections. Mexico, for example, now requires that antibiotics be dispensed only with a prescription. In response, larger pharmacy chains offer free medical consultations on premises.

The noun *receta,* which is used for "prescription," also means "recipe," revealing some history of pharmacotherapy. The verb *recetar* means "to prescribe." While medicines were traditionally called *medicamentos* or *remedios,* the expression *medicina* is now widespread.

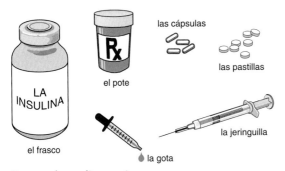

Formas de medicamentos

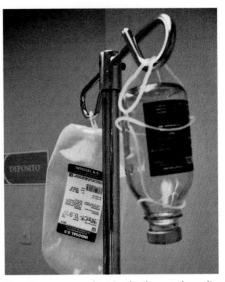

El suero es una solución de cloruro de sodio para hidratar al paciente por vía intravenosa.

Vocabulario: Formas de medicamentos

Las tabletas

la tableta, la pastilla	tablet, pill
la píldora, el comprimido	tablet, pill
la cápsula, la gragea	capsule
. . . masticable	. . . chewable
media tableta	half of a tablet
el frasco, la botella	pill bottle, bottle

Las inyecciones e infusiones

la inyección	injection
la jeringuilla	syringe
el suero, el intravenoso	IV
el suero / el intravenoso central	central IV line

Los líquidos

el jarabe	syrup
el elíxir	elixir
la gota	drop
la suspensión	suspension

Los medicamentos tópicos

la crema	cream, ointment
el ungüento	ointment, balm

The *ü* in *ungüento* is pronounced like English "w."

Otras formas

el aerosol	aerosol
el atomizador	atomizer
el gel	gel
el inhalador, la pompa (*slang*)	inhaler
el nebulizador (la máquina)	nebulizer (machine)
el parche	patch
el supositorio	suppository

Preguntas útiles

¿Es usted alérgico/a a algún medicamento?	Are you allergic to any medication?
¿Tiene usted alergia a algún medicamento?	Do you have an allergy to any medication?
¿Toma algún medicamento todos los días?	Do you take any medicine every day?
¿Necesita una receta nueva?	Do you need a new prescription?

Expresiones útiles

Hay que tomar media tableta.	You must take half a tablet.
Hay que darle dos pastillas.	You must give him/her two pills.

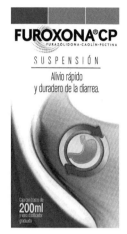

La Furoxona CP es una suspensión antidiarreica.

HACIA PRECISIÓN

 6.1 Ejercicio _____

Identifique las formas comunes de los siguientes medicamentos.

Modelo: La aspirina está disponible (*available*) en pastilla y pastilla masticable.

A. el acetaminofén
B. la leche de magnesia
C. el Pepto Bismol
D. la Visene
E. la insulina
F. el salbutamol
G. la guaifenesina
H. la hidrocortisona 2%
I. la nicotina
J. la Compazina
K. la vacuna para la varicela
L. el ibuprofeno

 6.2 Ejercicio _____

Haga expresiones completas con la forma correcta del verbo *tomar*.

A. ¿_____ (tomar) usted antiácidos por la noche?

B. Doña Violeta _____ (tomar) una aspirina todos los días.

C. ¿ _____ (tomar) tú medicamento para los ataques epilépticos?

D. Mi esposa y yo _____ (tomar) la vitamina B 12 (be doce) por la mañana.

E. El señor Altamirano _____ (tomar) un diurético para quitar el agua.

F. Los padres de Juan _____ (tomar) medicamento para la hipertensión.

G. Los pacientes _____ (tomar) antibióticos para curar las infecciones bacterianas.

HACIA FLUIDEZ

6.3 Actividad _____

Haga una encuesta (*survey*). Hable con cinco compañeros y pregúnteles si toman aspirina, vitaminas, antiácidos y ácido fólico. Pregúnteles también las horas que los toman. Después, hable de los resultados.

Modelo: ¿Toma usted una aspirina todos los días?
¿A qué hora la toma?
¿Qué toma cuando tiene dolor de cabeza?

Nombre	Aspirina	Vitamina	Antiácido	Ácido fólico

Estructura: Los imperativos con *favor de, hay que y tener que*

- In written Spanish, you can imply instructions by using the verb infinitive alone.

  Tomar las pastillas con leche.   Take the pills with milk.

- To make a gentle request, use *favor de* and a verb infinitive (the -*r* form).

  Favor de sentarse.   Please sit down.
  Favor de llamar a la clínica.   Please call the clinic.

- For a less personal request, use *hay que* or *es importante* and an infinitive. (*Hay* rhymes with the English word "buy" and means "there is" and "there are.") This tells something that ought to be done.

  Hay que tomar la medicina.   One must take the medicine.
  Es importante tomar mucha agua con el medicamento.
  Hay que tomar el medicamento a la misma hora todos los días.

- A stronger or more direct command is to tell the patient that he or she "has to" do something. For this, you may use *tener que* and an infinitive. In such two-verb combinations, the first verb is conjugated and the second verb is not.

Tienes que tomar la tableta. You have to take the pill.
Usted tiene que ir al laboratorio. You have to go to the laboratory.

- To clarify whether the patient understood the instruction, choose content-related questions that cannot be answered with "yes" or "no."

¿A qué hora toma el ibuprofeno?
¿Cuántas pastillas toma a las nueve?

HACIA FLUIDEZ

 6.4 Actividad _____

Explique las siguientes instrucciones. Escoja entre *favor de, hay que* y *tiene que.*

Modelo: Usar la nitroglicerina cuando le duele el pecho.
—Tiene que usar la nitroglicerina cuando le duele el pecho.

A. Llamar a la clínica mañana.
B. Esperar cinco minutos.
C. Comer más frutas y vegetales.
D. Tomar una aspirina de 81 miligramos todos los días.
E. Usar la insulina después de comer (*after eating*).
F. Tomar 2 acetaminofén cuando le duele la cabeza.
G. Hacer una cita en la clínica ambulatoria.
H. Usar el inhalador y llamar al 911 cuando tiene un episodio agudo del asma.

Answers
may vary.

Vocabulario: Instrucciones para la dosificación y vías de administración

Frequently, prescriptions follow this order: *medicamento—dosis—vía de administración—frecuencia—propósito* (name of medication, dosis, route of administration, frequency, and purpose).

—Tomar ibuprofeno, 400 mg por vía oral cada seis horas para el dolor.

La dosis

pastilla o tableta	pill
cucharadita	teaspoonful
cucharada	tablespoonful
inhalación	puff, inhalation
miligramo	milligram
mililitro	milliliter

La vía de administración

tomar, poner, inyectar, aplicar	to take, to put, to inject, to apply
por vía intravenosa, por suero	intravenously
por vía oral, por la boca	by mouth
por vía intramuscular	intramuscularly
por vía intradérmica	intradermically
por vía subcutánea	subcutaneously
por inhalación	by inhalation
debajo de la lengua	under the tongue
en el ojo derecho/izquierdo	in the right/left eye
en el oído derecho/izquierdo	in the right/left ear
por la nariz	in the nose
por el ano, por el recto	in the anus, in the rectum
por la vagina	in the vagina
en el área afectada	to the affected area

La frecuencia

una vez al día, diario	once per day, daily
. . . veces al día	. . . times a day
cada . . . horas	every . . . hours
a las 9 de la mañana/noche	at 9 a.m. / p.m.
por la mañana/noche	in the morning / at night
al acostarse	at bedtime

un día sí, un día no; en días alternos	every other day
todos los días	every day
por . . . días	for . . . days
media hora antes de comer	a half hour before eating
una hora después de comer	an hour after eating
con las comidas	with meals
con leche	with milk
con mucha agua	with plenty of water
cuando sea necesario	as needed
sin falta	without fail

El propósito

para la depresión	for depression
para el dolor	for pain
para dormir	for sleep
para la fatiga	for shortness of breath
para quitar la picazón	to take away the itching
para las alucinaciones ("las voces")	for hallucinations (for "voices")
para bajar el colesterol	to lower the cholesterol
para aliviar la ansiedad	to relieve the anxiety
para eliminar el agua	to eliminate water (retention)
para evitar el embarazo	to avoid pregnancy

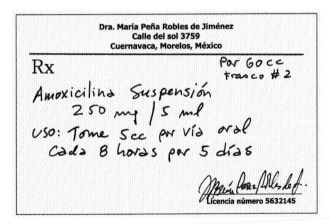

Dra. María Peña Robles de Jiménez
Calle del sol 3759
Cuernavaca, Morelos, México

Rx

Por 60 cc
frasco #2

Amoxicilina Suspensión
250 mg / 5 ml
USO: Tome 5cc por vía oral
Cada 8 horas por 5 días

Licencia número 5632145

 ## Estructura: El imperativo formal

- You learned several ways to give commands in the context of the pharmacy. Most were versatile and uncomplicated, because the verb representing the action remained in its infinitive form, except *tener que + infinitivo,* where *tener* must be conjugated.

infinitivo	Tomar las pastillas con leche.
favor de + infinitivo	Favor de llegar a tiempo.
hay que + infinitivo	Hay que tomar la tableta con mucha agua.
es importante + infinitivo	Es importante tomar el antibiótico por 5 días.
tener que + infinitivo	Tiene que tomar la medicina con comida.

- Spanish speakers also use direct commands, which are especially useful when a concise imperative is appropriate. When stitching a laceration, you might say, "Don't move!" During a physical exam you might say, "Breathe deeply!" and during an x-ray you might say, "Don't breathe." Here is how to make a formal (*usted*) command.
- Remove the *-o* from the first person singular form of the present tense and then add *-e* for verbs that end in *-ar* and *-a* for verbs that end in *-er* or *-ir*.

| respirar | ¡Respire profundamente! | Breathe deeply! |
| toser | ¡Tosa! / ¡No tosa! | Cough! / Don't cough! |

- This approach accommodates verbs that have an irregular first person singular (*yo*) form, such as *poner*. You'll learn about irregular verbs in chapter 9, and *poner* is one of them. To say, "Put the nitroglycerine under your tongue," think in two steps. The first person singular of *poner* ("to put") is *pongo;* and as the verb infinitive ends in *-er*, the formal command is *ponga*.

  Ponga la nitroglicerina debajo de la lengua.

- The formal command form of the verb *dar* is *dé*. The written accent differentiates it from the word *de* that you already know, as in *Soy de Puerto Rico*.

  Dé el jarabe al niño dos veces al día.

- Of course, native and fluent speakers do not have to think first about morphology. For novices, however, this shortcut may help: "Think *yo* and use the wrong letter." In chapter 12 you'll learn informal commands, which are used with children and with patients whom you address on a first-name basis.

HACIA PRECISIÓN

 6.5 Ejercicio_____

Dé las siguientes instrucciones en español. Para estar claro, escriba números árabes (1, 2, 3) en vez de (*instead of*) las palabras.

Modelo: Ibuprofen 600 mg, take 1 tablet by mouth 3 times a day.
          —Ibuprofeno 600 mg, tome 1 tableta por la boca 3 veces al día.

A. Take the medicine every day without fail.

_____

B. Amoxicilina (250 mg/5 ml), take 1 teaspoonful 3 times a day for 5 days.

_____

C. Guaifenesina, take 1 tablespoonful 4 times a day for congestion.

_____

D. Salbutamol, take 1 puff every 4 to 6 hours as needed for shortness of breath.

_____

E. Donepezilo, take 10 mg by mouth once a day in the morning.

_____

F. Ginkgo, take 160 mg by mouth at 8:00 a.m. and 8:00 p.m.

_____

G. Haloperidol, take 5 mg by mouth at 8:00 p.m.

_____

H. Acetaminophen, take 2 tablets every 4 to 6 hours as needed for pain.

_____

I. Mylanta, take 2 tablespoonfuls at bedtime.

_____

J. Omeprazole, take 1 capsule at 8:00 a.m.

_____

K. Isoniazid, take 1 tablet every day in the morning.

_____

L. Fluoxetine 20 mg, take 1 capsule in the morning.

_____

M. Phenytoin 100 mg, take 1 capsule 3 times a day.

_____

N. Loperamide, take 1 capsule every 2 to 3 hours as needed for diarrhea.

_____

6.6 Ejercicio _____

Escriba el imperativo formal de los siguientes verbos.

Infinitivo	Primera persona singular	Imperativo formal	Inglés
abrir	abro	¡Abra!	Open!
agitar	agito		Shake!
aplicar	aplico		Apply!
enjuagar*	enjuago		Rinse!
exhalar	exhalo		Exhale!
inhalar	inhalo		Inhale!
mantener**	mantengo		Hold!
oprimir	oprimo		Press!
poner	pongo		Put!
quitar	quito		Remove!

*To keep the "g" sound as in the English "go," add "u" to the Spanish *enjuague*.

**Mantener* is conjugated like *tener.*

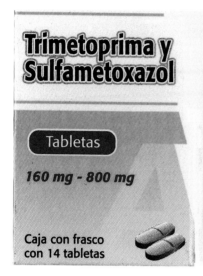

FORMULA:
Cada tableta contiene:
Trimetoprima .... 160 mg
Sulfametoxazol .... 800 mg
Excipiente cbp .... 1 tableta

VIA DE ADMINISTRACION: Oral.
DOSIS: La que el médico señale.
Consérvese el frasco bien tapado a temperatura ambiente a no más de 30°C y en lugar seco. Protéjase de la luz. Su venta requiere receta médica. No se administre durante el embarazo, lactancia, ni en niños menores de 3 meses. Este medicamento no deberá administrarse por períodos prolongados sin estricta vigilancia médica. No se deje al alcance de los niños.
Reg. No. 0310M79 SSA IV

La combinación de trimetoprima y sulfametoxazol es un antibiótico para combatir infecciones en el tracto urinario, el sistema digestivo y las vías respiratorias.

Vocabulario: Algunas clases de medicamentos

Palabras de frecuente uso

el analgésico/a, el calmante	analgesic
el antiácido	antacid
el antialérgico, el antihistamínico	antihistamine
el antibiótico	antibiotic
el antidepresivo	antidepressant
el antigripal	cold reliever
el antihipertensivo	antihypertensive
el antiinflamatorio no esteroide (AINES)*	nonsteroidal antiinflammatory drug (NSAID)
el antipirético, el antitérmico	antipyretic
el antitusígeno	cough suppressant
el broncodilatador	bronchodilator
el descongestionante	decongestant
el diurético	diuretic
el esteroide	steroid
el expectorante	expectorant

*The NSAIDs can be called *calmante, analgésico,* or *antipirético,* depending on the use. Some immigrants may not be familiar with brand names for certain medicines. They may be more familiar with generic names like *acetaminofén* or *ibuprofeno,* because pharmaceutical companies in the patient's country of origin may have their own brand names or may import generic medications. Paracetamol is a universal generic name for acetaminophen.

el laxante	laxative
la pastilla anticonceptiva	birth-control pill
la pastilla para dormir	sleeping pill
la vitamina	vitamin

Para completar su léxico

el anticoagulante	anticoagulant
el anticolinérgico	anticholinergic
el anticonvulsivo	anticonvulsive
el antidiarreico	antidiarrheal
el antiespasmódico	antispasmodic
el barbitúrico	barbiturate
la pastilla para bajar de peso	diet pill
el sedante, el calmante	sedative
el tranquilizante	tranquilizer

HACIA PRECISIÓN

 6.7 Ejercicio _____

Identifique la forma y la clase o el propósito de los siguientes productos. Favor de usar oraciones completas.

Modelo: Maalox
—Maalox es una suspensión. Es un antiácido. Es para aliviar la acidez estomacal.

A. acetaminofén
B. albuterol
C. penicilina
D. Coumadin
E. Tylenol
F. diazepam
G. carbamazepina
H. Ex-Lax
I. difenhidramina
J. ácido fólico
K. Pepto Bismol
L. Robitussin DM
M. crema hidrocortizona
N. phenobarbital

HACIA FLUIDEZ

6.8 Actividad _____

> Some complex instructions will still appear in English in keeping with our current level of proficiency.

The instructor will hand out two index cards to each student. On card one, write the class of a medication, e.g., *antibiótico*. On the other card, write a symptom or illness that might respond to that medication, e.g., *una infección en los oídos*. Next, the instructor should collect and redistribute the cards containing symptoms or illnesses. Students will then circulate in the room, speaking only Spanish, until they locate the student with the appropriate treatment for their condition.

Modelo: —Tengo una infección en los oídos. ¿Qué medicamento tienes?
—Tengo un antibiótico.

Here are some ideas for cards.

Card 1	*Card 2*
antidiarreico	diarrea
analgésico	dolor de cabeza
antiácido	acidez
antihistamínico	alergia
anticonvulsivo	convulsiones
antigripal	gripe
antihipertensivo	hipertensión
antitusígeno	tos
laxante	estreñimiento
pastilla para dormir	insomnia

6.9 Drama improvisado

Play "Scene Painting." One student goes to the front of the room and describes the space as a pharmacy. Identify the location of *el mostrador* (the counter), *el estante* (the shelving), and *el refrigerador* (the refrigerator). Take turns entering the pharmacy (respecting the locations of everything that is already established) and identifying and talking about things that you expect to see there. Practice anything that you have learned and be spontaneous.

Modelos: Aquí hay un estante alto. Los antibióticos están en el estante.
Los antibióticos no curan las enfermedades causadas por virus.

Aquí está el refrigerador. La insulina está en el refrigerador.
Es importante comer antes de usar la insulina.

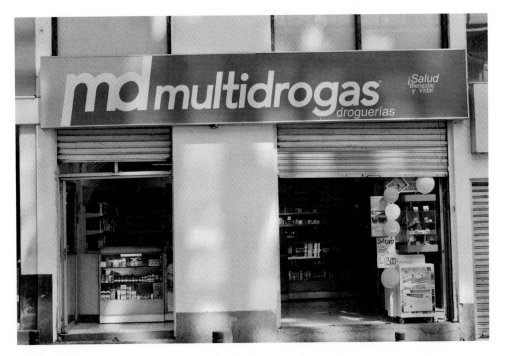

A las farmacias en Colombia las llaman droguería.

 Estructura: Los adjetivos demostrativos y los adjetivos afirmativos y negativos

- The demonstrative adjectives specify a particular person or thing. These are demonstrative adjectives:

	Singular	*Plural*	*Inglés*
Masculino	este	estos	this, these
Femenino	esta	estas	this, these

- The demonstrative adjective must agree in gender and number with the noun that it modifies.

Estas pastillas son para la diarrea.
Este medicamento es para el dolor.
Estos supositorios son para la nausea.
Esta inyección es para quitar las voces.

- These adjectives may be used in affirmative and negative sentences:

	Singular	*Plural*	*Inglés*
Masculino	alguno, algún	algunos	some, any
	ninguno, ningún*		none, not any
Femenino	alguna	algunas	some, any
	ninguna*		none, not any

- *Alguno* and *ninguno* drop the -*o* before a masculine singular noun, but *alguna* and *ninguna* keep the final -*a*.

   —¿Sufre usted de alguna enfermedad?
   —No. No sufro de ninguna enfermedad.
   —¿Es usted alérgico a algún medicamento?
   —No. No soy alérgico a ningún medicamento.

- In Spanish the double negative is necessary. Think in terms of agreement. In an affirmative sentence, use the affirmative adjective. In a negative sentence, use the negative adjective.

   —¿Toma algún medicamento todos los días?
   —No, no tomo ningún medicamento.

*The negative adjectives are almost always used in the singular form.

HACIA PRECISIÓN

6.10 Ejercicio _____

Use el adjetivo demostrativo apropiado (*este, estos, esta, estas*) para explicarle a don Ignacio los beneficios anticipados de sus medicamentos.

Don Ignacio, es muy importante usar _____ medicamentos en la manera indicada. _____ crema es para aliviar el dolor de la quemadura. En caso de fiebre, _____ pastillas son para quitar la fiebre. Si tiene mucho dolor, _____ pastillas son para el dolor. _____ jarabe es para la tos. Si está peor mañana, favor de llamar a _____ número de teléfono. Finalmente, _____ recetas son para comprar más medicamentos.

Ask about Medication Allergies and Educate Patients about Allergic Reactions

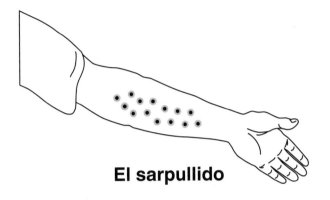

El sarpullido

Vocabulario: Las reacciones alérgicas

la alergia	allergy
el/la alergólogo/a	allergist
la anafilaxis	anaphylactic shock
el eccema	eczema
la epinefrina, la adrenalina	epinephrine, adrenaline
la falta de aire, la fatiga	shortness of breath
la hinchazón	swelling
la erupción (manchas rojas)	rash (red marks)
el jadeo	gasping
la picazón, la comezón	itch, itching
la raquiña (*slang*)	itching
el sarpullido, las ronchas	hives
el silbido	wheeze

Lectura: Los efectos secundarios

molesto	bothersome
bajar	to lower
mareo	dizziness
sequedad	dryness

Los doctores recetan los medicamentos para los beneficios de curar enfermedades o aliviar síntomas. Los medicamentos tienen efectos secundarios también. A veces los efectos secundarios son molestos pero desaparecen con el tiempo o con bajar la dosis. Los efectos secundarios incluyen náusea, mareo, indigestión, vómito, estreñimiento, diarrea, sequedad en la boca, dolor de cabeza, insomnio, irritabilidad y el sueño.

Muchas veces los efectos secundarios son benignos, pero algunas personas tienen una reacción alérgica. Algunas de las sustancias asociadas con las reacciones alérgicas son la aspirina, la cefalosporina, la eritromicina, la penicilina, la codeína y los cacahuates (*peanuts*). La reacción alérgica ocurre cuando el sistema inmunológico responde. La reacción alérgica más severa es la anafilaxis. Los síntomas de una reacción alérgica incluyen hinchazón, picazón, manchas rojas, inflamación en la garganta, asma, ritmo cardíaco irregular y/o dificultad para respirar. La dificultad para respirar siempre es una emergencia médica. Hay que llamar al doctor o al hospital inmediatamente si tiene una reacción alérgica después de tomar un medicamento.

Educate a Patient about Asthma

Lectura: El asma

El asma es una enfermedad crónica de los bronquios que causa inflamación en los pulmones y las vías respiratorias. Es una patología frecuente en la infancia, pero solo un 4 por ciento de los pacientes persiste con asma a los dieciocho años. El asma no es contagiosa. Durante un ataque (un episodio agudo) del asma, el paciente sufre de dificultad para respirar. Algunos síntomas incluyen:

la crisis de tos	coughing spell
los jadeos	gasping, panting
los silbidos	wheezing
la falta de aire, la fatiga	shortness of breath
la dificultad para respirar	shortness of breath
el pecho apretado	tight chest
la respiración silbante	wheezing
la dificultad para hablar	difficulty speaking
la comezón en la barbilla o garganta	itching in the chin or throat

El asma no tiene cura pero es posible controlar los síntomas con medicamentos que un doctor receta. Es necesario tener un cuidado médico regular para controlar el asma. Todas las personas que sufren de asma necesitan un medicamento de alivio rápido para usar durante un ataque. Muchas personas necesitan también usar todos los días un medicamento preventivo. Los medicamentos son en forma líquida, en forma de tableta o cápsula y en aerosol (para inhalar). Los antiinflamatorios son medicamentos preventivos y los broncodilatadores son para el tratamiento de episodios agudos.

cuidado medico
medical care

También hay que evitar las cosas que provocan los ataques. Algunas de las cosas que provocan los ataques son:

el polen y el polvo	pollen and dust
los ácaros del polvo	dust mites
las cucarachas	cockroaches

el moho	mold
la caspa de animal	animal dander
el humo	smoke
las alergias	allergies
las alfombras	carpets
los perfumes	perfumes
el frío	cold weather
el ejercicio físico	physical exercise
las infecciones virales	viral infections

Algunos episodios o ataques de asma son severos y son una emergencia médica de vida o muerte. Es necesario llamar al doctor o a la clínica si el efecto del medicamento de alivio rápido dura menos de cuatro horas (o si no quita la tos o la respiración silbante). Es importante tener un plan para ir al hospital cuando el medicamento no alivia los síntomas y la respiración está rápida y difícil.

HACIA FLUIDEZ

 6.11 Actividad _____

Haga y conteste estas preguntas con un compañero/a para confirmar su comprensión.

Las reacciones alérgicas

A. ¿Es posible aliviar un efecto secundario? ¿Cómo?
B. ¿Son todos los efectos secundarios una emergencia médica?
C. ¿Cuáles son los síntomas de una reacción alérgica?
D. ¿Cuál es la reacción alérgica más severa?
E. ¿Qué debo hacer si tengo una reacción alérgica después de tomar un medicamento?

El asma

F. ¿Qué tienen en común un ataque de asma y una reacción alérgica?
G. ¿Es el asma una enfermedad contagiosa?
H. ¿Cuáles son algunos de los alérgenos que provocan el asma?
I. ¿Qué es un medicamento preventivo?
J. ¿Qué es un medicamento de alivio rápido?
K. ¿Cuándo es necesario usar un medicamento de alivio rápido?
L. ¿Cuándo es necesario llamar al doctor o a la clínica?
M. ¿Cuándo es necesario ir rápidamente al hospital?

6.12 Actividad _____

Colabore con un/a compañero/a para exponer un drama (*present a skit*) donde un/a enfermero/a enseña a los padres de un niño con asma cómo prevenir los ataques. Haga un plan para ir al hospital cuando el medicamento de alivio rápido no alivia los síntomas de un episodio agudo.

 ## Ask Who Helps an Infirm Family Member

 ### Estructura: Los complementos indirectos y el verbo *dar* (*Indirect Objects and the Verb* Dar)

- Unlike the direct objects, which represent the person or thing that directly receives the action of the verb, the indirect objects indicate to whom or for whom the action is done. They are almost always necessary, as they help to identify the beneficiary of a transitive verb.
- The indirect objects are *me, te, le, nos*, and *les*.

Me duele el brazo.	My arm hurts (me).
Te cuido al niño.	I take care of the child for you.
Le escribo una receta.	I write you/him/her a prescription.
El radiólogo **nos** lee la placa.	The radiologist reads the film for us.
Les compro la medicina.	I buy the medicine for them.

- Notice that in the sentence *Te cuido al niño*, the verb is *cuidar*. The direct object is *el niño*, which tells who or what is being cared for. The indirect object is *te*, which tells for whom the child is being cared for. In the sentence, *Les compro la medicina*, the direct object is *la medicina*, because it is what is being bought. *Les* is the indirect object. It tells for whom the medicine is being purchased. Asking "what" of the verb identifies the direct object, while asking "to/for whom" identifies the indirect object.
- The indirect object *le* is less specific than *me, te,* and *nos. Le* can mean to or for "you," "him," or "her." Therefore, it is often clarified by adding *a* and a more specific designation of the beneficiary of the action.

El doctor **le** receta un medicamento **a Javier.**
La odontóloga **les** examina los dientes **a los niños.**

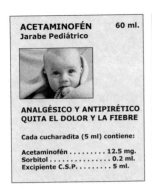
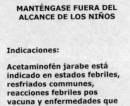

ACETAMINOFÉN   60 ml.
Jarabe Pediátrico

ANALGÉSICO Y ANTIPIRÉTICO
QUITA EL DOLOR Y LA FIEBRE

Cada cucharadita (5 ml) contiene:

Acetaminofén . . . . 12.5 mg.
Sorbitol . . . . 0.2 ml.
Excipiente C.S.P. . . . . 5 ml.

MANTÉNGASE FUERA DEL
ALCANCE DE LOS NIÑOS

Indicaciones:

Acetaminofén jarabe está
indicado en estados febriles,
resfriados communes,
reacciones febriles pos
vacuna y enfermedades que
producen dolor y fiebre.

Dosificación:

Niños de 1 a 3 años:
Según receta médica.

El acetaminofén pediátrico es para los niños con dolor o fiebre. No les dé aspirina para la fiebre.

- Study the following sentences, and note that the direct object pronouns represent the direct receiver of the action, and the indirect object pronouns represent the person to whom or for whom the action is being done.

Direct Objects	*Indirect Objects*
Los examino ahora.	**Le** examino los oídos **a usted**.
La pongo ahora.	**Le** pongo una inyección **a José**.

- *Dar* (to give) has an irregular form in the first person singular (*doy*), and is a verb that is frequently used in the context of the pharmacy. *Dar* commonly uses an indirect object to represent the person to/for whom something is given.

Le **doy** acetaminofén al bebé.	I give acetaminophen to the baby.
¿Le **da** comida sólida al bebé?	Do you give solid food to the baby?
¿Le **da** leche del pecho al bebé?	Do you give the baby breast milk?

- With instructions that use an infinitive form of the verb, you may attach the indirect object (as a suffix) to the infinitive. Where increased clarity is needed, add *a* and identify the person to whom the action is to be done.

Hay que **darle al niño** el jarabe cada cuatro horas sin falta.
Usted tiene que **darle a su madre** la insulina después de comer.

HACIA PRECISIÓN

6.13 Ejercicio _____

Complete las oraciones con el complemento indirecto y la forma correcta del verbo indicado.

Modelo: La enfermera _____ (tomar) la temperatura (a mí).
   —La enfermera __*me toma*__ la temperatura.

A. El doctor _____ (recetar) un medicamento a Juan.

B. La doctora _____ (preguntar) su historia médica a él.

C. Yo _____ (escribir) una carta a la compañía de seguros.

D. La anestesióloga _____ (explicar) el procedimiento (a mí).

E. El enfermero _____ (hablar) español con los pacientes.

F. Usted _____ (comprar) la medicina a sus padres.

G. La pediatra _____ (recetar) un antibiótico para mi bebé.

HACIA FLUIDEZ

 6.14 Actividad _____

Agregue el complemento indirecto apropiado a las siguientes oraciones.

Modelo: Receto un medicamento a su padre.
    —Le receto un medicamento a su padre.

A. Receto un medicamento a sus hijos.
B. Escribo una carta a usted.
C. Doy una aspirina a la paciente.
D. Enseño español a los estudiantes.
E. Tomo la temperatura al paciente cada cuatro horas.
F. Leo el libro a usted.
G. La doctora contesta la pregunta a nosotros.

 6.15 Actividad _____

La abuela de su compañero/a está enferma y necesita ayuda. Pregúntele quién le ayuda con lo siguiente. Su compañero/a contesta con datos adicionales.

Modelo: cocinar
    —¿Quién le cocina a tu abuela?
    —Mi madre le cocina todos los días.

A. ayudar con la casa
B. comprar la comida
C. hacer las citas médicas
D. recetar los medicamentos
E. enseñar a usar la insulina
F. examinar los pies para ver si hay úlceras
G. llamar al consultorio para hacer una cita con el doctor

Estructura: Los complementos directos e indirectos en combinación

- Recall that the direct objects represent the person or thing that directly receives the action of the verb, and the indirect objects indicate to whom or for whom the action of the verb is done. The direct objects are *me, te, lo/la, nos,* and *los/las.* The indirect objects are *me, te, le, nos,* and *les.*
- When direct and indirect objects are used together, the indirect object always goes first. The objects may be placed before a conjugated verb or as a suffix to a verb infinitive. It makes no difference which way you do this.

    La enfermera tiene que inyectar**me** la insulina.
    La enfermera **me la** tiene que inyectar.
    La enfermera tiene que inyectár**mela**.

- Never use two objects beginning with *l* together. Replace the indirect object *le* or *les* with *se* before the direct object *lo, la, los,* or *las.* For example, for "You have to give it to him every six hours":

    Se lo tiene que dar cada seis horas.
    Tiene que dár**selo** cada seis horas.

- In command forms, the direct and indirect objects are attached to the affirmative command as a suffix, and they precede the negative command as two separate words. Place the indirect object first, and when there are two objects beginning with "l," replace the indirect object with *se.*

    Tóme**selo** cuatro veces al día.
    No **se lo** tome antes de comer algo.

HACIA PRECISIÓN

6.16 Ejercicio _____

Use los complementos directos y los complementos indirectos en combinación para expresar las siguientes oraciones con menos palabras.

Modelo: Hay que dar el inhalador al niño cuatro veces al día si tiene fatiga.
            —Hay que dárselo cuatro veces al día si tiene fatiga.

A. Es importante poner a su madre un supositorio por la mañana.

_____

B. No dé la aspirina al niño si tiene fiebre.

_____

C. Dé el jarabe a la paciente a las ocho de la noche.

_____

D. Escriba a mí la receta nueva.

_____

E. No tome usted el medicamento si tiene irritación.

_____

F. Dé el medicamento al paciente con mucha agua.

_____

HACIA FLUIDEZ

6.17 Actividad _____

Observe el horario para los medicamentos de Juancito. Usted es enfermero/a y su compañero/a es el padre o la madre de Juancito. Pregúntale si le da los medicamentos a Juan y a qué hora se los da.

Modelo: —¿Cuántas veces al día le da la amoxicilina a Juancito y a qué hora se la da?
   —Se la doy tres veces al día, a las nueve de la mañana, a la una y a las nueve de la noche.

Medicamento	Hora de administración			
	9	*1*	*5*	*9*
Amoxicilina, 1 cucharadita	X	X		X
Acetaminofén, 2 cucharaditas	X			X
Robitussin, 1 cucharada	X	X	X	X
El inhalador, 2 inhalaciones	X			X

6.18 Actividad

Colabore con un/a compañero/a para planear y presentar un diálogo a la clase. Estas son algunas ideas.

A. Pregúntele a su compañero/a si toma algún medicamento diario y si tiene alergia a algún medicamento.
B. Su compañero/a es alérgico/a a algún medicamento. Pregúntele qué le pasa cuando toma el medicamento.
C. Explíquele a su compañero/a cómo usar un medicamento específico. Explíquele los posibles efectos secundarios.
D. Explíquele a su compañero/a los posibles problemas asociados con beber bebidas alcohólicas cuando toma un medicamento específico.
E. Explíquele a su compañero/a la vacuna para la gripe (*the flu vaccine*) y pregúntale si es alérgico/a a los huevos (*eggs*) o si ha tenido el síndrome de Guillain-Barré.

 6.19 Actividad

El/La profesor/a tiene un paquete grande de M&M's o Skittles. En este drama, los dulces son pastillas y cada color es un medicamento específico. Usted es enfermero/a y su compañero/a es paciente. Con su compañero/a, prepare y presente un diálogo donde le explica al / a la paciente cómo tomar el medicamento. Debe incluir el nombre del medicamento, el propósito de tomarlo, la dosis, la vía de administración, la frecuencia, los posibles efectos secundarios y qué debe hacer si tiene preguntas o problemas con el medicamento. Debe aprender los colores en español.

los rojos	the red ones	**los anaranjados**	the orange ones
los amarillos	the yellow ones	**los verdes**	the green ones
los azules	the blue ones	**los morados**	the purple ones
los marrones	the brown ones	**claros/oscuros**	light/dark

Explain How to Use a Pill Organizer

Lectura: El recordatorio de pastillas

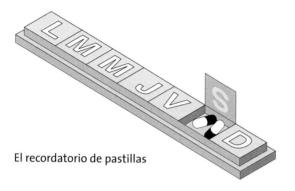

El recordatorio de pastillas

Aprenda estos verbos:

olvidar	to forget
vender	to sell
usar	to use
preparar	to prepare
poner	to put
corresponder	to correspond

El recordatorio de pastillas (también se llama el organizador de pastillas) es una caja que tiene siete compartimientos, uno para cada día de la semana. El recordatorio es para no olvidar tomar el medicamento. Las farmacias los venden. Use el organizador todos los días. Prepárelo el primer día de la semana, y ponga las pastillas de cada día en el compartimiento que corresponde al día. Por ejemplo, ponga las pastillas que usted toma los lunes, en el compartimiento que corresponde al lunes. Siempre tome el medicamento en la forma indicada.

HACIA FLUIDEZ

 6.20 Actividad _____ **caja** box

Usted es enfermero/a y su compañero/a es paciente. El/La paciente toma los siguientes medicamentos: metformina, 500 miligramos una vez al día para la diabetes tipo dos; atenolol, 50 miligramos una vez al día para la hipertensión; y levotiroxina, 100 microgramos en días alternos (un día sí y un día no) para el hipotiroidismo. Explíquele a su compañero/a cómo usar el recordatorio y el propósito de tomar los medicamentos.

6.21 Reciclaje _____

Escriba una receta de uno de los medicamentos en la actividad 6.20. Hay que incluir el nombre del medicamento, la dosis, la vía de administración, la frecuencia y el propósito.

 ## Exposición

 ### CHAPTER 6 SKILL: MAKING A PRESENTATION

You are going to role-play a pharmaceutical representative—but no free meals or other perks—and educate your classmates about your company's medication. First, listen as a sales rep describes her company's new pharmaceutical. Check off what information she includes in her presentation.

☐ nombre de marca	☐ nombre genérico	☐ clase de medicamento
☐ formas disponibles	☐ indicaciones	☐ contraindicaciones
☐ dosis disponibles	☐ dosificación por grupos de edades	☐ posibles efectos secundarios

Choose a medication with which you are familiar, and use the Internet to find a site that provides important information about the medication in Spanish. Write a presentation that you will give to your classmates. Make your presentation in class. Remember that you are selling, so be upbeat and enthusiastic about your product!

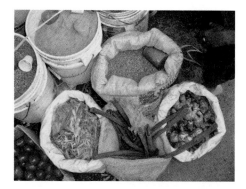 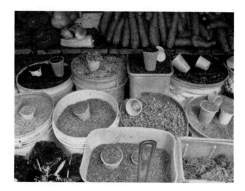

Phytotherapy is common in Latin America to the extent that it is important to know what the patient is taking and to review a list of contraindications or possible herb-drug interactions.

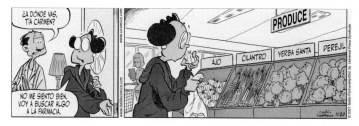

Baldo © 2007 Baldo Partnership. Dist. by Universal Uclick. Reprinted with permission. All rights reserved.

Cultural Note: *La confianza*

Now you can give medication instructions in Spanish. This may reduce errors and improve treatment adherence. However, when in doubt about the accuracy of your instructions or the patient's understanding, seek a qualified interpreter. Despite the accuracy of your instructions, you may miss cues about comprehension and the patient's cognitive capacity and competence to consent, even when the directions seem intuitive.

Amistad con todos, confianza con pocos
(Friendship with everyone, trust with only a few)

You may also improve treatment adherence by making a conscious effort to help the patient to address issues of trust. Some people believe—with good reason—that if you do not cross the language boundary, you will not earn the *confianza* of the patient. Being genuine and empathetic facilitates *confianza.* This may include having an authentic interest in Spanish and the patient's cultural perspective. *Confianza* is more than the literal translation, "confidence," implies. It combines trust and respect. When a health care provider earns the *confianza* of the patient, the patient will express feelings, listen more carefully, and be more likely to follow advice. Direct eye contact from the patient may be a sign of *confianza.* The health professional that earns *confianza* has communicated a genuine interest in the patient.

In many cultures, it is common to expect relationships to feel as if they were personal rather than business. Latinos call this *el personalismo.* In Latin America, one may build brand loyalty as much by making customer relationships feel personal as by advertising one's expertise and modern equipment. When a professional doesn't take a moment to greet each person in the room individually, a North American might assume the doctor is busy or has a lot of important things to do. A Latino in the same situation may feel that something is out-of-the-ordinary and attribute this to a lack of courtesy or respect. Practitioners should consider the possible adverse effects of maintaining strict relationship boundaries with customers from other cultures. Perhaps there is some personal information one might disclose—in the interest of making a relationship feel more natural to the patient—while not violating a necessary parameter of self-disclosure.

Courtesy and "small talk" are more conventional in Latino culture than in places where time and efficiency may be measured in patients per hour. It may take time to warm up. The Spanish-speaking patient may not mention his or her most urgent health concern first. He or she may wait until after discussing a subordinate concern and sensing the *confianza* needed before talking of more important or more intimate problems. It must be established that the practitioner has time to listen.

Communication styles may affect *confianza*. For example, Latinos tend to be "high-context" communicators. That is, they tend to focus as much on the nonverbal cues and context of a conversation as on the content. Saying coolly, "If you do not take the medication, you will get worse," without appropriate affect may dilute the message. The patient may think unconsciously, "He told me I'd get worse, but he did not appear very worried, so it will probably be okay."

Many Latinos who also speak English will prefer Spanish in times of distress. This is in part due to speaking Spanish at home or having spoken Spanish as a child. Coping mechanisms like "self talk" may be inseparable from one's native language. Some patients have denied that they speak English at all in the hopes of being assisted by a Spanish-speaking helper in whom they may sense more *confianza*. When English is a second language and the patient becomes psychotic, proficiency in English may diminish or disappear because of the psychotic disorganization. As the patient improves, the use of English also improves and can be a cognitive sign of recovery. Brain damage, as from a stroke, has been observed to disable a second language while leaving the first language intact.

Vocabulario del capítulo 6

Formas de medicamentos

Las tabletas

la tableta, la pastilla	tablet, pill
la píldora, el comprimido	tablet, pill
la cápsula, la gragea	capsule
. . . masticable	. . . chewable
media tableta	half of a tablet
el frasco, la botella	pill bottle, bottle

Las inyecciones e infusiones

la inyección	injection
la jeringuilla	syringe
el suero, el intravenoso	IV
el suero / el intravenoso central	central IV line

Los líquidos

el jarabe	syrup
el elíxir	elixir
la gota	drop
la suspensión	suspension

Los medicamentos tópicos

la crema	cream, ointment
el ungüento	ointment, balm

Otras formas

el aerosol	aerosol
el atomizador	atomizer
el gel	gel
el inhalador, la pompa (*slang*)	inhaler
el nebulizador (la máquina)	nebulizer (machine)
el parche	patch
el supositorio	suppository

Instrucciones para la dosificación y vías de administración

La dosis

pastilla o tableta	pill
cucharadita	teaspoonful
cucharada	tablespoonful

inhalación	puff, inhalation
miligramo	milligram
mililitro	milliliter

La vía de administración

tomar, poner, inyectar, aplicar	to take, to put, to inject, to apply
por vía intravenosa, por suero	intravenously
por vía oral, por la boca	by mouth
por vía intramuscular	intramuscularly
por vía intradérmica	intradermically
por vía subcutánea	subcutaneously
por inhalación	by inhalation
debajo de la lengua	under the tongue
en el ojo derecho/izquierdo	in the right/left eye
en el oído derecho/izquierdo	in the right/left ear
por la nariz	in the nose
por el ano, por el recto	in the anus, in the rectum
por la vagina	in the vagina
en el área afectada	to the affected area

La frecuencia

una vez al día, diario	once per day, daily
. . . veces al día	. . . times a day
cada . . . horas	every . . . hours
a las 9 de la mañana/noche	at 9 a.m./p.m.
por la mañana/noche	in the morning / at night
al acostarse	at bedtime
un día sí, un día no; en días alternos	every other day
todos los días	every day
por . . . días	for . . . days
media hora antes de comer	a half hour before eating
una hora después de comer	an hour after eating
con las comidas	with meals
con leche	with milk
con mucha agua	with plenty of water
cuando sea necesario	as needed
sin falta	without fail

El propósito

para la depresión	for depression
para el dolor	for pain
para dormir	for sleep
para la fatiga	for shortness of breath
para quitar la picazón	to take away the itching

para las alucinaciones ("las voces")	for hallucinations (for "voices")
para bajar el colesterol	to lower the cholesterol
para aliviar la ansiedad	to relieve the anxiety
para eliminar el agua	to eliminate water (retention)
para evitar el embarazo	to avoid pregnancy

Verbos asociados con las recetas

abrir	to open
agitar	to shake
aplicar	to apply
enjuagar	to rinse
exhalar	exhale
inhalar	inhale
mantener	maintain
oprimir	to press
poner	to put, to place
quitar	to remove

Algunas clases de medicamentos

analgésico/a, el calmante	analgesic
el antiácido	antacid
el antialérgico, el antihistamínico	antihistamine
el antibiótico	antibiotic
el anticoagulante	anticoagulant
el anticolinérgico	anticholinergic
el anticonvulsivo	anticonvulsive
el antidepresivo	antidepressant
el antidiarreico	antidiarrheal
el antiespasmódico	antispasmodic
el antigripal	cold reliever
el antihipertensivo	antihypertensive
el antiinflamatorio no esteroide (AINES)	nonsteroidal antiinflammatory drug (NSAID)
el antipirético, el antitérmico	antipyretic
el antitusígeno	cough suppressant
el barbitúrico	barbiturate
el broncodilatador	bronchodilator
el descongestionante	decongestant
el diurético	diuretic
el esteroide	steroid
el expectorante	expectorant
el laxante	laxative

la pastilla anticonceptiva	birth-control pill
la pastilla para bajar de peso	diet pill
la pastilla para dormir	sleeping pill
el sedante, el calmante	sedative
el tranquilizante	tranquilizer
la vitamina	vitamin

Las reacciones alérgicas

la alergia	allergy
la anafilaxis	anaphylactic shock
el eccema	eczema
la epenefrina, la adrenalina	epinephrine, adrenaline
la falta de aire	shortness of breath
la hinchazón	swelling
la erupción (manchas rojas)	rash (red marks)
el jadeo	gasping
la picazón, la comezón	itch, itching
la raquiña (*slang*)	itching
el sarpullido, las ronchas	hives
el silbido	wheeze

El asma

la crisis de tos	coughing spell
los jadeos	gasping, panting
los silbidos	wheezing
la falta de aire, la fatiga	shortness of breath
la dificultad para respirar	shortness of breath
el pecho apretado	tight chest
la respiración silbante	wheezing
la dificultad para hablar	difficulty speaking
la comezón en la barbilla o garganta	itching in the chin or throat
el polen y el polvo	pollen and dust
los ácaros del polvo	dust mites
las cucarachas	cockroaches
el moho	mold
la caspa de animal	animal dander
el humo	smoke
las alergias	allergies
las alfombras	carpets
los perfumes	perfumes
el frío	cold weather
el ejercicio físico	physical exercise
las infecciones virales	viral infections

Los colores

amarillo	yellow
anaranjado	orange
azul	blue
blanco	white
claro/oscuro	light/dark
marrón	brown
morado	purple
negro	black
rojo	red
verde	green

El organizador de pastillas

olvidar	to forget
vender	to sell
usar	to use
preparar	to prepare
poner	to put
corresponder	to correspond

Preguntas útiles

¿Es usted alérgico/a a algún medicamento?	Are you allergic to any medication?
¿Tiene usted alergia a algún medicamento?	Do you have an allergy to any medication?
¿Toma algún medicamento todos los días?	Do you take any medicine every day?
¿Necesita una receta nueva?	Do you need a new prescription?

Expresiones útiles

Hay que tomar media tableta.	You must take half a tablet.
Hay que darle dos pastillas.	You must give him/her two pills.

Chapter 7
La nutrición y las dietas

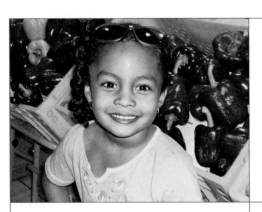

Communication Goals

Vocabulary

Structure

Cultural Note

Website   www.yalebooks.com/medicalspanish
Video   *Trama: Una dieta para Francisco; Demostración: Los grupos alimenticios*
Audio   The USDA Food Groups *Mi plato; Las dietas especiales; Exposición*
Electronic Workbook

B y the end of this chapter you will know the names of common foods in Spanish and be able to ask patients about their dietary habits and preferences. You will be able to give basic instructions for low-fat, low concentrated sugar, weight-reducing, and clear-liquids diets.

 ## Ask Patients about Food Preferences

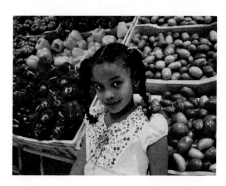

A Naura le gustan los vegetales. Aquí hay ajíes y tomates. Foto cortesía del Dr. Jorge Amarante

 ### Vocabulario: Mi plato del USDA

Granos: «Consuma la mitad en granos integrales»

el pan	bread
las pastas	pasta
el arroz (el arroz integral)	rice (whole-grain rice)
el cereal cocido	cooked cereal
el cereal seco	dry cereal
la tortilla	tortilla

In Mexico a *tortilla* is an unleavened corn cake. In the Caribbean region it is an omelet.

Verduras: «Varíe sus verduras»

los vegetales, las verduras	vegetables, green vegetables
el ají, el pimiento	pepper
la calabaza	squash
la cebolla	onion
los guisantes	peas
la lechuga	lettuce
el plátano de cocinar	plantain
el repollo	cabbage
la zanahoria	carrot

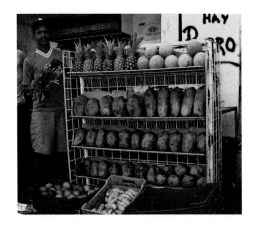

Enfoque en las frutas. Hay piña, melón, papaya, naranja y banana.

Frutas: «Enfoque en las frutas»

la banana, el guineo,	
el banano, el plátano*	banana
la ciruela	prune
el mango	mango
la manzana	apple
el melón	melon
la naranja, la china (Caribe)	orange
la papaya	papaya
la piña	pineapple
el tomate, el jitomate	tomato
la toronja	grapefruit
la uva	grape

*The fruit that is eaten raw (excluding *el plátano de cocinar*) may be called *el guineo* in Puerto Rico and the Dominican Republic; *el banano* in Central America and Colombia; and *el plátano* in Cuba.

Leche: «Coma alimentos ricos en calcio»

el mantecado, el helado	ice cream
la leche baja en grasa	low-fat milk
la leche descremada	fat-free (no-fat) milk
el queso bajo en grasa	low-fat cheese
el yogur bajo en grasa	low-fat yogurt

Carnes y frijoles «Escoja proteínas bajas en grasa»

la carne de res	beef
el cerdo	pork
los frijoles, las habichuelas	beans, pea beans
el huevo	egg
la manteca de cacahuate	peanut butter
el pescado	fish
el pollo	chicken

Aceites «Los aceites no son un grupo de alimentos, pero son parte de una buena dieta»

el aceite	oil
el aceite de maíz, de oliva, de soja	corn, olive, soybean oil
las grasas	fats
la manteca	lard
la mantequilla	butter
la margarina	margarine
la mayonesa	mayonnaise

Expresiones útiles

Debe comer más vegetales.	You should eat more vegetables.
Debe comer menos grasa.	You should eat less fat.
No debe usar mucha sal.	You should not use a lot of salt.
En vez de comer dulces, coma frutas.	Instead of eating candy, eat fruit.

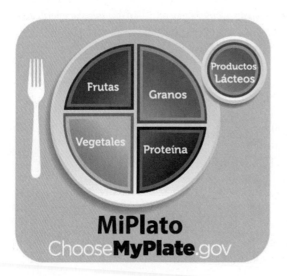

"Choose My Plate" replaced the USDA pyramid.

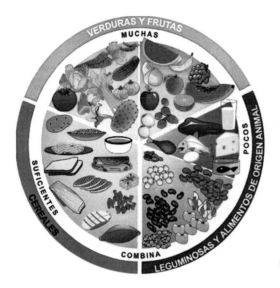

El plato del bien comer

 Estructura: Verbos como *gustar*

- The verb *disgustar* means "To disgust." Like the verb *doler,* which you know from chapter 3, it is most frequently used in the third person (singular and plural), and it is used with indirect objects (*me, te, le, nos, les*). For example,

  Me disgustan las arañas.   Spiders disgust me.
  A Luisa le disgustan las anchoas.   Anchovies disgust Luisa.

- The verb *gustar* is the opposite of *disgustar* and means "to please." It may be confusing to English speakers because the meaning-based translation of *Me gusta el café* is "I like coffee." The literal translation, "Coffee pleases me" explains why we use the form *gusta.* That which pleases is the subject of the verb *gustar.*

  Me gusta el café.   I like coffee.
  ¿Te gusta el café?   Do you like coffee?
  A Luisa le gusta el té.   Luisa likes tea.
  No nos gusta la cerveza.   We don't like beer.
  A los bebés les gusta la leche.   Babies like milk.

- If the subject (that which pleases) is plural, use the third person plural form of the verb.

  Me gustan las comidas.   I like the meals.
  ¿Le gustan las uvas?   Do you like grapes?

- We can also react to an activity by following the verb *gustar* with a verb infinitive.

  No me gusta cocinar.   I do not like to cook.
  ¿Qué le gusta comer?   What do you like to eat?

- Other verbs that are used like *gustar* include, for example,

  interesar (*to interest*)   Me interesa la medicina.
  importar (*to matter*)   Nos importan los pacientes.
  aburrir (*to bore*)   Me aburre la televisión.
  fascinar (*to fascinate*)   A Juan le fascina comer.
  molestar* (*to annoy*)   Me molesta la comezón.

  *OJO: false cognate

Vocabulario: Las comidas

el desayuno	breakfast	**desayunar**	to eat breakfast
el almuerzo	lunch	**almorzar**	to eat lunch
la cena	supper, dinner	**cenar**	to eat supper/dinner
la comida	meal, dinner	**la merienda**	snack
la bebida	beverage	**el alimento**	food

El desayuno

el huevo	egg
el pan tostado, la tostada	toast
el tocino	bacon
el panqueque	pancake
la salchicha	sausage
la fruta	fruit
el cereal	cereal
la toronja	grapefruit
la avena	oatmeal

El almuerzo

el emparedado, el sándwich (Caribe)	sandwich
el jamón	ham
el queso	cheese
la sopa	soup
la ensalada	salad
las papas fritas	french fries

La cena

el arroz	rice
la papa	potato
el pan	bread
las pastas	pasta
la carne	meat
los frijoles, las habichuelas	beans
el pollo	chicken
la carne de res	beef
el cerdo	pork
el pescado	fish
el vegetal, la verdura	vegetable

Las bebidas

el café	coffee
el té	tea
la leche	milk
el refresco, la gaseosa	soft drink
el chocolate	hot chocolate, hot cocoa
el agua*	water
el jugo de naranja, —de china (Caribe)	orange juice
el jugo de manzana	apple juice
el jugo de ciruela	prune juice
el jugo de tomate	tomato juice
la cerveza	beer
el vino	wine

Agua, like *asma* and *área,* are feminine nouns that are used with the masculine definite article (*el*). Adjectives take their feminine form, however (*el agua está fría*).

Preguntas útiles

¿Toma usted bebidas alcohólicas?	Do you drink alcoholic beverages?
¿Toma café descafeinado?	Do you drink decaffeinated coffee?

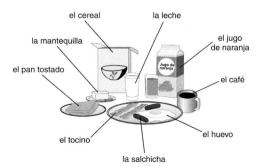

el cereal · la leche · la mantequilla · el jugo de naranja · el pan tostado · Jugo de naranja · el café · el tocino · el huevo · la salchicha

¿Qué le gusta comer para el desayuno?
(¿Con qué le gusta desayunar?)

HACIA PRECISIÓN

7.1 Ejercicio

Complete las siguientes oraciones con el vocabulario nuevo.

A. _____ (el pollo, la carne de res) es carne roja.

B. _____ (el pescado, el cacahuate) es del océano.

C. _____ (el mantecado, el melón) es rico en calcio.

D. La avena es buena para _____ (la fiebre, la picazón).

E. Para consumir bacteria beneficiosa, coma _____ (yogur, cerdo).

F. Para tener más fibra en la dieta, coma _____ (pan, pan integral).

G. Para tener más vitamina A, coma _____ (carne de res, zanahorias).

H. Un ingrediente principal de la ensalada es _____ (la lechuga, la manteca).

I. _____ (la ciruela, el huevo) es posible futuro madre o padre de familia.

J. Para bajar el colesterol, coma _____ (avena, tocino).

7.2 Ejercicio

Complete las frases siguientes en una manera lógica como el modelo.

Modelo: A mí _____ me gustan _____ (gustar) las frutas.

A. A mí _____ (aburrir) trabajar en una oficina.

B. A mis padres _____ (fascinar) cuidar a su nieto.

C. A mí _____ (interesar) cocinar sin mucha grasa.

D. A los estudiantes _____ (fascinar) aprender el español.

E. A nuestro profesor _____ (importar) hablar dos idiomas.

F. A nosotros _____ (gustar) comer arroz con pollo y ensalada.

7.3 Ejercicio

En el diagrama, escriba algunos de los alimentos que usted asocia con el desayuno, el almuerzo y la cena. Organícelos (*Organize them*) por sus grupos alimenticios.

	Desayuno	*Almuerzo*	*Cena*
Granos	_____	_____	_____
	_____	_____	_____
Verduras	_____	_____	_____
	_____	_____	_____
Frutas	_____	_____	_____
	_____	_____	_____
Leche	_____	_____	_____
	_____	_____	_____
Carnes y frijoles	_____	_____	_____
	_____	_____	_____

HACIA FLUIDEZ

 7.4 Actividad

Entreviste (*Interview*) a sus compañeros/as. Circule en la clase y pregúntales sobre sus gustos. Después comparta los resultados de la encuesta. En este ejercicio hable en el registro informal (tú).

Modelo: tomar café por la mañana
—¿Te gusta tomar café por la mañana?
—Sí, me gusta tomar café por la mañana.
(o)
—No, no me gusta el café. No lo tomo por la mañana.

A. tomar jugo de ciruela con el desayuno
B. comer huevos todos los días
C. comer una banana con el almuerzo
D. comer un emparedado (sándwich) para el almuerzo
E. tomar cerveza con la cena
F. tomar bebidas alcohólicas todos los días
G. tomar café por la tarde
H. comer la toronja con sal

7.5 Drama improvisado _____

Let's play "Categories," which you may recall from chapter 1. Form a circle, everybody holding one finger up. The first person makes eye contact with a person across the circle and states the name of a food (*la toronja,* for example). That person lowers his or her finger, makes eye contact with another, and states the name of a different food. Continue until everyone has a food (no duplicates), with the first person being last to receive one. Recall who said what to you and what you said to whom. Next, go through the list in that same order multiple times. Make eye contact with your receiver prior to speaking. When you have perfected this list, a student starts a second list. When you have perfected the second list, do both lists simultaneously.

  7.6 Drama improvisado _____

As a variation of "Categories" to practice vocabulary, a leader asks for lists of five items. For example, the leader says, *Kevin, dime* (tell me) *cinco frutas.* After Kevin says each item, the class counts. Kevin says *mango* and the class says *uno.* Kevin says *naranja,* and the class says *dos.* After five items, everyone says (in energetic, percussive tones) *cinco frutas.* In addition to food groups, options include categories such as *cinco comidas que contienen mucha grasa.* Another idea is to recycle vocabulary from previous chapters, for example, *cinco especialidades médicas.*

  7.7 Drama improvisado _____

Play "*Fruta, vegetal, grano o proteína.*" The entire class stands in a large circle. One student stands in the center of the circle, points to a student in the circumference, says either *fruta, vegetal, grano,* or *proteína,* and slowly approaches that

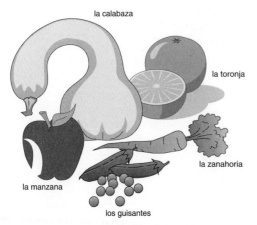

la calabaza

la toronja

la zanahoria

la manzana

los guisantes

Varíe sus verduras y enfóquese en las frutas.

student with an arm outstretched. The student in the circle must say a food that is in the chosen category before the first student touches him or her. If he or she cannot do so, he or she switches places with the student in the center.

 ## Estructura: Los verbos *querer* y *preferir* para expresar gustos y preferencias

- "I like coffee" is *Me gusta el café.* "I want coffee" is *Quiero café. Querer* is an irregular *-er* verb. The first *e* changes from *e* to *ie* except in the first person plural.

yo	**Quiero** una ensalada.
tú	¿**Quieres** un vaso de leche?
él, ella, usted	¿**Quiere** tomar la pastilla con agua o con jugo?
nosotros/as	**Queremos** comer una dieta balanceada.
ellos, ellas, ustedes	Mis padres **quieren** bajar de peso.

- Like *gustar,* the conjugated form of the verb *querer* can precede a noun or another verb. The second verb is not conjugated.

Quiero tomar un vaso de agua.
¿**Quieres cenar** en la cafetería?

- *Preferir* is an irregular *-ir* verb. Like *querer,* the first *e* changes from *e* to *ie* except in the first person plural. Also like *querer,* its conjugated form can precede an unconjugated verb (the infinitive).

yo	**Prefiero** el arroz a las papas.
tú	¿**Prefieres** el arroz o las papas?
él, ella, usted	Sandra **prefiere** la leche al refresco.
nosotros/as	Sergio y yo **preferimos** beber leche.
ellos, ellas, ustedes	Mis padres **prefieren** tomar té.

- The phrase *Si Dios quiere* means "God willing." Some Spanish-speakers may prefer this over a more direct "yes" or "no" when talking about plans.

HACIA FLUIDEZ

 7.8 Actividad_____

Practique el vocabulario nuevo. Ofrezca (*Offer*) alimentos específicos a un/a compañero/a. Su compañero/a decide qué le gusta comer y qué prefiere comer para el desayuno, el almuerzo y la cena.

> Modelo: desayuno, huevos
> —Para el desayuno, ¿quiere huevos?
> —Sí, quiero huevos (Sí, los quiero).
> (o)
> —No, no quiero huevos. Prefiero pan tostado y café.

 7.9 Actividad_____

Use el verbo *preferir* para preguntarle a un/a compañero/a sobre sus preferencias.

> Modelo: café o té
> —¿Prefiere usted café o té?
> —Bueno, me gusta el café, pero prefiero el té.

A. la leche fría o el chocolate
B. el pollo o la carne de res
C. las papas o el arroz
D. el tocino o la salchicha

E. la sopa o la ensalada
F. el vino o la cerveza
G. las frutas o los vegetales
H. el pescado o el cerdo

 7.10 Drama improvisado_____

Con un/a compañero/a, prepare un drama para exponer. Usted invita a su compañero/a a comer. Su compañero/a tiene hambre pero es quisquilloso/a (*a picky eater*). La última línea (*last line*) debe ser, «Para una buena hambre no hay pan duro» (*"For a good hunger, there's no such thing as stale bread"*).

> Modelo: Carlos: Tengo hambre. Necesito comer.
> María: ¿Quieres arroz con habichuelas?
> Carlos: No me gusta el arroz. Prefiero comer una hamburguesa.
> María: No hay hamburguesa en la casa. ¿Quieres una ensalada?
> Carlos: No me gusta la ensalada. Prefiero papas fritas.
> María: Carlos, coma la ensalada. Para una buena hambre no hay pan duro.

Educate Patients about Special Diets

Vocabulario: Las dietas especiales

la nutrición	nutrition	**la dieta**	diet
comer	to eat	**ayunar**	to fast
seguir*	to follow	**la dieta balanceada**	balanced diet
la sal	salt	**el sodio**	sodium
la grasa	fat	**el colesterol**	cholesterol
el azúcar	sugar	**la fibra**	fiber
la proteína	protein	**el almidón**	starch
el líquido claro	clear liquid	**el calcio**	calcium
el carbohidrato	carbohydrate	**el peso**	weight
la libra	pound	**la onza**	ounce
la caloría	calorie	**el gramo**	gram

*Seguir is an irregular verb. The command form is ¡Siga! as in ¡Siga una dieta balanceada!

Preguntas útiles

¿Come bien el/la niño/a?	Does the child eat well?
¿Tiene usted buen apetito?	Do you have a good appetite?
¿Cuánto pesa usted?	How much do you weigh?
¿Ha bajado de peso recientemente?	Have you lost weight recently?
¿Ha subido de peso recientemente?	Have you gained weight recently?
¿Cuánto mide usted?	How tall are you?

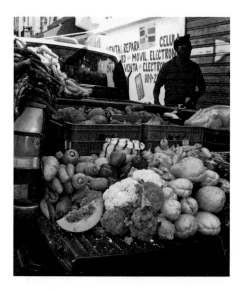

Coma de cuatro a cinco porciones del grupo de verduras diaria. Hay zanahoria, ají, calabaza, coliflor, bróculi, chayote y berenjena.

Estructura: El verbo *deber*

The verb *deber* is a regular verb ending in *-er.* It is useful for discussing diets because it expresses what one should or should not do.

yo	**Debo** comer porciones más pequeñas.
tú	No **debes** comer mucha grasa.
él, ella, usted	Usted no **debe** comer comida rápida.
nosotros/as	**Debemos** comer una dieta balanceada.
ellos, ellas, ustedes	Los pacientes no **deben** comer mucha sal.

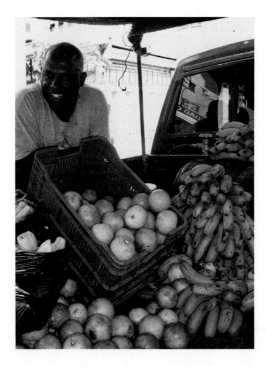

Debe comer más frutas y vegetales para la fibra y las vitaminas.

HACIA FLUIDEZ

 ## 7.11 Actividad _____

Use el verbo *deber* y el vocabulario nuevo para escribir sugerencias útiles y después comparta estas sugerencias con el grupo.

Modelo: Debe consumir mucha fibra. Las frutas son ricas en fibra.
No debe comer mucha grasa. La carne roja tiene mucha grasa.

Lectura: Un plan para bajar de peso

Para tener una dieta saludable y balanceada, debe comer todos los días comidas de cada grupo de alimentos. También es importante tener un equilibrio entre lo que come y su actividad física. Una dieta balanceada tiene de siete a ocho porciones del grupo de los granos (los granos integrales son preferidos), de cuatro a cinco porciones (400 gramos) de los grupos de las frutas y los vegetales, de dos a tres del grupo de las proteínas (con menos de origen animal) y no mucha grasa.

Para bajar de peso, es importante comer una dieta balanceada, hacer ejercicio regularmente, comer menos calorías y no comer mucha grasa ni azúcar. Para comer menos calorías, debe comer menos porciones o comer porciones más pequeñas.

Lectura: La dieta baja en grasa y colesterol

Una persona con el colesterol alto no debe comer mucha grasa. El coco, los aceites y las proteínas de animal tienen grasa y suben el colesterol en la sangre. Las personas con el colesterol alto deben tomar leche descremada o baja en grasa.

Información nutricional	
Porciones por recipiente 22	
Tamaño de la porción 2/3 taza (55g)	
Cantidad por porción	
Calorías	**50**
% del valor nutricional diario	
Grasa total 1g	**1%**
Grasa saturada 0g	**0%**
Grasas *trans* 0g	
Colesterol 0mg	**0%**
Sodio 115mg	**5%**
Carbohidratos total 37g	**13%**
Fibras dietéticas 0g	
Azúcares total 12g	
Incluye 10g azúcares añadidas	**22%**
Proteína 3g	
Vitamina D 2mcg	**10%**
Potasio 235 mg	**6%**

Los porcentajes de valores diarios se basan en una dieta de 2.000 calorías. Sus valores diarios pueden ser mayores o menores según sus necesidades de calorías.

No deben comer más de tres huevos a la semana. Los alimentos que son preferidos incluyen los panes y cereales, las tortillas de maíz, el arroz, los frijoles y todas las frutas y vegetales. No coma la carne de res más de tres veces a la semana. Coma porciones pequeñas y quite la grasa antes de cocinarla. También quite la piel del pollo antes de cocinarlo. Debe comer pescado grasoso, como el atún, el salmón y las sardinas. Las grasas permitidas son el aceite de maíz, el aceite de oliva y el aceite de soja (*soy*). El aceite de maíz puede bajar el colesterol.

subir	to raise
quitar	to take away
bajar	to lower

Lectura: La dieta baja en azúcares concentradas

nivel level   Las personas que tienen un nivel alto de triglicéridos en la sangre y las personas que sufren de la diabetes deben seguir una dieta baja en azúcares concentradas. La diabetes es una enfermedad que afecta el metabolismo del cuerpo, o la capacidad de procesar los alimentos. Las personas que tienen diabetes tienen demasiada (*too much*) glucosa en la sangre. La diabetes es una de las *enfermedades crónicas no transmisibles*. Para controlar la diabetes hay que hacer ejercicio regularmente, comer una dieta balanceada, controlar el peso y evitar las azúcares concentradas. La obesidad y el consumo excesivo de azúcar pueden causar la diabetes tipo dos.

Si su doctor receta una medicina para controlar la diabetes, hay que tomarla en la manera indicada. Con respecto a la dieta, no debe dejar de comer ninguna de las comidas (*don't skip meals*). Coma las comidas a la misma hora y coma la misma porción todos los días, especialmente si usa medicamento para bajar la glucosa. Coma alimentos ricos en fibra como granos, frutas y vegetales. Escoja carbohidratos complejos (*complex carbohydrates*) naturales, como plátanos, frijoles, tubérculos, arroz integral y cereales y harinas integrales. Evite los carbohidratos refinados (*refined carbohydrates*), como cereales azucarados, pan blanco y harina blanca. Debe consumir menos sal, grasa, azúcar y alcohol. Los siguientes alimentos tienen mucha azúcar. Evítelos (*Avoid them*).

el azúcar de caña	cane sugar
el dulce / los dulces	candy
la miel de abeja	honey
el almíbar, el sirope	syrup
el pastel, el bizcocho (Caribe)	cake
la leche condensada	condensed milk
la gaseosa, el refresco (Caribe)	soft drinks

Azúcar has ambiguous gender. The masculine form is more common in Spain, and the feminine form in the Americas, where when singular, the article *el* is used and an adjective is feminine.

HACIA PRECISIÓN

7.12 Ejercicio _____

El señor López tiene el colesterol muy alto. Él tiene varias preguntas. Favor de contestarle las siguientes preguntas.

A. ¿Debo cocinar con manteca?   No, no debe _____.

B. ¿Debo comer pollo y pescado?   Sí, debe_____.

C. ¿Debo comer mucho coco (*coconut*)?   _____.

D. ¿Debo tomar leche baja en grasa?   _____.

E. ¿Debo comer queso bajo en grasa? _____.

F. ¿Debo comer papas fritas? _____.

G. ¿Debo usar aceite de maíz? _____.

H. En vez de la carne de res, ¿qué debo comer? _____.

I. ¿Cómo debo preparar el pollo para cocinar? _____.

7.13 Ejercicio _____

El señor Vega tiene diabetes y los triglicéridos altos. También tiene muchas preguntas. Favor de contestarle las siguientes preguntas.

A. ¿Debo usar mucha azúcar cuando cocino? No, no debe _____.

B. ¿Debo comer ensalada? Sí, debe_____.

C. ¿Debo beber vino? _____.

D. ¿Debo comer muchos dulces? _____.

E. ¿Debo comer frijoles? _____.

F. ¿Debo usar leche condensada? _____.

G. ¿Debo tomar refrescos dietéticos? _____.

H. ¿Debo usar azúcar artificial? _____.

7.14 Ejercicio _____

Escriba una dieta balanceada para una persona que sufre de diabetes.

El desayuno   El almuerzo

_____   _____

_____   _____

_____   _____

_____   _____

La cena   La merienda (Snack)

_____   _____

_____   _____

_____   _____

_____   _____

Teach Patients How to Prepare for a Colonoscopy

Vocabulario: La colonoscopia, la dieta de líquidos claros y la dieta blanda

el agua	water
los líquidos transparentes	transparent liquids
los refrescos claros	clear soda
el café o té sin leche	coffee or tea without milk
el jugo de manzana	apple juice
el caldo transparente	transparent broth
la gelatina de sabor artificial	artificially flavored gelatine
los laxantes	laxatives
el citrato de magnesio	magnesium citrate
el bisacodilo	bisacodyl
evitar	to avoid
suplementos con hierro	iron supplements

A soft diet may be indicated as an intermediate step between a clear-liquids diet and a regular diet or for persons who require choking precautions. This vocabulary will help.

la dieta blanda, la dieta de puré	soft diet (purée diet)
la dieta corriente	regular diet
los frijoles majados	mashed beans
el puré de . . .	purée of . . .
papa, arroz, manzana	potato, rice, apple

HACIA PRECISIÓN

7.15 Ejercicio_____

Complete estas instrucciones para una colonoscopia. Incluya ejemplos de lo que debe y no debe comer y tomar. Comparta sus instrucciones con sus compañeros. Note: usted decide la fecha y la hora del procedimiento.

Su colonoscopia es el _____ a las _____ de la

_____. No _____ (deber) tomar aspirina, antiinflamatorios, anti-

coagulantes o suplementos con hierro después del _____. El día antes de la prueba, _____ (tomar) de ocho a diez vasos de agua u otro líquido transparente, como el jugo de manzana, el café negro sin _____, el caldo _____ y la gelatina de sabor artificial. _____ (Tomar) bisacodilo 5 mg, 4 comprimidos por vía _____ a las ocho de la mañana y siga una dieta de _____ _____. No _____ (consumir) comida sólida y no _____ (deber) tomar ningún producto lácteo. A las seis de la tarde, _____ (tomar) diez onzas de citrato de magnesio. A las nueve de la noche, tome otras diez onzas de _____ de _____. Siga una dieta de _____ _____ toda la _____. No tome nada por dos horas antes de la colonoscopía.

LAS COMPRAS

jugo de manzana
salchicha
helado
tocino
sal
toronja
té
avena
pescado
arroz
zanahoria
yogur
coco
gelatina
banana

HACIA FLUIDEZ

 7.16 Actividad _____

Consulte la lista de las compras y aconseje (*advise*) a los siguientes pacientes sobre lo que deben y no deben comprar.

> Modelo: la señora Acevedo, la dieta baja en sal
> —Señora Acevedo, usted debe comprar las zanahorias pero no compre las salchichas. Coma frutas y vegetales frescos.

A. la señora Blanco Peña, la dieta baja en grasa y colesterol
B. Pedrito Jiménez, la dieta de líquidos claros
C. la señora Medina Ortiz, la dieta para bajar de peso
D. doña Olga, la dieta baja en azúcares concentradas

 7.17 Drama improvisado _____

Arrange seats as if at a dinner party and have spontaneous conversation around the imaginary table. (Miming and handling imaginary dinnerware will add to the reality.) Without previous planning, address a classmate in a way that establishes your relationship with him or her. When a classmate addresses you in this way, accept this information about yourself and respond accordingly. Conversation topics may include food likes and dislikes, special diets, dysfunctional family relationships, and anything that you create.

> Modelo: —Quiero más papas, por favor.
> —Mamá, vas a tener una colonoscopia mañana.
> —Sí, tengo una colonoscopia mañana pero tengo hambre hoy. Me gustan las papas cuando las preparo con mucha mantequilla.

 ## Educate Parents about Feeding

Vocabulario: La alimentación del bebé

la alimentación	feeding
complementario/a	supplementary
el vaso plástico	plastic cup

la lactancia	lactation
la leche materna	mother's milk
la leche artificial, fórmula	formula
el recién nacido	newborn

Lectura: La alimentación: ¿Cómo come el bebé? ¿Come bien?

Durante los primeros seis meses, el bebé debe tomar solo leche materna y debe tomarla a demanda (cuando el bebé quiere). Normalmente toma cada dos a tres horas. No necesita agua u otros líquidos. El bebé no necesita leche artificial (fórmula), aunque el pediatra puede (*can*) recomendarla por una razón médica, si la madre tiene problemas con la lactancia o por el estilo de vida (*lifestyle*) de la madre.

Después de los seis meses y hasta los doce meses, la leche materna es una buena opción, y el bebé puede tomar agua en vaso plástico también. A los seis meses debe tomar veinticuatro onzas al día o tomar leche del pecho de cuatro a cinco veces al día. A los seis meses se puede introducir otros alimentos. Se llama *la alimentación complementaria*. Debe introducir los alimentos nuevos cada tres o cinco días para poder detectar las alergias. No debe tomar bebidas azucaradas como el jugo (zumo) de frutas y no debe añadir sal ni azúcar a la comida.

HACIA PRECISIÓN

 7.18 Ejercicio_____

¿Cierto o falso? Lea las siguientes declaraciones y escoja entre cierto y falso.

A. Es ideal introducir la fórmula durante los primeros seis meses.
B. Si toma fórmula, el bebé debe tomar mucha agua también.
C. Los bebés deben comer en horas específicas.
D. Los bebés no necesitan fórmula si toman leche materna sin problema.
E. Debe introducir un alimento nuevo todos los días para poder detectar las alergias.
F. Si el bebé no come bien debe añadir un poco de sal o azúcar a la comida.

HACIA FLUIDEZ

 7.19 Drama improvisado _____

Play the game "*Afortunadamente, desafortunadamente.*" Take turns adding to a string of statements. Start with *Tengo hambre* or *Tengo sed.* The next statement begins with *afortunadamente,* the statement after that begins with *desafortunadamente,* and so on.

> Modelo: —Tengo sed.
> —Afortunadamente, tenemos café.
> —Desafortunadamente, el café está frío y no me gusta el café frío.
> —Afortunadamente, hay cerveza.
> —Desafortunadamente, esta noche tengo que trabajar.

 7.20 Drama improvisado _____

Con un/a compañero/a, prepare un drama sobre las dietas para presentar a la clase. La última línea debe ser, «Por la boca muere el pez» (*The fish dies because of his mouth*).

> Modelo: Carlos: María, ¿Qué quieres comer?
> María: Quiero comer helado.
> Carlos: Pero mi amor, tienes diabetes y no debes comer dulces.
> María: Quiero comer salchicha.
> Carlos: Pero tienes el colesterol alto y no debes comer grasa.
> María: No me importa la dieta.
> Carlos: Por la boca muere el pez.

 7.21 Reciclaje _____

Food and drink can be comforting, which can make dieting little more than wishful shrinking. Recycle the comfort idioms that use the verb *tener* that you learned in chapter 3. Find out what a partner likes or prefers to eat or drink when he or she feels hungry, thirsty, hot, cold, afraid, or in a hurry.

> Modelo: —¿Qué prefieres tomar o comer cuando tienes miedo?
> —Cuando tengo miedo prefiero tomar café descafeinado y comer espinacas como Popeye.

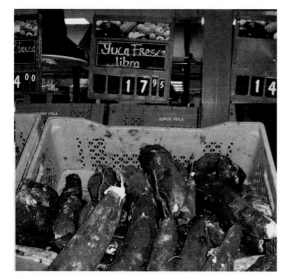

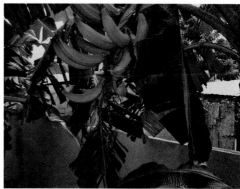

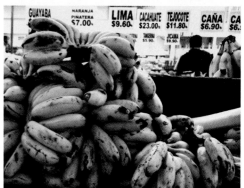

above: La yuca

above right: El plátano

right: La banana («el guineo» en Puerto Rico y la República Dominicana)

Exposición

 CHAPTER 7 SKILL: EXPLAINING INFORMATION AND DESCRIBING

For this presentation, imagine you are assisting a patient with a lifestyle disease to optimize his or her health through diet. Follow these steps.

1. Listen to the sample presentation from the audio program and take notes about the patient based on what you hear. You may hear the following information:
    *   the patient's name, age, height, and weight
    *   the medical condition
    *   several specific foods that the patient likes and dislikes
    *   types of food to consume and avoid
2. Next, imagine a new patient, make up the kind of information that you heard in the audio, and write it down.

3. From the information that you have created, prepare a narrative in which you explain a dietary intervention to your patient. In the narrative, explain the lifestyle disease, the purpose of the diet, the foods to consume and to avoid, and the ways in which you have considered the patient's likes, dislikes, and preferences.
4. Create a sample menu for one day using the information that you wrote down in step 3.
5. Review your profile with a classmate. Your instructor may ask you to submit your description for feedback, to present it to the whole group, or to post it on your class website.

Cultural Note: Diet and Regional Foods

Lo que no mata, engorda (¡y lo que engorda, mata!)

Hispanic cuisine includes many starchy vegetables. In some areas, this may be due to their availability as compared to other foods. Although they are like vegetables in their vitamin content, their carbohydrate content is more similar to bread than to vegetables. They include rice, lima beans (*habas*), corn, *plátano,* and winter squash (*calabaza*).

Yuca and *plátano* are two starchy vegetables that you may not know. *Yuca* is a root that may be boiled (and topped with sautéed onions with vinegar!) or grated, pressed, and fried. Before the Encounter, the native people made a cake called *casave* by grating and pressing the *yuca,* adding salt, and cooking it on a hot rock. (To make *casave* at home, grate the *yuca,* press out all the juice through cheesecloth, add salt, and cook it on a dry cast-iron pan. The raw juice contains cyanide, which has caused toxicity in people who process it in large quantity without precautions.) The colonists took *casave* back to Spain because it did not spoil on the long voyages.

The Encounter refers to the meeting of Europeans and indigenous people in America and replaces the word discovery in this context.

Plátano is a vegetable that looks like a large, fat banana but has a flavor of its own (although when very ripe it tastes like a sweet potato). Fried, crushed, and refried it makes *tostones,* a real favorite in the Caribbean, but not good for low-fat diets. Other roots and tubers like *batata, yautía, malanga,* and *ñame* are carbohydrates that are boiled alone or in sauces and stews. Although these are complex carbs, people on a strict diabetic diet might be instructed to be careful and consistent with carbohydrates.

Más cura la dieta que la receta
(The diet cures more than the prescription)

Epidemiologically, Latinos born outside of the United States have lower incidents of obesity and obesity-exacerbated illnesses such as hypertension and type 2 diabetes. After five years in the United States, however, they begin to close the gap with Latinos born in the United States and with a sample of all native-born North Americans. A recent study found that Latinos here less than five years had a 16 percent rate of obesity, and after five years in the United States, this had increased to 22 percent. Latinos born in the United States and U.S. citizens in general had a 30 percent rate of obesity. There were similar progressions for hypertension and type 2 diabetes.

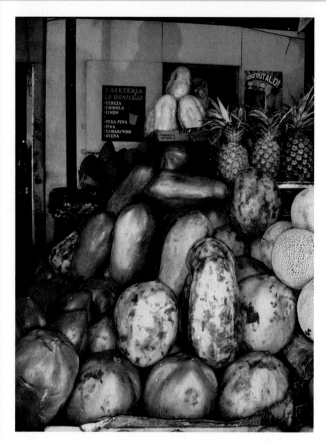

Para la merienda, vamos a comer frutas. Hay zapote, papaya, piña y melón.

Vocabulario del capítulo 7

Los grupos alimenticios

Granos

el pan	bread
las pastas	pasta
el arroz (el arroz integral)	rice (whole-grain rice)
el cereal cocido	cooked cereal
el cereal seco	dry cereal
la tortilla	tortilla

Verduras

los vegetales, las verduras	vegetables, green vegetables
el ají, el pimiento	pepper
la calabaza	squash
la cebolla	onion
los guisantes	peas
la lechuga	lettuce
el plátano de cocinar	plantain
el repollo	cabbage
la zanahoria	carrot

Frutas

la banana, el guineo	banana
la ciruela	prune
el mango	mango
la manzana	apple
el melón	melon
la naranja, la china	orange
la papaya	papaya
la piña	pineapple
el tomate, el jitomate	tomato
la toronja	grapefruit
la uva	grape

Leche

el mantecado, el helado	ice cream
la leche baja en grasa	low-fat milk
la leche descremada	fat-free (no-fat) milk
el queso bajo en grasa	low-fat cheese
el yogur bajo en grasa	low-fat yogurt

Carnes y frijoles

la carne de res	beef
el cerdo	pork
los frijoles, las habichuelas	beans, pea beans
el huevo	egg
la manteca de cacahuate	peanut butter
el pescado	fish
el pollo	chicken

Aceites

el aceite	oil
el aceite de maíz, de oliva, de soja	corn, olive, soybean oil
las grasas	fats
la manteca	lard
la mantequilla	butter
la margarina	margarine
la mayonesa	mayonnaise

Verbs like *Gustar*

gustar	to please	**interesar**	to interest
importar	to matter	**aburrir**	to bore
fascinar	to fascinate	**molestar**	to annoy

Las comidas

el desayuno	breakfast	**desayunar**	to eat breakfast
el almuerzo	lunch	**almorzar**	to eat lunch
la cena	supper, dinner	**cenar**	to eat supper, dinner
la comida	meal, dinner	**la merienda**	snack
la bebida	beverage	**el alimento**	food

El desayuno

el huevo	egg
el pan tostado, la tostada	toast
el tocino	bacon
el panqueque	pancake
la salchicha	sausage
la fruta	fruit
el cereal	cereal
la toronja	grapefruit
la avena	oatmeal

El almuerzo

el emparedado, el sándwich (Caribe)	sandwich
el jamón	ham

el queso	cheese
la sopa	soup
la ensalada	salad
las papas fritas	french fries

La cena

el arroz	rice
la papa	potato
el pan	bread
las pastas	pasta
la carne	meat
las habichuelas	beans
el pollo	chicken
la carne de res	beef
el cerdo	pork
el pescado	fish
el vegetal, la verdura	vegetable

Las bebidas

el café	coffee
el té	tea
la leche	milk
el refresco, la gaseosa	soft drink
el chocolate	hot chocolate, hot cocoa
el agua	water
el jugo de naranja, — de china (Caribe)	orange juice
el jugo de manzana	apple juice
el jugo de ciruela	prune juice
el jugo de tomate	tomato juice
la cerveza	beer
el vino	wine

Las dietas especiales

la nutrición	nutrition	**la dieta**	diet
comer	to eat	**ayunar**	to fast
seguir	to follow	**la dieta balanceada**	balanced diet
la sal	salt	**el sodio**	sodium
la grasa	fat	**el colesterol**	cholesterol
el azúcar	sugar	**la fibra**	fiber
la proteína	protein	**el almidón**	starch
el líquido claro	clear liquid	**el calcio**	calcium
el carbohidrato	carbohydrate	**el peso**	weight
la libra	pound	**la onza**	ounce
la caloría	calorie	**el gramo**	gram

La colonoscopia, la dieta de líquidos claros y la dieta blanda

el agua	water
los líquidos transparentes	transparent liquids
los refrescos claros	clear soda
el café o té sin leche	coffee or tea without milk
el jugo de manzana	apple juice
el caldo transparente	transparent broth
la gelatina de sabor artificial	artificially flavored gelatine
los laxantes	laxatives
el citrato de magnesio	magnesium citrate
el bisacodilo	bisacodyl
evitar	to avoid
suplementos con hierro	iron supplements
la dieta blanda, la dieta de puré	soft diet (purée diet)
la dieta corriente	regular diet
los frijoles majados	mashed beans
el puré de . . .	purée of . . .
papa, arroz, manzana	potato, rice, apple

La alimentación del niño

la alimentación	feeding
complementario/a	supplementary
el vaso plástico	plastic cup
la lactancia	lactation
la leche materna	mother's milk
la leche artificial, fórmula	formula
el recién nacido	newborn

Preguntas útiles

¿Toma usted bebidas alcohólicas?	Do you drink alcoholic beverages?
¿Toma café descafeinado?	Do you drink decaffeinated coffee?
¿Come bien el/la niño/a?	Does the child eat well?
¿Tiene usted buen apetito?	Do you have a good appetite?
¿Cuánto pesa usted?	How much do you weigh?
¿Ha bajado de peso recientemente?	Have you lost weight recently?
¿Ha subido de peso recientemente?	Have you gained weight recently?
¿Cuánto mide usted?	How tall are you?

Expresiones útiles

Debe comer más vegetales.	You should eat more vegetables.
Debe comer menos grasa.	You should eat less fat.
No debe usar mucha sal.	You should not use a lot of salt.
En vez de comer dulce, coma frutas.	Instead of eating candy, eat fruit.

Chapter 8
El examen físico

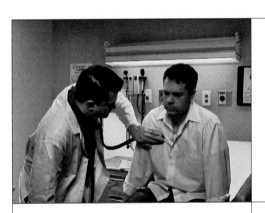

Communication Goals

Vocabulary

Structure

Cultural Note

Website   www.yalebooks.com/medicalspanish

Video   *Trama: El examen físico; Demostración: La pulmonía*

Audio   *El examen físico; Exposición*

Electronic Workbook

By the end of this chapter you will know the Spanish terms necessary to conduct the physical exam portion of a history and physical. You will be able to ask how long various symptoms have been present, to ask what makes things better or worse, to describe bowel habits, and to explain and schedule referrals for common tests. If this class can be held in an exam room, this may help you form kinesthetic memory cues and to think of the questions and expressions that you most frequently use in this setting.

Clarify the Chief Complaint

Vocabulario: El motivo de la consulta

el motivo de la consulta	the chief complaint
¿Qué le pasa?	What is happening (to you, him, her)?
¿Qué tiene?	What is the matter?
¿En qué le puedo ayudar?	How can I help you?

Expresiones de tiempo

¿Con qué frecuencia?	How often?
nunca, jamás	never
casi nunca	almost never
de vez en cuando	once in a while
Va y viene.	It comes and goes.
a veces	at times
una o dos veces al día	once or twice a day
a menudo	often
frecuentemente	frequently
siempre	always
Es continuo.	It's continuous.
¿Desde cuándo?	Since when?
desde esta mañana	since this morning
desde anoche	since last night
desde ayer	since yesterday
desde el lunes	since Monday
desde hace tres días	since three days ago
desde la semana pasada	since last week
¿Cuánto tiempo hace?	How long has it been?
Hace una hora.	It's been an hour.
Hace dos días.	It's been two days.

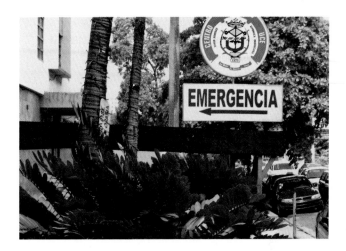

¿Cuánto tiempo dura?	How long does it last?
Dura de una a dos horas.	It lasts for one or two hours.
Dura varios días.	It lasts for several days.

Estructura: ¿Cuánto tiempo hace?

- The verb *hacer* means "to do" and "to make," and is irregular in the first person singular.

yo	**Hago** la cena a las ocho de la noche.
tú	**¿Haces** ejercicio todos los días?
él, ella, usted	Mi mamá **hace** un pastel delicioso.
nosotros/as	¿Qué **hacemos** hoy?
ellos, ellas, ustedes	Mis amigos no **hacen** nada hoy.

- *Hacer* is also used in expressions of time. In such expressions, it is used in the third person singular.

¿Cuánto tiempo hace?	How long has it been?
Hace dos días.	It has been two days.
¿Hace mucho tiempo?	Has it been a long time?
Hace poco tiempo.	It has been a short time.
No hace mucho tiempo.	It has not been a long time.

- Use *¿Cuánto tiempo hace que . . . ?* with a verb phrase to ask how long a symptom or condition has been going on.

  ¿Cuánto tiempo hace que usted tiene diabetes?
  ¿Cuánto tiempo hace que le duele el brazo?

- Use *hace* + period of time + *que* + verb phrase to declare how long the symptom or condition has been going on.

Hace dos años que tengo diabetes.
Hace una semana que me duele el brazo.

		dos horas				me duele la cabeza.
Hace	+	tres días	+	que	+	se me hinchan los tobillos.
		cuatro meses				tomo atorvastatina.

HACIA FLUIDEZ

 8.1 Actividad

Pregúntale a un/a compañero/a cuánto tiempo hace que tiene los siguientes síntomas. Responda ad lib.

Modelo: Me duele la espalda.
—¿Cuánto tiempo hace que le duele la espalda?
—Hace tres días que me duele la espalda.

A. Tengo fiebre.
B. Estoy enfermo.
C. Tengo hipertensión.
D. Me duele la garganta.
E. Tengo rigidez en el cuello.
F. Toso mucho.
G. Estoy mareado.
H. Mi hijo tiene gripe.
I. Tengo dolor de cabeza.
J. Mi suegra tiene dolor del pecho.

 8.2 Actividad

Prepare un diálogo con un/a compañero/a para presentar a la clase. Pregúntale qué le pasa (el motivo de la consulta), la frecuencia del síntoma, cuánto tiempo hace, desde cuándo y cuánto tiempo duran los episodios. Use el formulario para clarificar el motivo de la consulta y organizar su presentación. Aquí hay ideas para el motivo de la consulta.

Tengo ardor en el estómago.	My stomach burns.
Tengo sudores por la noche.	I have night sweats.
Se me hinchan los tobillos.	My ankles get swollen.
Me duele el pecho.	My chest hurts.
Sangro por la nariz.	My nose bleeds.

1. Motivo de la consulta:

_____.

2. Frecuencia:

_____.

3. Cuánto tiempo hace:

_____.

4. Desde cuándo:

_____.

5. Duración:

_____.

Un chiste

Doctor:	¿Qué le pasa?
Paciente:	Tengo amnesia total.
Doctor:	¿Desde cuándo tiene amnesia?
Paciente:	Desde el sábado ocho de mayo del 2019 a las dos en punto de la tarde.
Doctor:	¡Caramba!

Vocabulario: ¿Qué le mejora?

Verbos

ayudar	to help
mejorar	to improve
empeorar	to worsen
sentirse	to feel

Preguntas útiles

¿Qué le ayuda?	What helps you?
¿Qué le mejora?	What makes you better?
¿Qué le empeora?	What makes you worse?
¿Qué le hace sentir mejor?	What makes you feel better?
¿Qué le hace sentir peor?	What makes you feel worse?

Expresiones útiles

El ibuprofeno me ayuda.   Ibuprofen helps me.
Comer fritura me empeora.   Eating fried food makes me worse.

Vocabulario: Las materias fecales

heces, materias fecales	feces
defecar, evacuar, ensuciar	to move one's bowels
hacer pupú	to "go poop" (juvenile)
¿Tiene diarrea o estreñimiento?	Do you have diarrhea or constipation?
¿Con qué frecuencia evacua?	How often to you move your bowels?
¿De qué color es la materia fecal?	What color is the stool?
¿Hay sangre?	Is there blood?
¿Cómo son las heces	How are the stools?
(las materias fecales)?	
¿Son . . .	Are they . . .
. . . blancas?	. . . white?
. . . verdosas?	. . . greenish?
. . . como la brea?	. . . like tar?
. . . flotantes?	. . . floating?
. . . blandas?	. . . soft?
. . . líquidas?	. . . liquid?
. . . mocosas?	. . . with mucus?
. . . duras y secas?	. . . hard and dry?

HACIA FLUIDEZ

 8.3 Actividad _____

Prepare un diálogo con un/a compañero/a para presentar a la clase. Usted es gastroenterólogo/a y su compañero/a sufre de estreñimiento. Clarifique el problema, por ejemplo cuánto tiempo hace y cómo son las heces fecales. Después hable de posibles remedios. Algunos remedios generales para el estreñimiento son:

comer papaya
hacer ejercicio todos los días
beber mucha agua u otros líquidos
tomar el tiempo necesario para evacuar
tomar laxantes solamente si el médico lo indica
comer más frutas, verduras y granos porque son ricos en fibra
tomar dos cucharadas de hidróxido de magnesia y un vaso de agua al acostarse

Conduct a Physical Examination

Estructura: El verbo *ir* para hablar del futuro

- The verb *ir* is an irregular verb and means "to go." These are the forms of the verb in the present tense.

yo	**Voy** a la clínica todos los viernes.
tú	¿**Vas** al dentista cada seis meses?
él, ella, usted	¿**Va** usted a la farmacia hoy?
nosotros/as	**Vamos** a la cafetería para comer.
ellos, ellas, ustedes	Mis hijos **van** a la casa de su abuela.

- To tell where one is going, use the correct form of the verb, the preposition *a,* and the name of a place.

Voy a la clínica.	I am going to the clinic.
Mi madre va a México.	My mother is going to Mexico.

- To tell what is going to happen in the near future, use the correct form of the verb *ir,* the preposition *a,* and a verb infinitive. Here the preposition does not translate literally.

Usted va a estar bien.	You are going to be fine.
Voy a llamar al cirujano.	I am going to call the surgeon.

- *Vamos* also means "Let's." Its use highlights collaboration without "talking down to" as it might seem in English.

Vamos a ver.	Let's see.
Vamos a esperar.	Let's wait; let's hope.
Vamos a tomarle la temperatura.	Let's take your temperature.

Estructura: Las contracciones *al* y *del*

- As you have learned, the preposition *a* means "to." When followed by the definite article *el,* the two are contracted to form the word *al.* There is no contraction with *la, las,* or *los.*

Voy a la clínica.	I go (I'm going) to the clinic.
Voy **al** hospital.	I go (I'm going) to the hospital.

- The "personal *a*" also contracts with the definite article *el.*

Examino **al** señor Ulloa ahora.	I'll examine Señor Ulloa now.

- The preposition *de* means "of" or "from" and is used to express possession as well. When *de* is followed by the definite article *el,* the two are contracted to form the word *del.* There is no contraction with *de la, de las,* or *de los.*

Le llamo de la clínica.	I'm calling (you, him, her) from the clinic.
Le llamo **del** hospital.	I'm calling (you, him, her) from the hospital.
¿Cuál es el teléfono **del** Sr. Vega?	What is Sr. Vega's telephone number?

HACIA FLUIDEZ

 8.4 Actividad _____

Observe la foto de la Clínica Chan Aquino. ¿Qué servicios ofrecen? Pregúntale a su compañero/a cuál es su propósito para ir a la clínica.

Modelo: —Voy a la clínica Chan Aquino.
　　　　　—¿Para qué va a la clínica?
　　　　　—Voy a la clínica para una biopsia de la piel.

Algunos de los servicios incluyen:
　　cirugía cardiovascular　　radiografía del pecho
　　evaluación psicológica　　análisis de sangre
　　electrocardiograma　　　examen físico infantil

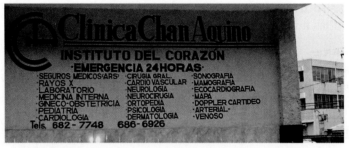

 8.5 Actividad _____

La madre de su compañero/a tiene una cita en la clínica mañana. Pregúntale los detalles de los planes, por ejemplo el motivo de la consulta, con quién va, la hora que van a ir, la hora que van a regresar. Su compañero/a debe responder ad lib.

regresar to return

Modelo: —Mi mamá va a la clínica mañana.
　　　　　—¿Por qué va ella a la clínica? / ¿Para qué va ella a la clínica?
　　　　　—Ella va porque le duele la garganta.

¿Por qué? Why (*cause*)?
¿Para qué? Why (*purpose*)?

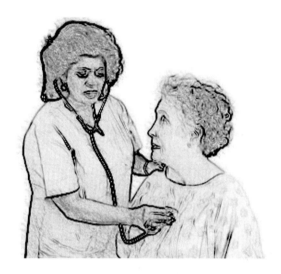

Escuchar (auscultar)

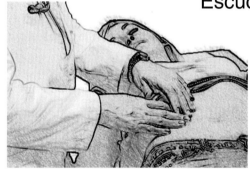

Tocar (palpar)

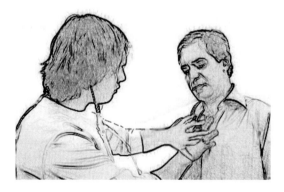

Dar golpecitos (percutir)

Vocabulario: El examen físico

mirar	to look, to look at
mirar la garganta	to look at the throat
escuchar, auscultar	to listen, to listen to, to auscultate
escuchar los pulmones	to listen to the lungs
escuchar el corazón	to listen to the heart
el estetoscopio	stethoscope
tocar, presionar, palpar	to touch, to press, to palpate
percutir, dar golpecitos	to percuss, to tap on
medir al bebé*	to measure the baby
pesar al niño (a la niña)	to weigh the child
tomar la temperatura	to take the temperature
tomar la tensión arterial	to take the blood pressure
medir el oxígeno en la sangre	to measure the blood oxygen
sacar sangre para un análisis	to draw blood for a test
hacer un electrocardiograma	to take an electrocardiogram
hacer un examen digital de la próstata	to do a digital exam of the prostate
poner un suero	to establish an IV
poner una inyección	to give an injection
poner una venda, curita	to put on a bandage, band-aid
poner puntos	to suture
sacar puntos	to remove stitches

*Bebé is assigned masculine gender regardless of the sex of the baby.

Medir is an irregular verb (mido, mides, mide, medimos, miden). Many of these verbs use the indirect object pronoun to represent the patient. Recall that these pronouns may be placed either before the conjugated verb or as a suffix attached to the infinitive. It makes no difference which.

La doctora **le** va a mirar los ojos.   La doctora va a mirar**le** los ojos.

> When treating a minor injury, a mother may say, *Sana, sana, culito de rana; si no te sanas hoy, te sanas mañana* (Heal, heal, toad's little tail; if you don't heal today, you'll heal tomorrow).

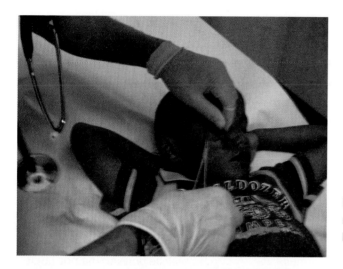

El doctor le pone puntos al niño. La cortadura va a sanar bien.

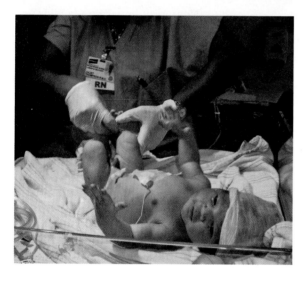

La enfermera mide al recién nacido. Es su primer examen físico. Foto cortesía de Otoniel Acevedo Medina.

HACIA PRECISIÓN

8.6 Ejercicio_____

En la foto, la enfermera mide al bebé. ¿Qué más le hace al bebé en su primer examen físico? Escriba una «x» en las actividades que son parte del primer examen físico infantil. Después comparta con la clase los resultados.

A. _____ ponerle puntos

B. _____ escucharle el corazón

C. _____ pesarle

D. _____ ponerle un suero

E. _____ examinarle la próstata

F. _____ escucharle los pulmones

G. _____ tomarle la temperatura

H. _____ sacarle sangre para un análisis

8.7 Ejercicio _____

Identifique las oraciones de la columna «B» que van frecuentemente con las oraciones de la columna «A» durante un examen físico. Escriba en la columna «B» la letra que corresponde de la columna «A».

<table>
<tr><td colspan="2" align="center">A</td><td align="center">B</td></tr>
</table>

A. Voy a mirarle los ojos.	_____ Respire profundamente.
B. Voy a percutirle el pecho.	_____ ¿Le duele cuando lo presiono?
C. Voy a mirarle la garganta.	_____ ¡Golpecitos!
D. Voy a tocarle el cuello.	_____ Mueva la cabeza hacia la derecha.
E. Voy a escucharle los pulmones.	_____ Acuéstese boca arriba por favor.
F. Voy a presionarle el abdomen.	_____ ¿Tiene problemas con la vista?
G. Voy a hacerle un electrocardiograma.	_____ Abra la boca y diga «a-a-a-a».
H. Tenemos que examinarle los testes.	_____ Vire la cabeza y tosa.

HACIA FLUIDEZ

 8.8 Actividad _____

Con un/a compañero/a tomen turnos para ser médico y paciente. El/La médico le pregunta al / a la paciente qué le pasa y el/la paciente le dice el motivo para la consulta. Después, el/la médico debe usar el vocabulario nuevo para decirle qué va a hacer para investigar el problema.

Modelo: —¿Qué le pasa?
          —Sufro del corazón. Tengo taquicardia.
          —Voy a escucharle el corazón.

Aquí hay unos motivos de consulta.
  A. Tengo fiebre.
  B. Tengo una cortadura.
  C. Me duele mucho la garganta.
  D. Sufro de asma y tengo la respiración corta.
  E. Hace cinco días que tengo puntos en la pierna.
  F. Necesito la vacuna antitetánica (*tetanus vaccine*).
  G. Mi papá tiene pulmonía y necesita antibióticos.
  H. Estoy aquí para chequearme la glucosa en la sangre.
  I. Mi bebé no come mucho y está demasiado chiquito.
  J. Sufro de la presión alta. Me duele la cabeza y estoy mareado.

8.9 Actividad _____

Un/a estudiante escribe cuatro columnas en la pizarra (*board*). Las columnas son: mirar, auscultar, palpar y percutir. El resto de los estudiantes deben escribir palabras, frases y oraciones asociadas con cada columna. Por ejemplo, en la columna *auscultar* escriba *Voy a escucharle la arteria carótida* o *¿Toma medicamento para bajar el colesterol?*

HACIA FLUIDEZ

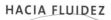 *EC activity?*

 (8.10 Actividad) _____

Use esta guía (*guide*) para demostrar un examen físico con un/a compañero/a. Su compañero/a debe contestar las preguntas ad lib.

> Practice language while miming movements. Pretend to palpate.

Guía: El motivo de la consulta

Favor de quitarse la ropa y ponerse la bata del hospital. No se quite el calzoncillo. Voy a volver pronto. ¿Qué le pasa? ¿Cuánto tiempo hace que usted tiene (el problema, los síntomas)? ¿Desde cuándo? ¿Con qué frecuencia? ¿Qué tiempo dura/n (el problema, los síntomas)? ¿Qué mejora el problema? ¿Qué lo empeora?

la bata	robe
el calzoncillo	underpants

Los medicamentos actuales

¿Toma usted algún medicamento todos los días? ¿Quién le receta el medicamento? ¿Cuántos miligramos toma? ¿Cuántas pastillas toma? ¿Cuántas veces al día toma el medicamento? ¿Es usted alérgico/a a algún medicamento? ¿Qué pasa cuando lo toma? ¿Tiene efectos secundarios?

El examen físico

Voy a mirarle los ojos. Míreme la nariz. Mire a ese punto de luz. ¿Tiene problema de la vista? ¿Usa lentes? Voy a mirarle los oídos. ¿Le duelen los oídos? Voy a mirarle la nariz y la garganta. Abra la boca, saque la lengua y diga «a-a-a-h». Voy a tocarle el cuello.

Voy a escucharle los pulmones y el corazón. Respire profundamente por la boca. Otra vez. Tosa. Tosa otra vez. ¿Hay flema cuando tose? ¿De qué color es la flema? ¿Es de un color claro, amarillo o verdoso? ¿Hay sangre cuando tose? ¿Le duele cuando tose? ¿Tiene dolor de pecho? ¿Es un dolor fuerte (punzante, quemante, pesado)? ¿Tiene a veces los tobillos hinchados?

¿Tiene dolor de estómago? ¿Le duele el abdomen? ¿Tiene diarrea? ¿Tiene estreñimiento? ¿Hay sangre cuando orina? ¿Hay sensación de ardor cuando orina? ¿Hay picazón? ¿Hay una secreción blanca? ¿Tiene relaciones sexuales?

acostarse to lie down   Favor de acostarse. ¿Le duele cuando presiono aquí?

A Word That Says a Lot: *Así*

You can boast that using only one Spanish word, you can teach someone how to tie shoelaces or to button a shirt. What word is that useful and versatile? When you are not sure how to verbalize an instruction, simply demonstrate the action you want the patient to perform and say the word *así*, which in this context means "in this way" or "like this."

Vocabulario: Exámenes especiales para mujeres y hombres

Palpar los senos o los testes

Prior to palpating the breasts or testes, tell the patient, *Tenemos que examinarle los senos* or *Tenemos que examinarle los testes (los testículos).* The use of *tenemos que* highlights necessity as the motivator; *examinar* is a clinical term; and the first person plural demonstrates partnership.*

Here are some useful questions and expressions.

Hombres

Tengo que examinarle la próstata a través del ano con el dedo, usando un guante. Ponga los codos en la camilla. Tengo que introducir un dedo para palparle la próstata. Es un poco incómodo, pero terminamos rápido. Tengo que examinarle los testes. Baje el calzoncillo. Vira la cabeza y tosa.

Mujeres

Tenemos que examinarle los senos. Ponga las manos en las caderas. Levante los brazos arriba de la cabeza. Favor de acostarse. Voy a palparle los senos. ¿Cuántos

---

*This expression helps you avoid novice-speaker faux pas such as, *Voy a tocarle los senos* or *Quiero palparle los testes.*

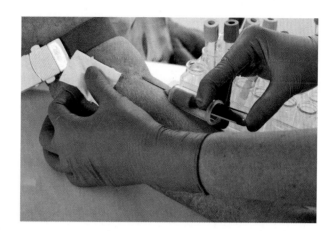

«Tengo que sacarle sangre para hacer un análisis».

años tenía cuando menstruó por primera vez? ¿Cuántos años tenía cuando nació su primer hijo? ¿Tiene secreciones del seno?

 ## Schedule Follow-up Tests

Vocabulario: Algunos análisis y procedimientos

El laboratorio

la biopsia	biopsy
el análisis de orina	urine test
el análisis de sangre	blood test
el análisis de glucosa en la sangre	blood glucose test
el cultivo de las heces fecales	stool culture
la concentración de alcohol en la sangre	blood alcohol level

Los imágenes diagnósticos

la radiografía, los rayos equis	x-ray
la placa	film, x-ray
la tomografía computarizada	CT scan
el ecograma, el sonograma, el ultrasonido	echogram, sonogram, ultrasound
el mamograma	mammogram
el angiograma	angiogram
las imágenes por resonancia magnética	MRI

Pruebas de los órganos

la broncoscopia	bronchoscopy
la espirometría	spirometry
el electrocardiograma	EKG
la prueba de estrés	stress test
la supervisión Holter	Holter monitor
el electroencefalograma	EEG
la colonoscopia	colonoscopy
la endoscopia	endoscopy

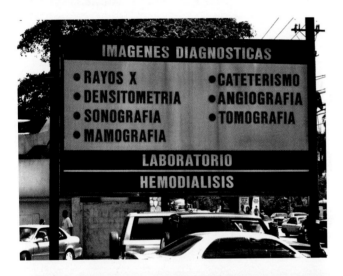

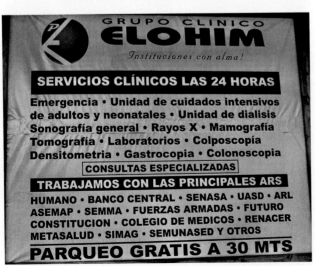

HACIA PRECISIÓN

 8.11 Ejercicio _____

Identifique las pruebas por su nombre después de leer las descripciones.

A. Es una radiografía, o una placa de una vena o arteria. Antes de hacerla, se introduce un catéter en una vena o arteria. Se inyecta una solución, o medio de contraste. La prueba es para descubrir si hay enfermedad en una vena, una arteria o un órgano.

_____

B. Es una grabadora portátil para grabar información del ritmo cardíaco durante un tiempo, como un electrocardiograma.

grabadora portátil
portable recorder

_____

C. Son para hacer unas imágenes muy específicas de una parte del cuerpo sin usar rayos equis.

_____

D. Es un procedimiento en que se introduce un tubo o un catéter por la nariz o por la boca para examinar los bronquios o los pulmones.

_____

E. Es una prueba en la cual un patólogo examina una muestra de tejido con un microscopio para descubrir si hay cáncer u otra enfermedad.

muestra de tejido
tissue sample

The word *o* changes to *u* before words that begin with *o* or *ho*.

_____

F. Es un examen de rayos equis de los senos para descubrir si hay tumores o quistes.

quiste cyst

_____

G. Es una prueba en la cual el paciente exhala en un instrumento que mide cuánto aire entra y sale de los pulmones para medir la capacidad respiratoria de los pulmones.

_____

H. Es una exploración del interior del intestino grueso con un colonoscopio.

_____

HACIA FLUIDEZ

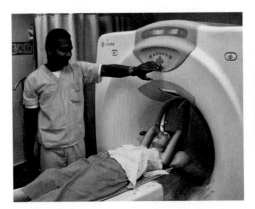 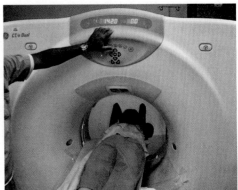

 8.12 Actividad

Vea las fotos de la niña que necesita una tomografía computarizada. Usted es técnico/a de radiografía y su compañero/a es un/a paciente que sufre de dolores de cabeza persistentes. Demuestre (*Demonstrate*) una entrevista donde usted se presenta al / a la paciente y le explica el procedimiento.

Vocabulario: Haciendo citas

de/por* la mañana	in the morning
de/por la tarde	in the afternoon/evening
de/por la noche	in the nighttime
tan pronto que sea posible	as soon as possible
de una vez	at once
mañana	tomorrow
pasado mañana	the day after tomorrow
la semana que viene	next week
dentro de dos semanas	within two weeks
el mes que viene	next month
el año que viene	next year

*Use *de* when a specific time is mentioned, as in *Puedo venir a las cinco de la tarde.* Use *por* when a specific hour is not mentioned, as in *Necesito una cita por la tarde.*

Preguntas útiles

¿Es posible venir mañana?	Is it possible to come tomorrow?
¿Puede venir el lunes a las cinco?	Can you come on Monday at five?

HACIA FLUIDEZ

8.13 Actividad

Usted es recepcionista y su compañero/a es un/a paciente que necesita varios de los siguientes análisis o procedimientos. Haga una cita (*Make an appointment*) para la fecha y la hora conveniente para la clínica y el/la paciente y dentro del tiempo especificado.

A. sacar los puntos (dentro de dos semanas)
B. hacer un análisis de sangre (dentro de una semana)
C. una endoscopia (dentro de un mes)
D. un electroencefalograma (mañana)
E. un angiograma (la semana que viene)
F. un análisis de orina (dentro de una semana)
G. un electrocardiograma (dentro de dos semanas)

8.14 Actividad

Vea el vocabulario de *análisis y procedimientos*. Usted es enfermero/a y su compañero/a es un/a paciente que necesita un análisis o procedimiento específico. Explíquele el procedimiento y después comparta su conversación con la clase.

Modelo: análisis de glucosa en la sangre
—Usted necesita un análisis de glucosa en la sangre. Tenemos que sacarle una gota de sangre del dedo para determinar cuánta glucosa, o azúcar, hay en la sangre.

Say What Is Happening Right Now

Estructura: El presente del progresivo

- To describe actions that are currently in progress (in progress as you are speaking), use the appropriate form of the verb *estar* and the present participle of the verb that represents the action.
- Form the present participle by adding the suffix *-ando* to verbs that end in *-ar* and the suffix *-iendo* to verbs that end in *-er* and *-ir*.

Estoy hablando con el enfermero. I am talking with the nurse.
El paciente está esperando. The patient is waiting.

- Several of the verbs that you already know take irregular forms in the present participle.

leer   **La doctora está leyendo el expediente médico.**
dormir   **La paciente está durmiendo en este momento.**

- Frequently this follows the phrase *en este momento,* for example, *En este momento estoy examinando a un paciente.*

HACIA PRECISIÓN

 8.15 Ejercicio _____

Indique qué están haciendo las siguientes personas en este momento.

Modelo: escribir una receta, yo
         —Estoy escribiendo una receta.

A. preparar una ensalada de fruta, Mamá

_____

B. recetar algo para el dolor, yo

_____

C. trabajar en la clínica ambulatoria hoy, nosotros

_____

D. llegar al hospital ahora, el cardiólogo

_____

E. mejorar, tú

_____

F. percutir el pecho, la doctora

_____

HACIA FLUIDEZ

 8.16 Drama improvisado _____

Play "What are you doing?" (This is fun!) Form a circle with one student in the middle. This student mimes an activity, for example taking someone's blood pressure. A student in the circle asks, *¿Qué estás haciendo?* The student in the middle uses the present progressive tense to say that he or she is doing something other than what he or she is doing, for example, *Estoy midiendo al bebé.* The student who asks the question then takes the center of the circle and must mime measuring a baby until another student asks, *¿Qué estás haciendo?* and the play continues in the same way when the new student in the middle says something other than what he or she is doing. Here are some of the verbs that you have learned.

caminar	cocinar	estudiar	examinar	sacar
llamar	recetar	tomar	comer	percutir
leer	escuchar	palpar	mirar	hacer

 8.17 Reciclaje _____

This form can be downloaded from the website.

Vea la fotografía del doctor y su paciente. ¿Qué está diciendo el doctor? Use el formulario *Historia clínica* (p. 236) para demostrar el examen con un/a compañero/a. Note las siguientes abreviaturas: tensión arterial (TA), frecuencia cardíaca (FC) y frecuencia respiratoria (FR).

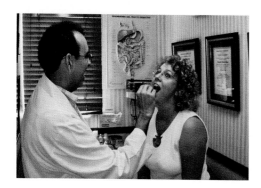

«Voy a mirarle la garganta».

 8.18 Reciclaje _____

Vea los cuatro letreros (*signs*) (p. 237) y conteste las siguientes preguntas.

A. ¿A qué hora es el grupo de autoayuda?
B. ¿Quién me puede operar las cataratas?
C. ¿Quién trabaja en el departamento de maternidad?
D. ¿Está abierto los martes el consultorio del Dr. Padilla Desgarennes?
E. ¿A qué hora cierra el consultorio del Dr. Blas Salinas?
F. ¿Cuál es el número de teléfono del gastroenterólogo?

Historia clínica

Fecha de consulta: _____

Apellidos: _____   Nombres: _____

Fecha de nacimiento: _____   Lugar de nacimiento: _____

Sexo: _____   Nacionalidad: _____   Teléfono: _____

Motivo de la consulta: _____

Historia familiar: _____

Antecedentes médicos: _____

Medicamentos actuales: _____

Alergias: _____

Tabaco, alcohol, drogas: _____

       Último uso: _____

PA _____ / _____   FC _____   FR _____   Altura _____   Peso _____

Pulmones: _____

Corazón: _____

Abdomen: _____

Impresión diagnóstica: _____

Tratamiento: _____

_____

_____
Firma

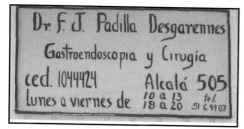
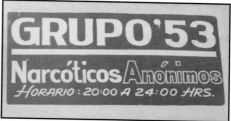
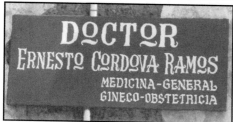
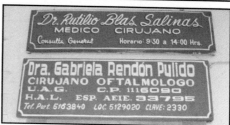

 ## Exposición

 ### CHAPTER 8 SKILL: CREATING A CASE PRESENTATION

You are going to listen to the recording of a doctor presenting a case in morning rounds and then create a case presentation of your own.

1. Listen to the sample case on the audio program. While you listen, look at the following form and take note of which categories of information are provided. Is there some information included in the presentation that is not in the form below? Take notes on what categories the form may be missing.

2. Adapt the form so that it reflects all the information in the audio case presentation.

Nombre del paciente: _____ Sexo: _____ Edad: _____

Temperatura: _____ Frecuencia cardíaca: _____ Tensión arterial: _____

Frecuencia respiratoria: _____ Historia médica: _____

_____

Medicamentos actuales y dosis: _____

Síntoma: _____

Cuánto tiempo hace:_____ Frecuencia:_____

Cuánto tiempo dura: _____

Pruebas o procedimientos que necesita: _____

_____

3. Fill out the revised form, using different information than what is presented in the recording.
4. Now create a case presentation based on that information and present it to the class.

Cultural Note: A Dynamic Process

Bien se está San Pedro en Roma ("Saint Peter is best off in Rome"—
a saying similar to "There's no place like home")

Al son que le toquen, bailen ("Dance to the song that is played"—
a saying similar to "When in Rome, do as the Romans do")

Culture is dynamic, and frontiers are disappearing. Culture is both imported and exported. Groups are penetrated by outside cultures' products and media, such as the Internet, television, and advertisements. People export culture as they migrate. Then they acculturate gradually, generally in three generations, although children tend to do it faster. The host culture, or receiving culture, is changed also. As the world shrinks, flattens, and globalizes, cultures encounter situations that are easily assimilated and others that are not, forcing them to adapt. Immigrants and others who have cross-cultural experiences may decide that there are aspects of both cultures that they like and dislike. They may either consciously or unconsciously cling to—or reject— specific aspects of their culture of origin while embracing aspects of the host culture. An immigrant to the United States whose children assimilate at a faster pace may lament, *Mis hijos están americanizados.*

Language competency is an essential component of acculturation. Families may resist acculturation by recognizing that the way to preserve cultural views and traditions is to speak Spanish at home. Children, on the other hand, may resist speaking Spanish, as a way to avoid appearing different among peers. This may create intergenerational communication gaps. The same children may one day regret not speaking Spanish and decide to take classes in order to rediscover their heritage or connect with elderly family members.

Children learn to navigate both worlds skillfully. (For example, Creole languages generally emerge in one generation as children translate for their families and foreign occupiers, creating an enduring combination of first language structure and second language lexicon.) Families eventually choose what parts of culture to preserve and what to leave behind in order to assimilate more comfortably. With some experience, families and individuals may function very successfully in both cultures. For example, a wedding planned by a Latin-American family might not begin at the time printed on the invitation. This is because it must not begin until the bride is ready and all guests have arrived. The same family, when scheduling a business appointment, may insist *Empezamos a la una, hora americana* ("We'll start at one o'clock, American time"), to encourage punctuality.

During the process of acculturation individuals may feel lonely, frustrated, and incompetent to function in the new society. Parents may struggle with communicating with their children's teachers or pediatrician. They may not understand why their children would rather play with friends than go to Tío Alfredo's birthday party and wonder why neighbors do not collaborate in rearing each other's children. Elderly persons may feel less valued and respected than in their culture of origin. Temporary relief is available in enclaves or neighborhoods that keep the cultural identity of their members while coexisting with the surrounding dominant culture. These enclaves also provide great opportunities for host culture members to have cross-cultural experiences.

Models for comparing health across ethnic groups have focused on genetics and racial differences, on cultural lifestyles (diet and exercise, for example), on socioeconomic status, and on proximity to pathogens (living in cities, for example). Although each view has merit, controlling socioeconomic factors in health care access (literacy, insurance, transportation, and the linguistic competency of the patient and provider) can ameliorate some of the health disparity between groups.

Vocabulario del capítulo ocho

El motivo de la consulta

el motivo de la consulta	the chief complaint
¿Qué le pasa?	What is happening (to you, him, her)?
¿Qué tiene?	What is the matter?
¿En qué le puedo ayudar?	How can I help you?

Expresiones de tiempo

¿Con qué frecuencia?	How often?
nunca, jamás	never
casi nunca	almost never
de vez en cuando	once in a while
Va y viene.	It comes and goes.
a veces	at times
una o dos veces al día	once or twice a day
a menudo	often
frecuentemente	frequently
siempre; Es continuo.	always; It's continuous.
¿Desde cuándo?	Since when?
desde esta mañana	since this morning
desde anoche	since last night
desde ayer	since yesterday
desde el lunes	since Monday
desde hace tres días	since three days ago
desde la semana pasada	since last week
¿Cuánto tiempo hace?	How long has it been?
Hace una hora.	It's been an hour.
Hace dos días.	It's been two days.
¿Cuánto tiempo dura?	How long does it last?
Dura de una a dos horas.	It lasts for one or two hours.
Dura varios días.	It lasts for several days.

¿Qué le mejora?

ayudar	to help
mejorar	to improve
empeorar	to worsen
sentirse	to feel

Las materias fecales

heces, materias fecales	feces
defecar, evacuar, ensuciar	to move one's bowels
hacer pupú	to "go poop" (juvenile)

¿Tiene diarrea o estreñimiento?	Do you have diarrhea or constipation?
¿Con qué frecuencia evacua?	How often do you move your bowels?
¿De qué color es la materia fecal?	What color is the stool?
¿Hay sangre?	Is there blood?
¿Cómo son las heces	How are the stools?
(las materias fecales)?	
¿Son . . .	Are they . . .
. . . blancas?	. . . white?
. . . verdosas?	. . . greenish?
. . . como la brea?	. . . like tar?
. . . flotantes?	. . . floating?
. . . blandas?	. . . soft?
. . . líquidas?	. . . liquid?
. . . mocosas?	. . . with mucus?
. . . duras y secas?	. . . hard and dry?

El examen físico

mirar	to look, to look at
mirar la garganta	to look at the throat
escuchar, auscultar	to listen, to listen to, to auscultate
escuchar los pulmones	to listen to the lungs
escuchar el corazón	to listen to the heart
el estetoscopio	stethoscope
tocar, presionar, palpar	to touch, to press, to palpate
percutir, dar golpecitos	to percuss, to tap on
medir al bebé	to measure the baby
pesar al niño (a la niña)	to weigh the child
tomar la temperatura	to take the temperature
tomar la tensión arterial	to take the blood pressure
medir el oxígeno en la sangre	to measure the blood oxygen
sacar sangre para un análisis	to draw blood for a test
hacer un electrocardiograma	to take an electrocardiogram
hacer un examen digital de la próstata	to do a digital exam of the prostate
poner un suero	to establish an IV
poner una inyección	to give an injection
poner una venda, curita	to put on a bandage, band-aid
poner puntos	to suture
sacar puntos	to remove stitches

Algunos análisis y procedimientos
El laboratorio

la biopsia	biopsy
el análisis de orina	urine test

el análisis de sangre	blood test
el análisis de glucosa en la sangre	blood glucose test
el cultivo de las heces fecales	stool culture
la concentración de alcohol en la sangre	blood alcohol level

Los imágenes diagnósticos

la radiografía, los rayos equis	x-ray
la placa	film, x-ray
la tomografía computarizada	CT scan
el ecograma, el sonograma, el ultrasonido	echogram, sonogram, ultrasound
el mamograma	mammogram
el angiograma	angiogram
las imágenes por resonancia magnética	MRI

Las pruebas de los órganos

la broncoscopia	bronchoscopy
la espirometría	spirometry
el electrocardiograma	EKG
la prueba de estrés	stress test
la supervisión Holter	Holter monitor
el electroencefalograma	EEG
la colonoscopia	colonoscopy
la endoscopia	endoscopy

Haciendo citas

de/por la mañana	in the morning
de/por la tarde	in the afternoon/evening
de/por la noche	in the nighttime
tan pronto que sea posible	as soon as possible
de una vez	at once
mañana	tomorrow
pasado mañana	the day after tomorrow
la semana que viene	next week
dentro de dos semanas	within two weeks
el mes que viene	next month
el año que viene	next year

Preguntas útiles

¿Qué le ayuda?	What helps you?
¿Qué le mejora?	What makes you better?
¿Qué le empeora?	What makes you worse?
¿Qué le hace sentir mejor?	What makes you feel better?

¿Qué le hace sentir peor?	What makes you feel worse?
¿Es posible venir mañana?	Is it possible to come tomorrow?
¿Puede venir el lunes a las cinco?	Can you come on Monday at five?

Expresiones útiles

El ibuprofeno me ayuda.	Ibuprofen helps me.
Comer fritura me empeora.	Eating fried food makes me worse.

Chapter 9

«¿Qué pasó?»

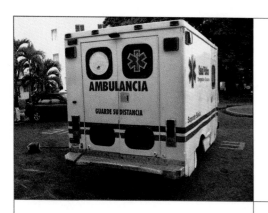

Communication Goals

Vocabulary

Structure

Cultural Note

Website   www.yalebooks.com/medicalspanish

   Video   *Trama: Memorias de México; Demostración: Dolor terrible*

   Audio   *Tiempos pasados; Antes de la cirugíu; Palabras tranquilizadoras; Ejercicio 9.16;
      Exposición*

   Electronic Workbook

Ⅰn this chapter you will talk about things that occurred in the past. You will learn to ask, "What happened?" and "Did you take your medicine?" You will be able to ask, "When was the last time that you . . . ?" You'll also be able to ask about the context of the chief complaint: "What was going on when this happened?" Contextual themes will incorporate pre-surgical interviews, heart disease, cardiac rehabilitation, and the work of visiting nurses and paramedics.

Ask What Happened

Vocabulario: Tiempos pasados

esta mañana	this morning
hoy	today
anoche	last night
ayer	yesterday
anteayer	the day before yesterday
el jueves pasado	last Thursday
la semana pasada	last week
el mes pasado	last month
el año pasado	last year

lunes	martes	miércoles	jueves	viernes
anteayer	ayer	hoy	mañana	pasado mañana

Estructura: El pretérito de los verbos regulares

- Now you'll be able to describe actions that were completed in the past. Like the present tense, form the preterit past tense by changing the form of the verb according to the subject (who or what did the action). The first and third persons have written accents that guide you to stress that syllable when speaking. The other forms are stressed on the next-to-last syllable. Here are the forms of the verb *tomar* in the preterit. Verbs ending in *-ar* that follow this pattern of endings are called "regular verbs."

yo	**Tomé** la aspirina esta mañana.
tú	¿**Tomaste** el antiácido antes de comer?
él, ella, usted	¿**Tomó** usted mucha agua con el medicamento?
nosotros/as	Raúl y yo **tomamos** el autobús para llegar.
ellos, ellas, ustedes	Mis hijos **tomaron** las vitaminas esta mañana.

- Similarly, form the preterit of regular verbs ending in -*er* and -*ir* by changing the form of the verb according to the subject. Here are the forms of the verb *comer* in the preterit. Verbs ending in -*er* and -*ir* that follow this pattern are called "regular verbs."

yo	**Comí** arroz con pollo anoche.
tú	¿**Comiste** bien?
él, ella, usted	Juan no **comió** nada.
nosotros/as	Ada y yo **comimos** mucho en la cafetería.
ellos, ellas, ustedes	Mis hijos **comieron** el almuerzo en la escuela.

- The first person plural (*nosotros*) form for all regular verbs (-*ar*, -*er*, and -*ir*) is the same in both the present and the preterit tenses. Tell them apart by the context.

  Nosotros siempre tomamos café por la mañana (*present tense*).
  Ayer tomamos café antes de ir al hospital (*past tense*).

HACIA PRECISIÓN

 9.1 Ejercicio_____

Complete las siguientes oraciones con la forma correcta del verbo entre paréntesis. Use el pretérito.

A. Anoche mis tíos y mis primos nos _____ (visitar).

B. Ellos _____ (llegar) a las cinco de la tarde.

C. Mis padres _____ (cocinar) mucha comida deliciosa.

D. Mi hermano y yo _____ (comer) ensalada, carne y arroz.

E. Después de comer, yo _____ (estudiar) para la clase de español.

F. En la noche mi tía _____ (sufrir) de acidez.

G. A las ocho mi tío le _____ (comprar) un antiácido para mi tía.

H. Mi tía se _____ (tomar) el antiácido con un vaso de agua.

9.2 Ejercicio _____

Complete las siguientes preguntas con la forma correcta del pretérito del verbo entre paréntesis. Después practique las preguntas con un/a compañero/a.

nacer
to be born
tragar
to swallow

A. ¿En qué año _____ (nacer) usted?

B. ¿A usted le _____ (escribir) la doctora una receta nueva?

C. ¿Por cuántos años _____ (vivir) sus padres con usted?

D. ¿Cuántas botellas de vino _____ (beber) los enfermeros en la fiesta?

E. ¿_____ (ver*) tú el accidente ayer?

F. ¿A qué hora _____ (salir) tú de tu casa esta mañana?

G. ¿_____ (cuidar) bien los enfermeros a tu padre en el hospital?

H. ¿_____ (tragar) doña María la pastilla grande sin problema?

*When *ver* is used in the preterit, the accents are not written.

HACIA FLUIDEZ

 9.3 Actividad _____

Usted es un/a enfermero/a que visita a sus pacientes en sus casas. Su compañero/a es su paciente. Vea la lista de «Quehaceres para hoy» (p. 249) y pregúntele al / a la paciente **qué hizo** (*what he or she did*) o no hizo hoy.

Modelo: tomar el antibiótico
—¿Tomó usted el antibiótico?
—Sí, tomé el antibiótico.
(o)
—No, no lo tomé.

 9.4 Actividad _____

Pregúntele a un/a compañero/a si las siguientes personas hicieron o no (*did or did not do*) lo que el doctor les recomendó.

Modelo: el paciente, tomar el medicamento hoy
—¿Tomó el paciente el medicamento hoy?
—Sí, el paciente tomó el medicamento hoy.
(o)
—No, el paciente no tomó el medicamento hoy.

A. tú, tomar la aspirina esta mañana
B. su madre, tomar la codeína anoche
C. usted, usar la insulina
D. los niños, usar el inhalador
E. Maribel, comer cinco porciones de frutas hoy
F. el señor Vega, tomar el antibiótico hoy
G. ustedes, tomar las vitaminas con el desayuno
H. la paciente, usar el oxígeno
I. Juan, comprar el jarabe
J. la doctora, escribir la receta para mi hermano

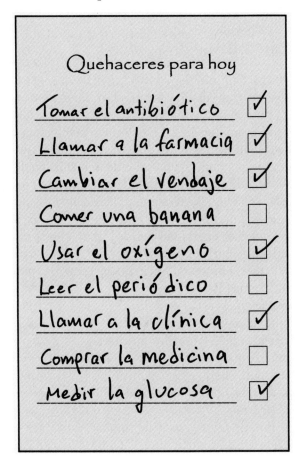

 9.5 Actividad _____

Es una telenovela y ustedes son actores. En esta telenovela, el protagonista Rafaelito toma una sobredosis de su medicamento, su novia Isabela llama al 9–11 y Pedro el paramédico es el héroe del día. Escoja tres actores y juntos lean el texto de la telenovela en voz alta. **Exageren** las emociones. Mientras leen, tienen que conjugar los verbos (entre paréntesis) en el pretérito del pasado.

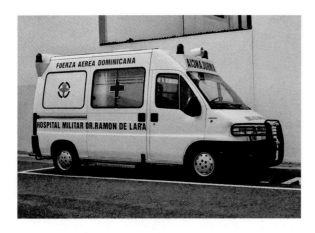

Llámenos al teléfono nueve-once si nos necesita.

Isabela: Rafaelito es mi novio y lo amo. Lo amo mucho pero es un hombre difícil y no puedo vivir con él.

Rafaelito: Isabela es mi novia y la amo. La amo muchísimo pero ella dice que no puede vivir conmigo. No puedo vivir sin ella. Quiero morir. Hace diez minutos que (tomar) una sobredosis de mis medicamentos.

Isabela: Ay, Rafaelito, mi amor, mi vida, mi corazón. (Tomar) una sobredosis porque no quieres vivir sin mí. Pero Rafaelito, no vas a morir, porque (llamar) al nueve-once y la ambulancia va a llegar pronto.

Pedro: Soy Pedro el paramédico. Estoy aquí y todo va a estar súper bien. ¿Quién (llamar) al nueve-once?

Isabela: Yo (llamar) porque mi novio (tomar) pastillas para quitarse la vida.

Pedro: Señor, ¿qué (tomar) usted?

Rafaelito: Pastillas. Aquí está la botella. Son para los nervios.

Pedro: ¿Cuántas pastillas (tomar) usted?

Rafaelito: (Tomar) todas. Como diez pastillas.

Pedro: ¿Cuánto tiempo hace que usted las (tomar)?

Rafaelito: Hace media hora, más o menos.

Pedro: ¿(Tomar) bebidas alcohólicas también?

Rafaelito: No. No bebo.

Pedro: ¿(Vomitar)? ¿Tiene deseo de vomitar?

Rafaelito: No. No (vomitar), pero tengo mucho sueño.

Pedro: Vamos a llevarlo al hospital. Usted va a estar súper bien.

Isabela: Pedro, tú (salvar) a mi novio. Eres buenísimo. ¿Cuál es tu número de teléfono?

Pedro: Llámeme si me necesita. Mi teléfono es nueve-once. Con su permiso, en este momento tengo que salvar una vida. Hasta luego.

9.6 Drama improvisado _____

Practice verbs in the past tense with another game of "Three-headed Person." Space permitting, form a circle. Otherwise choose a pattern for taking turns while seated in the classroom, for example, up and down rows. Recall that a discrete sentence usually has a subject and a predicate. The first person states a subject (for example, *yo, usted, Juan, mis padres, la uróloga*). The next person supplies the verb, conjugated in the preterit according to the subject. The third person provides an ending that tells more about the subject. Then the class repeats the whole sentence in loud and percussive tones.

> Modelo: —La psicóloga
> —examinó
> —a mi padre.
> —La psicóloga examinó a mi padre.

 ## Estructura: El pretérito de algunos verbos irregulares

The verbs *ser, ir, estar, tener, decir,* and *poner* are among those that have irregular morphology in the preterit past tense. This means they do not follow the same pattern as regular verbs.

- The verbs *ser* and *ir* use the same forms in the preterit. They are differentiated by the context of the sentence.

yo	**Fui** estudiante de medicina por un año. (Ser)
tú	¿**Fuiste** a la clínica ayer? (Ir)
él, ella, usted	Hoy es domingo. Ayer **fue** sábado. (Ser)
nosotros/as	**Fuimos** a la clínica para consultar con el neurólogo. (Ir)
ellos, ellas ustedes	Los niños no **fueron** pacientes de esta clínica. (Ser)

- Recall that the verb *estar* (to be) is used to talk about location, feelings, and conditions. Here are the forms of *estar* in the preterit.

yo	**Estuve** enfermo anoche.
tú	**Estuviste** en la clínica ayer.
él, ella, usted	Mi esposa **estuvo** en el hospital el lunes.
nosotros/as	**Estuvimos** en casa anoche.
ellos, ellas, ustedes	Los niños **estuvieron** enfermos con gripe.

- The verb *tener* (to have) uses forms that are very similar to the verb *estar*. Recall that *tener que* + infinitive means "to have to." In the preterit, we can talk about things that we *had* as well as things that we *had to do* in the past.

yo	**Tuve** fiebre anoche.
tú	**Tuviste** un ataque epiléptico.
él, ella, usted	Ana **tuvo** que tomar la nitroglicerina para quitar el dolor.
nosotros/as	Mi hermano y yo **tuvimos** que cuidar a nuestro padre.
ellos, ellas, ustedes	Mis padres **tuvieron** que llamar una ambulancia.

- The verb *decir* (to say, to tell) normally requires the indirect object pronoun, which indicates to whom something was said. (You can review indirect object pronouns in chapter 6.)

yo	Le **dije** a la enfermera que mi mamá sufre de azúcar.
tú	¿Qué le **dijiste** a tu mamá anoche, Paquito?
él, ella, usted	El pediatra me **dijo** que el niño no tiene infección.
nosotros/as	Le **dijimos** a Rosa que ella debe ir al consultorio.
ellos, ellas, ustedes	Los pacientes **dijeron** que la cafetería debe servir arroz.

- The verb *poner* (to put, to place) will be helpful in the context of the pharmacy and the emergency department (*poner una inyección, poner un suero y poner puntos*). It often requires an indirect object.

yo	Me **puse** la nitroglicerina debajo de la lengua.
tú	¿Le **pusiste** la vacuna antitetánica al paciente?
él, ella, usted	La doctora me **puso** dieciocho puntos en la cara.
nosotros/as	Nosotros nos **pusimos** la insulina después del desayuno.
ellos, ellas, ustedes	Los enfermeros les **pusieron** sueros a los pacientes.

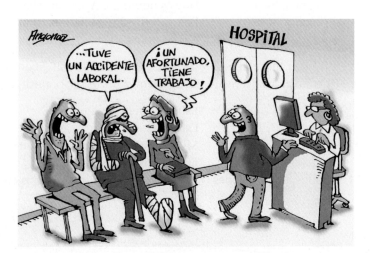

Cortesía del humorista
Pepe Angonoa

HACIA PRECISIÓN

 9.7 Ejercicio_____ _____

Indique si los verbos en las siguientes oraciones son formas de *ir* o *ser*.

A.	Ayer **fue** miércoles.	IR	SER
B.	La prueba de Pap **fue** negativa.	IR	SER
C.	La semana pasada **fui** a la clínica.	IR	SER
D.	**Fui** estudiante de medicina en el 2014.	IR	SER
E.	El enfermero **fue** a la cafetería para comer.	IR	SER
F.	El cirujano que me operó **fue** el doctor Pérez.	IR	SER
G.	Mi madre y yo **fuimos** al consultorio el martes.	IR	SER
H.	Mis hijos **fueron** a Chile para visitar a sus abuelos.	IR	SER

 9.8 Ejercicio _____

Una madre pasó una noche difícil. Complete el párrafo con la forma correcta de los verbos *ser, ir, estar, tener, recetar, decir* o *poner* en el pretérito.

Anoche el bebé _____ (estar) enfermo. Mi pobre bebé _____ (tener) una fiebre alta. Su temperatura _____ (estar) en cuarenta grados. Nosotros _____ (ir) al hospital. El doctor que nos atendió _____ (ser) el doctor Vargas. Yo _____ (estar) muy nerviosa. La enfermera le _____ (poner) un suero. El doctor me _____ (decir) que _____ (ser) una infección de los oídos y nos _____ (recetar) un antibiótico.

9.9 Ejercicio _____

Estos son los planes que el doctor Aquino tuvo para el enero pasado. Haga oraciones para decir qué hizo (*what he did*) y cuándo.

Modelo: 3 de enero
—El tres de enero el doctor Aquino y Ana comieron en la casa de Javier.

3 de enero	comer en la casa de Javier con Ana
5 de enero	visitar a doña Mercedes en Boston
11 de enero	trabajar en la clínica desde las ocho hasta las cinco
13 de enero	el doctor Aquino y don Máximo ir a la clase de inglés

14 de enero	consultar con el anestesiólogo
15 de enero	no comer nada, beber líquidos claros y tomar citrato de magnesio
16 de enero	tener una colonoscopia
17 de enero	ir al consultorio de la doctora Muñoz Domínguez para un examen físico
30 de enero	ir de vacaciones a Venezuela

HACIA FLUIDEZ

 9.10 Actividad _____

Usted es un/a enfermero/a que visita a sus pacientes en sus casas. Su compañero/a es su paciente. Pregúntele al / a la paciente si *tuvo que* hacer lo siguiente.

Modelo: tomar la nitroglicerina
      —¿Tuvo usted que tomar la nitroglicerina?
      —Sí, tuve que tomar la nitroglicerina.
      (o)
      —No, no tuve que tomar la nitroglicerina.

A. usar insulina
B. ir a la clínica
C. usar el oxígeno
D. cambiar el vendaje
E. llevar a su esposo/a al hospital
F. tomar una pastilla para el dolor
G. llamar a la compañía de seguros médicos

 9.11 Actividad _____

Lea la carta que doña Silvestrina le escribió a su hijo en los Estados Unidos y con un/a compañero/a contesten las siguientes preguntas.

A. ¿Cómo se llama la madre de Felipe, y cómo está ella?
B. ¿Qué le pasó a doña Silvestrina?
C. ¿Tuvo fiebre?
D. ¿Cuál fue la temperatura?
E. ¿Cuántos días estuvo en el hospital?
F. ¿Qué tratamiento le dieron?
G. ¿Quién cuidó a doña Silvestrina?

9 de enero de 2013

Querido hijo,

¿cómo estás? Espero que bien. Estoy mejor, gracias a Dios. Estuve en el hospital por 3 días. Tuve una fiebre de 40 grados y tu hermana me llamó la ambulancia.

Tuve una pulmonía la cual dijo la doctora es una infección de los pulmones. Me dieron antibióticos por suero y eso me ayudó a quitar la infección y la fiebre.

Los doctores y enfermeros me cuidaron bien. Fueron muy amables.

Escríbeme pronto. Gracias por el dinero que me enviaste. Que Dios te bendiga.

Tu madre que te quiere mucho.

Silvestrina Robles de Jiménez

P.d. tu hermana te manda saludos

Give Test Results

El resultado de una prueba puede ser positivo o negativo. Como son adjetivos, tienen género y número. Por ejemplo,

> Su prueba de tuberculosis fue *positiva*.
> Las placas de su pecho fueron *negativas*.
> El resultado de su radiografía fue *negativo*.

HACIA PRECISIÓN

9.12 Ejercicio _____

Informe al paciente de sus resultados. Si todo está bien, añada (*add*) «Todo está bien. Gracias a Dios». Si no, añada «Tenga confianza. Todo va a estar bien».

Modelo: la placa del pecho (negativa)
—Tenemos el resultado de la placa del pecho. Fue negativa, gracias a Dios.

A. la biopsia   (positiva)
B. el análisis de sangre   (negativo)
C. el electrocardiograma   (negativo)
D. la prueba de tuberculosis   (positiva)
E. la tomografía computarizada   (negativa)
F. la prueba del SIDA (*AIDS*)   (negativa)
G. la prueba de Papanicolaou   (negativa)
H. el sonograma de la vesícula biliar (*gall bladder*)   (negativo)

 ## Conduct a Pre-surgery Interview

 ### Vocabulario: Antes de la cirugía

¿Cuándo fue la última vez que . . . ?	When was the last time that . . . ?*
usar alcohol o drogas	to use alcohol or drugs
orinar	to urinate
evacuar, defecar	to move one's bowels
menstruar	to menstruate
empezar su período	to start your menses
beber algo	to drink something
comer algo	to eat something
¿Tiene/Usa usted . . . ?	Do you have / Do you use . . . ?
una peluca	a wig
un diente flojo	a loose tooth
un prótesis	a prosthesis
una dentadura postiza	dentures
lentes o lentes de contacto	glasses or contact lenses
problemas con el corazón	heart problems
problemas con los pulmones	lung problems

*Modelo: ¿Cuándo fue la última vez que usted usó cocaína?

Preguntas útiles

¿Cuándo comenzó su último período?
¿Está usted alérgico/a a algún medicamento?
¿Cuándo fue la última vez que usted / el niño evacuó?

HACIA FLUIDEZ

 9.13 Actividad _____

Con un/a compañero/a, prepare y presente a la clase una entrevista pre-quirúr-gica (*presurgical interview*). Usted es anestesiólogo/a y su compañero/a es un/a paciente que llegó para tener una colecistectomía.

Nombre: _____ Alergías: _____

Historia médica: _____

Prótesis: _____

Diente flojo: _____ Lentes de contacto: _____

Alcohol/drogas: _____

La última vez que:

Bebió: _____ Comió: _____ Evacuó: _____

Orinó: _____ Comenzó el período: _____

 ## Vocabulario: Palabras tranquilizadoras

Todo va a estar bien.	Everything is going to be fine.
Por favor, cálmese.	Please calm down.
No tenga miedo.	Don't be afraid.
Tenga confianza.	Have trust.
No se preocupe.	Don't worry (formal).
No te preocupes.	Don't worry (informal).
No va a doler.	It's not going to hurt.
Va a mejorar.	It's going to get better.
Hay que seguir adelante.	One must go on.

 9.14 Actividad _____

Observe el dibujo (p. 258) de la sala de emergencias. Hable de los pacientes que esperan al doctor y decida a quién el doctor debe de atender primero y quién debe ser segundo y tercero. Después presenten una entrevista entre uno/a de los pacientes y el/la enfermero/a de clasificación (*triage nurse*) para identificar el motivo de la consulta y llegar a una definición más específica del problema.

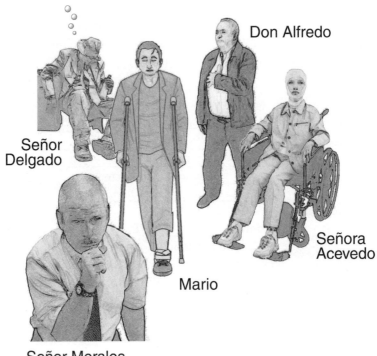

Sala de emergencias

Don Alfredo

Señor
Delgado

Señora
Acevedo

Mario

Señor Morales

9.15 Actividad

Usted es paramédico y su compañero/a es paciente. Con su compañero/a, prepare y presente a la clase una entrevista donde el paramédico llega al lugar (*location*) de una emergencia y determina qué pasó. Aquí hay posibles preguntas.

¿Qué le pasó?
¿Perdió la conciencia?
¿Tiene dificultad para respirar?
¿Tiene deseo de vomitar?
¿Es usted alérgico/a a algún medicamento?
¿Toma usted algún medicamento todos los días?
¿Qué otros problemas de salud tiene usted?
¿Cuál es el nombre de su doctor?

Ask What Was Happening

Estructura: El imperfecto del pasado

- You have been practicing the preterit tense, which is used to narrate actions that were completed in the past. In contrast, the imperfect tense describes past conditions and actions without freezing them in time. For example,

¿Qué pasó?   What happened?
¿Qué pasaba cuando eso pasó?   What was going on when that happened?

- Here are the forms of the verbs in the imperfect. Verbs ending in *-er* and *-ir* share the same verb endings, while verbs ending in *-ar* have their own set of forms.

	Tomar	*Comer*	*Vivir*
yo	tomaba	comía	vivía
tú	tomabas	comías	vivías
él, ella, usted	tomaba	comía	vivía
nosotros/as	tomábamos	comíamos	vivíamos
ellos, ellas, ustedes	tomaban	comían	vivían

- A few verbs are irregular in the imperfect. Here are two of them.

	Ser	*Ir*
yo	era	iba
tú	eras	ibas
él, ella, usted	era	iba
nosotros/as	éramos	íbamos
ellos, ellas, ustedes	eran	iban

Cuando era niño, mi abuela me **hacía** té de manzanilla.
When I was a child, my grandmother made me chamomile tea.

Antes, yo **tomaba** una cerveza de cuarenta onzas todas las noches.
I used to drink a 40-ounce beer every night.

Yo siempre **comía** fritura sin pensar en el colesterol.
I always would eat fried food without thinking about cholesterol.

Cuando **vivíamos** en Chile, **tomábamos** té de orégano para el estómago.
When we lived in Chile, we drank oregano tea to calm the stomach.

- Use the imperfect to describe the following.

  o Habitual actions when the duration or the starting and stopping times are not specified

    Antes, **fumaba** dos paquetes de cigarrillos todos los días.
    Cuando **me enfermaba** mi abuela **me preparaba** un té.

  o Actions that were in progress or in the background

    ¿Qué **hacía** usted cuando el dolor empezó?
    Mientras **caminaba** en el parque me **dolían** las rodillas.

  o How things *used to* be

    Mis padres **eran** estrictos con nosotros.
    Antes, los doctores **tenían** más tiempo para hablar con los pacientes.

  o Time and age in the past

    Eran las cuatro de la mañana cuando tomé la nitroglicerina.
    Cuando **tenía** cinco años me sacaron las amígdalas.

- The verb *ir* can indicate past intentions when used in the imperfect and combined with another verb.

  Iba a darle aspirina al niño para el dolor, pero tenía fiebre también.
  I was going to give aspirin to the child for the pain, but he had fever, too.

Un chiste

Una mujer murió y su esposo, el viudo, estaba en la funeraria con un amigo. El hombre lloraba inconsolablemente. Tenía mucha baba (mucho moco) en la barbilla. Cuando llegó otra persona su amigo le dijo, «Mira, la baba». El hombre le respondió, «Sí, lavaba y cocinaba».

HACIA PRECISIÓN

     9.16 Ejercicio _____

Complete el párrafo con la forma correcta de los verbos. Use formas del imperfecto.

Cuando yo _____ (ser) niño, mi familia _____ (vivir) en Puerto Rico. Mis abuelos _____ (vivir) con nosotros. Mi abuela _____ (saber) mucho de las plantas medicinales. Cuando yo _____ (tener) gripe, ella me _____ (hacer) té de hojas de limón y naranja. Cuando _____ (tener) gases en la barriga, me _____ (preparar) té de anís. Mis padres no me _____ (dar) remedios caseros. Ellos me _____ (llevar) a la farmacia, y el farmacéutico nos _____ (vender) un jarabe o una pastilla. No me _____ (gustar) los jarabes. _____ (preferir) las tisanas de mi abuelita.

HACIA FLUIDEZ

 9.17 Actividad _____

Con un/a compañero/a haga y conteste las siguientes preguntas. Comparta con la clase información interesante. Note que aquí vamos a practicar el registro informal (*tú*).

A. ¿Dónde vivían tus padres cuando eran niños?
B. Cuando tenías cinco años, ¿dónde vivías?
C. ¿Qué idiomas hablaban tus padres en casa?
D. ¿Qué te gustaba comer cuando eras niño/a?
E. ¿Te enfermabas mucho cuando eras niño/a?
F. ¿Ibas al doctor frecuentemente?
G. ¿Sabía tu abuela mucho de remedios caseros?
H. ¿Qué tomabas tú cuando eras niño/a y estabas resfriado/a?
I. Cuando eras estudiante, ¿te enfermabas de las enfermedades que estudiabas?

 9.18 Actividad _____

Vea las placas de caderas. Escoja una de las placas y explique la historia del paciente a la clase o a un/a compañero/a. Las siguientes preguntas son una guía.

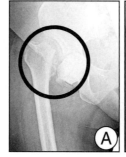 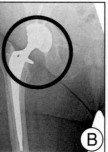 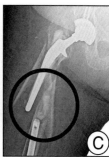

¿Dónde estaba cuando se le fracturó la cadera?
¿Qué hacía? (¿Qué estaba haciendo?)
¿Qué síntomas tenía?
¿Quién le llevó al hospital?
¿Le reemplazaron la cadera? ¿Cuándo?
Si tuvo un reemplazo, ¿qué pasó después?
¿Cuánto tiempo pasó en un centro de rehabilitación?

reemplazar to replace

Note que algunas preguntas usan el pretérito del pasado y otras usan el imperfecto.

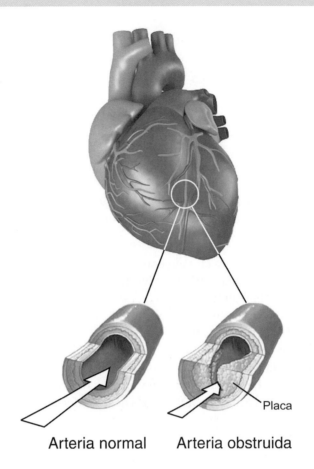

Arteria normal   Arteria obstruida

Placa

 ## Educate a Patient about Heart Disease

Vocabulario: Enfermedades del corazón

la angina de pecho (estable, inestable)	angina (stable, unstable)
la arritmia	arrhythmia
la fibrilación auricular	atrial fibrillation
la enfermedad arterial coronaria	coronary artery disease
la cardiopatía isquémica	ischemic heart disease
el infarto de miocardio	myocardial infarction
la miocarditis	miocarditis
la insuficiencia cardíaca	congestive heart failure
la valvulopatía	valve disease

Lectura: El infarto de miocardio

Los pulmones hacen posible el paso de oxígeno desde el aire a la sangre. Las arterias coronarias llevan la sangre oxigenada al corazón. Las arterias coronarias pueden tener una acumulación de colesterol que se llama placa. Si la placa interfiere con el flujo de la sangre, unas células del miocardio (el tejido muscular del corazón) pueden morir por falta de oxígeno. Esto es un infarto de miocardio. Los síntomas pueden incluir

tejido muscular
muscle tissue

- dolor del pecho
- ansiedad, palpitaciones o dificultad para respirar
- mareo, náuseas o vómitos y
- sudor excesivo

A veces el dolor del pecho corre hacia la mandíbula o hacia un brazo, típicamente el brazo izquierdo. El dolor puede ser pesado, aplastante o como un intenso ardor de indigestión. Un ataque cardíaco es una emergencia médica de vida o muerte. Veinte mil personas mueren de problemas cardíacos todos los años. El paciente que tiene cualquier síntoma de un ataque debe llamar al 911 inmediatamente para recibir una intervención rápida. En la ambulancia y/o en el centro de emergencias empiezan tratamientos de primeros auxilios y un examen físico. El tratamiento inmediato puede incluir

- administración de oxígeno
- sueros y medicamentos por vía intravenosa
- nitroglicerina y/o morfina para reducir el dolor
- aspirina u otro medicamento anticoagulante y
- electrochoque para corregir arritmias

En el hospital, mientras dan los tratamientos de primeros auxilios y hacen el examen físico, llaman a un cardiólogo. Los exámenes especializados que hacen un cardiólogo incluyen

- el angiograma coronario
- el ecocardiograma
- la prueba de esfuerzo con ejercicio
- la prueba de esfuerzo nuclear y
- la tomografía computarizada o resonancia magnética del corazón.

Para hacer el angiograma el cardiólogo inyecta un tinte especial (radioisótopos) y hace radiografías para observar el flujo de la sangre en el corazón. El ecocardiograma usa ultrasonido para tomar imágenes del corazón. La prueba de esfuerzo es para saber cómo funciona el corazón durante el ejercicio, o la tolerancia del corazón al ejercicio. Para hacer la prueba de esfuerzo nuclear, inyectan radioisótopos en la sangre para tomar imágenes del flujo de sangre. Dependiendo de los resultados, el cardiólogo o un cirujano cardiovascular puede recetarle medicamento, una dieta especial o un procedimiento o cirugía. Los tratamientos incluyen

- medicamentos anticoagulantes (para disolver el coágulo)
- una dieta saludable para el corazón
- la angioplastia
- un *stent* (por su nombre en inglés)
- la cirugía de revascularización coronaria (CABG)

estrecho/a	narrow
malla	mesh
desvío	detour

La angioplastia es un procedimiento para abrir vasos sanguíneos estrechos o bloqueados. Durante este procedimiento, el cardiólogo puede dejar un *stent,* o un pequeño tubo de malla metálica que se expande adentro de la arteria para mantenerla abierta. La cirugía de revascularización coronaria es para crear una nueva vía para llevar sangre al corazón. El cardiólogo toma una vena o arteria de otra parte del cuerpo y la usa para hacer un desvío alrededor de la parte bloqueada de la arteria. Muchas de las personas que han sufrido un ataque cardíaco participan en un programa de rehabilitación cardíaca que incluye clases, ejercicio y grupos de apoyo.

HACIA PRECISIÓN

 9.19 Ejercicio _____

Lea las pistas y definiciones más abajo y escriba las letras correspondientes al lado de la terminología indicada.

_____ grupo de apoyo   _____ *stent*

_____ placa   _____ palpitaciones

_____ malla metálica   _____ dolor pesado del pecho

_____ ecocardiograma   _____ electrocardiograma

_____ dieta saludable para el corazón

A. Es una sensación en que el corazón está latiendo muy rápido o con un ritmo irregular.
B. Es un plan de comer que usualmente está bajo en grasa.
C. Es la acumulación de colesterol en una arteria que puede reducir el flujo de sangre.

D. Varios pacientes que han sufrido problemas de salud similares se reúnen para hablar de sus experiencias, compartir sentimientos y ayudarse el uno al otro a superar (*to succeed*) emocionalmente.

E. Es la sensación de tener mucha presión en el pecho y de no poder tomar aire.

F. Es una prueba que usa ultrasonidos para dar una imagen del corazón.

G. Es un pequeño tubo de malla metálica que expande adentro de la arteria para mantener la arteria abierta.

H. Es una prueba que evalúa el ritmo y la función del corazón a través de la actividad eléctrica del corazón.

I. También se usa este material en las puertas y ventanas para evitar los mosquitos en la casa.

HACIA FLUIDEZ

 9.20 Actividad_____

Busca un/a cardiólogo/a de México en Internet. Hable en la clase sobre los detalles que él o ella publicó en su página. Por ejemplo, ¿Cómo se llama? ¿Dónde ha estudiado? ¿Dónde está su consultorio? ¿Cuáles son los días y horas de servicio? ¿Qué formas de pago acepta? ¿Acepta algún plan médico? ¿Cuáles patologías cardíacas menciona? ¿Cuáles pruebas diagnósticas ofrece? ¿Cuáles cirugías o procedimientos ofrece?

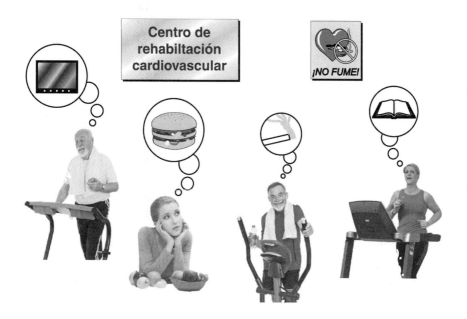

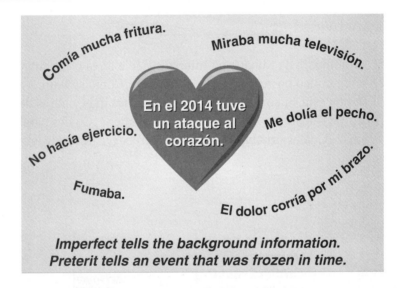

9.21 Actividad

The scene from the *Centro de rehabilitación cardiovascular* (p. 265) shows that one's actual behavior may be healthier than one's thoughts. These patients are thinking about their old habits despite their changed behavior. Hold a cardiac rehabilitation group therapy session. Use the imperfect tense to tell about your former life as a heart attack waiting to happen, the preterit tense to recount your heart attack, and the present tense to tell about your new habits. Here's an example.

> Antes, comía mucha fritura y no hacía ejercicio. En el 2014 tuve un ataque al corazón. Ahora como frutas y vegetales, voy al gimnasio todos los días y tomo una aspirina por la mañana.

Comía mucha fritura.

Miraba mucha televisión.

No hacía ejercicio.

En el 2014 tuve un ataque al corazón.

Me dolía el pecho.

Fumaba.

El dolor corría por mi brazo.

Imperfect tells the background information.
Preterit tells an event that was frozen in time.

Factores asociados con el corazón

Here are some things that may be associated with heart health, either for good or for bad.

tener sobrepeso, estar obeso/a	bajar de peso
comer más frutas y verduras	hacer ejercicio regularmente
dejar de fumar	tomar una aspirina todos los días
controlar la diabetes	controlar la hipertensión
comer fritura, comer dulces	cocinar con mucha sal
quitar la grasa de la carne	lidiar (*cope*) con el estrés
mirar mucha televisión	pasar mucho tiempo en el sofá

9.22 Drama improvisado_____

Create a meeting of a self-help group like Alcoholics Anonymous or Weight Watchers. Use discretion, as you'll not know who may be a member in real life. Use the imperfect tense to tell what your life was like before you made a commitment to solving your problem, the preterit tense to say what happened to change your ways, and the present tense to describe your current behavior. Here is an example.

> Mi nombre es Bárbara y soy alcohólica. Antes, bebía todas las noches y trasnochaba. No llegaba a mi casa hasta las cuatro de la mañana. No podía levantarme temprano para ir a trabajar. En el 2006 me enfermé de la diabetes y dejé de beber. Ahora voy a las reuniones de Alcohólicos Anónimos, paso más tiempo en la casa con mi familia y bebo café negro sin azúcar.

Factores asociados con el alcoholismo

Here is a word bank to facilitate your communication if you choose alcoholism as the problem. You have already learned vocabulary related to a healthy diet, exercise, and weight control in previous chapters.

trasnochar	to stay up all night
estar ebrio/a	to be intoxicated
estar borracho/a	to be drunk
manejar ebrio/a	to drive while intoxicated
sobrio/a	sober
pelear	to argue, fight
pasar tiempo en los bares	to spend time in bars
malgastar dinero	to spend money unwisely
dejar de beber	to give up drinking

HACIA FLUIDEZ

 9.23 Reciclaje __ _____

Observe las imágenes de la «Visita al doctor». Usted es la paciente. Use el vocabulario del examen físico y la gramática del tiempo pasado para decirle a un amigo qué pasó en su visita al doctor. Si necesita ideas, estas preguntas le van a ayudar.

¿Por qué fue usted al consultorio?   ¿Le tomó la temperatura?
¿Qué síntomas tenía usted?   ¿Cómo estuvo su presión arterial?

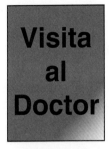
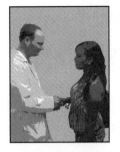
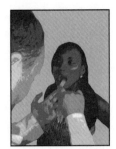

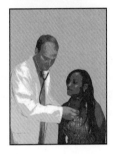
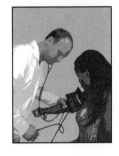
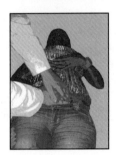

¿Le miró los oídos?   ¿Le escuchó el intestino?
¿Le percutió el pecho?   ¿Qué fue el diagnóstico?
¿Qué parte del cuerpo le palpó? ¿Le recetó un medicamento?

 Exposición

 CHAPTER 9 SKILL: NARRATING IN THE PAST

You are going to listen to a patient tell about a recent injury and then write your
own narration that tells about a different injury that happened in the past.

1. Use the chart that follows to organize the information that you hear. Write
    down the specific information in Spanish, and indicate by drawing a circle
    to show whether the preterit tense (P) or imperfect tense (I) was used when
    providing the information. **OJO:** The information you hear may not follow the
    order shown in the chart.

P I ¿Cuándo fue?	P I ¿Qué tipo de accidente fue?
P I ¿Dónde estaba?	P I ¿Qué hacía?
P I ¿Qué pasó?	P I ¿Qué pasó después?
P I ¿Cuál fue el diagnóstico?	P I ¿Cuál fue el tratamiento?

2. Now decide what injury you want to describe. Jot down notes about that injury, answering the questions from the chart.
3. Write your narration, using forms of the preterit and imperfect as needed. Remember that you will use preterit forms to describe completed actions and imperfect forms to talk about background information or ongoing and habitual actions in the past.
4. Present your narration to the class.

Cultural Note: *Remedios caseros*

A grandes males, grandes remedios
(Big problems call for big solutions)

Pythagoras said, "Before calling the doctor, call a friend." A Latino might advise, *Antes de llamar al médico llame a la abuelita o al farmacéutico.* Not long ago, one's *abuela* was the first line of medical defense. She always knew what *remedio casero,* or home remedy, to recommend. When Abuela's *tisana* (botanical infusion) did not work, then the family would consult with the pharmacist, who might have recommended and sold a drug that in many countries would require a doctor's prescription. If that did not work, the family would consult a physician. This particular pathway may have sprung from tradition, finances, or the availability of a health care provider.

In most of the Spanish-speaking world, herbal remedies are available at open-air markets, neighborhood grocers, and botanical shops (*botánicas*), although travelers may bring remedies when returning from abroad. Dried plants pass customs in a way that live plants with soil do not. The U.S. Food and Drug Administration does not regulate herbal remedies. Although a remedy that is made from a fresh or dried plant is commonly referred to as *un té,* this is a generalization of "tea," which is the name of a more specific group of plants. The proper name for such remedies is *una tisana* or *una infusión.*

The dawning of the age of antibiotics and the widespread use of medications that either block or enhance (agonize) neurotransmitters led many to attribute illness to microbes or chemical imbalances. Another worldview attributes illness to an imbalance in the body or spirit. Forces that may be out of balance have been described as yin and yang and hot and cold among others. Many Latinos think of certain botanical remedies as being *hot* and others as *cold.* These are general terms that include a small percentage of

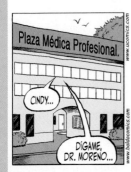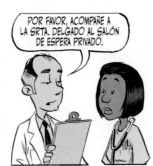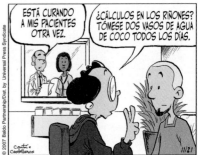

botanical remedies. "Hot" remedies include ginger, cinnamon, rosemary, and citrus leaves (*jengibre, canela, romero y hojas de los árboles cítricos*) and help restore balance when we suffer from "cold" disorders such as a cold or a depressed affect. "Cold" remedies include anise, chamomile, linden flower, and oregano (*anís, manzanilla, flor de tilo y orégano*) and help restore balance when we suffer from "hot" disorders such as dyspepsia, "nerves," or insomnia.

In general, many home remedies are effective either for their own medicinal properties, for their placebo effect, for the comfort they conjure, or a combination of these. However, when there is a more effective agent available, the use of a home remedy may delay medical care at the patient's peril. Although phytotherapy is generally considered safe and effective, it may be helpful to know what a patient is taking and to review a list of contraindications or possible herb-drug interactions. Interactions may include the capacity of the herb to slow the absorption of a drug (suspected of fibrous herbs such as psyllium), to affect the drug's elimination, to synergize its effect, or to add to its hepatotoxicity. For example, *sábila* (aloe vera) and *nopal* (prickly pear cactus) may synergize other antihyperglycemic agents.

The availability of antibiotics without a prescription in Latin America and other areas of the world may have contributed to the emergence of antibiotic-resistant microbes. An antibiotic that loses its efficacy may have to be taken off the market for as long as 45 years prior to regaining its effectiveness. In 2010 Mexico banned the sale of antibiotics and antiviral drugs without a doctor's prescription. To adjust to this, larger pharmacies have employed physicians who offer free consultations at the pharmacy. These consultations are not usually informed by laboratory and other tests, but the measure is intended to prolong the efficacy of antibiotics.

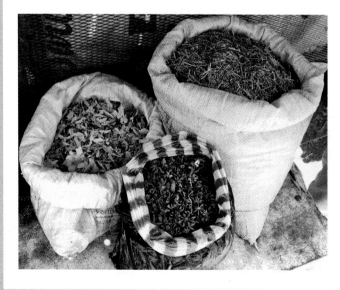

Flor de tilo (izquierda, para dormir), manzanilla (derecha, para los nervios) y anís (centro, para el estómago)

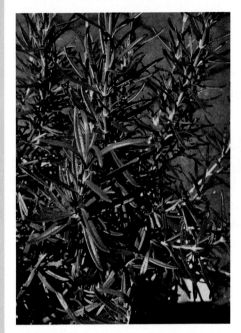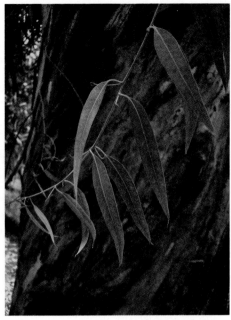

El romero (izquierda) alivia problemas calientes. El eucalipto (derecha) puede tener efectos mucolíticos. El aceite de eucalipto puede ser tóxico cuando no está diluido.

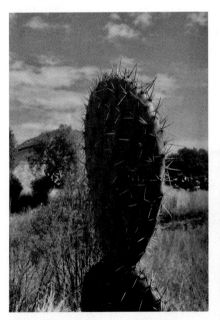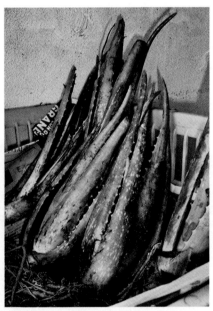

El nopal (izquierda) y la sábila (derecha) pueden tener efectos antihiperglucémicos y aumentar los efectos de medicamentos que bajan la glucosa.

Vocabulario del capítulo 9

Tiempos pasados

esta mañana	this morning
hoy	today
anoche	last night
ayer	yesterday
anteayer	the day before yesterday
el jueves pasado	last Thursday
la semana pasada	last week
el mes pasado	last month
el año pasado	last year

Antes de la cirugía

¿Cuándo fue la última vez que . . . ?	When was the last time that . . . ?
usar alcohol o drogas	to use alcohol or drugs
orinar	to urinate
evacuar, defecar	to move one's bowels
menstruar	to menstruate
empezar su período	to start your menses
beber algo	to drink something
comer algo	to eat something
¿Tiene/Usa usted . . . ?	Do you have / Do you use . . . ?
una peluca	a wig
un diente flojo	a loose tooth
un prótesis	a prosthesis
una dentadura postiza	dentures
lentes o lentes de contacto	glasses or contact lenses
problemas con el corazón	heart problems
problemas con los pulmones	lung problems

Palabras tranquilizadoras

Todo va a estar bien.	Everything is going to be fine.
Por favor, cálmese.	Please calm down.
No tenga miedo.	Don't be afraid.
Tenga confianza.	Have trust.
No se preocupe.	Don't worry (formal).
No te preocupes.	Don't worry (informal).
No va a doler.	It's not going to hurt.
Va a mejorar.	It's going to get better.
Hay que seguir adelante.	One must go on.

Enfermedades del corazón

la angina de pecho (estable, inestable)	angina (stable, unstable)
la arritmia	arrhythmia
la fibrilación auricular	atrial fibrillation
la enfermedad arterial coronaria	coronary artery disease
la cardiopatía isquémica	ischemic heart disease
el infarto de miocardio	myocardial infarction
la miocarditis	miocarditis
la insuficiencia cardíaca	congestive heart failure
la valvulopatía	valve disease

Factores asociados con el corazón

tener sobrepeso, estar obeso/a	bajar de peso
comer más frutas y verduras	hacer ejercicio regularmente
dejar de fumar	tomar una aspirina todos los días
controlar la diabetes	controlar la hipertensión
comer fritura, comer dulces	cocinar con mucha sal
quitar la grasa de la carne	lidiar con el estrés
mirar mucha televisión	pasar mucho tiempo en el sofá

Factores asociados con el alcoholismo

trasnochar	to stay up all night
estar ebrio/a	to be intoxicated
estar borracho/a	to be drunk
manejar ebrio/a	to drive while intoxicated
sobrio/a	sober
pelear	to argue, fight
pasar tiempo en los bares	to spend time in bars
malgastar dinero	to spend money unwisely
dejar de beber	to give up drinking

Preguntas útiles

¿Cuándo comenzó su último período?

¿Está usted alérgico/a a algún medicamento?

¿Cuándo fue la última vez que usted / el niño evacuó?

Chapter 10

Padecimientos e historia médica

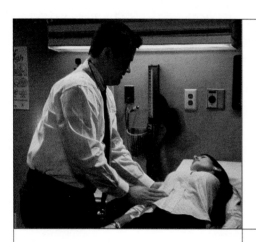

Communication Goals

Vocabulary

Structure

Cultural Note

Website   www.yalebooks.com/medicalspanish

Video   *Trama: La colecistitis; Demostración: La sonografía*

Audio   *Padecimientos y la historia abreviada; El cáncer; Exposición*

Electronic Workbook

B y the end of this chapter you will know how to ask about medical history, including illnesses, surgeries, and immunizations. You will learn the names of internal organs, to talk about illnesses and diseases, and to prepare patients for various surgeries.

Ask about Current Medical Conditions

The vocabulary in this chapter is organized in the order that the words might appear during a history and physical exam. Beginning with an abbreviated history, we proceed to illnesses organized by a review of systems, and a list of tropical and infectious diseases. Then we provide additional lexicon and more elaborate practice on cancer, tuberculosis, tropical diseases, and pandemic flu. Let's begin with the abbreviated history, because some practitioners consider these diseases to be too dangerous to miss.

padecimiento
malady, chronic
condition

Vocabulario: Padecimientos y la historia abreviada

La cabeza

la epilepsia	epilepsy
la convulsión, el ataque epiléptico	convulsion, seizure
el golpe en la cabeza	closed head injury
la amnesia	amnesia
la concusión	concussion
la pérdida de conocimiento	loss of consciousness

La enfermedad cardiovascular

la angina de pecho	angina pectoris
el ataque al corazón	heart attack
el infarto cardíaco, el infarto de miocardio	coronary infarction
la trombosis cardíaca	coronary thrombosis
la hipertensión, la presión alta	hypertension
la insuficiencia cardíaca	congestive heart failure

Otros padecimientos

el asma	asthma
el cáncer	cancer
la diabetes	diabetes
la hepatitis	hepatitis
la ictericia, la piel amarillenta	jaundice, yellowish skin
los ojos amarillentos	yellowish eyes
problemas de los riñones	kidney problems
la insuficiencia renal	kidney failure
. . . aguda, crónica	. . . acute, chronic
la fiebre reumática	rheumatic fever
la tuberculosis	tuberculosis

Preguntas útiles

¿Padece del corazón?	Do you have heart problems?
¿Padece de los riñones?	Do you have kidney problems?
¿Ha tenido problemas con el hígado?	Have you had liver problems?
¿Tuvo alguna vez un golpe en la cabeza?	Have you had a head injury?

 Estructura: El verbo *padecer*

- The verb *padecer* means "to suffer from," and is used to speak of illnesses or conditions from which the patient suffers. In the present indicative tense *padecer* is irregular in only the first person singular (*yo*). It is used with the preposition *de.*
- These are the forms of the verb *padecer* in the present tense.

yo	**Padezco** de leucemia.
tú	**¿Padeces** de diabetes?
él, ella, usted	¿De qué **padece** usted?
nosotros/as	Mi hermano y yo **padecemos** de asma.
ellos, ellas, ustedes	Mis padres **padecen** del corazón.

- *Sufrir* can also be used to identify current medical conditions. Like *padecer,* it is used with the preposition *de. Sufrir* is a regular verb ending in *-ir.*

  —¿Sufre de alguna enfermedad o problema médico?
  —Hace cinco años que sufro de artritis reumatoide.

HACIA PRECISIÓN

 10.1 Ejercicio _____

Haga oraciones completas usando sujetos de la columna «A», la forma correcta del verbo *sufrir* o *padecer* y complementos de la columna «B».

Modelo: los niños / asma
—Los niños padecen de asma. Los niños sufren de asma.

A	B	
los niños	artritis	_____.
los pacientes	asma	_____.
la paciente	angina	_____.
mis padres	anemia	_____.
mi hijo	diabetes	_____.
yo	enfisema	_____.
Roselín y Ashley	hepatitis C	_____.
usted	cólera	_____.
mi hermana y yo	cataratas	_____.

 10.2 Ejercicio _____

Seleccione las palabras entre paréntesis que mejor completen las oraciones.

A. La tuberculosis del pulmón es (un virus, una bacteria).
B. La piel amarillenta es un síntoma de (hepatitis, tuberculosis).
C. Los pacientes que sufren de (asma, epilepsia) tienen convulsiones.
D. Los pacientes con hiperglucemia padecen de (diabetes, angina de pecho).
E. Los tobillos hinchados son un síntoma de (diabetes, insuficiencia cardíaca).
F. Si un tumor es (benigno, maligno), el paciente tiene cáncer.
G. La fatiga, o la falta de aire, es un síntoma de (asma, epilepsia).
H. Un análisis del esputo (*sputum*) puede confirmar un diagnóstico de (angina, tuberculosis).
I. La causa principal de la enfermedad valvular del corazón es (la fiebre reumática, el infarto cardíaco).

Vocabulario: Padecimientos y el repaso de sistemas

Learning new words involves using them and elaborating on them. An additional way to aid the process of memorization is to organize the information to be memorized. Some well-known methods suggest using "pegs" such as categories to organize the list to be memorized. For this we'll use the review of systems that is often used in a history and physical exam. We won't necessarily repeat the medical conditions that were part of the abbreviated history, above.

El sistema neurológico

la espina bífida	spina bifida
la hemorragia cerebral, el derrame*	hemorrhage
el infarto cerebral	cerebral infarct
la jaqueca, la migraña	migraine
la parálisis cerebral	cerebral palsy
el tumor cerebral	brain tumor

El sistema respiratorio

la amigdalitis**	tonsillitis
la bronquitis crónica	chronic bronchitis
la enfermedad pulmonar obstructiva crónica (EPOC)	COPD
el enfisema	emphysema
la pulmonía, la neumonía	pneumonia
la tuberculosis	tuberculosis

El sistema cardiovascular

el aneurisma	aneurysm
las hemorroides	hemorrhoids
la hipercolesterolemia	hypercholesterolemia
la hiperlipidemia	hyperlipidemia
la hipertensión, la hipotensión	hypertension, hypotension
el soplo cardíaco	heart murmur

Derrame refers to a leak or overflow. It is not a medical term, but may be used for hemorrhage.

**Here *amígdala* refers to "tonsil" and other organs formed by the union of various lymph nodes, and not the "amygdala" (*amígdala cerebral*) that is a structure in the brain.

El sistema gastrointestinal

el cálculo biliar (la piedra biliar)	gallstone
la cirrosis hepática	cirrhosis of the liver
el cólico, el empacho*	colic, indigestion
el pólipo	polyp
el reflujo esofágico, la acidez	esophageal reflux
la úlcera	ulcer

El sistema genitourinario

el agrandamiento de la próstata	BPH
el cálculo (las piedras) en el riñón	renal calculus (stones)
la endometriosis	endometriosis
la infección del aparato urinario	urinary tract infection
la nefritis	nephritis

El sistema endocrinológico

la hiperglucemia, la hipoglucemia	hyperglycemia, hypoglycemia
el hipertiroidismo, el hipotiroidismo	hyperthyroidism, hypothyroidism
la obesidad	obesity

El sistema esqueleto muscular

la artritis reumatoide	rheumatoid arthritis
la distrofia muscular	muscular dystrophy
la esclerosis múltiple	multiple sclerosis
la ciática	sciatica
la osteoporosis	osteoporosis

La piel

la catarata	cataract
el eccema	eczema
la irritación del pañal	diaper rash
la melanoma	melanoma
los piojos	head lice
la psoriasis	psoriasis
la sarna	scabies

*A folk explanation attributes *empacho* to food sticking to the walls of the intestine. A parent may report, *El niño está empachado,* and pinch and pull at the abdomen to help "dislodge" the food.

Problemas de la sangre

la anemia	anemia
la hemofilia	hemophilia
la leucemia	leukemia
el linfoma	lymphoma
la anemia drepanocítica	sickle cell anemia

HACIA FLUIDEZ

 10.3 Actividad _____

Esta actividad se juega similar al *Jeopardy*. Diga en voz alta una definición o una pista (*clue*) para una de las enfermedades. La clase debe adivinar (*guess*) la enfermedad de la lista de vocabulario.

Modelo: Es una inflamación del hígado [definición].
  —¿Qué es la hepatitis?
  Un tratamiento común es ponerse nitroglicerina debajo de la lengua [pista].
  —¿Qué es la angina de pecho?
  Uno en quinientos africano-americanos la tiene [pista].
  —¿Qué es la anemia drepanocítica?

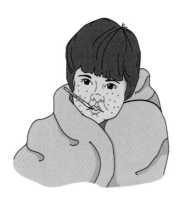

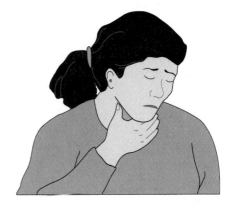

el sarampión   la paperas

Vocabulario: Las enfermedades infecciosas y tropicales

Where you want a more complete history-taking interview, you may ask about some of the following diseases. Venereal infectious diseases are included in chapter 12.

el cólera	cholera
la conjuntivitis	conjunctivitis
la culebrilla	herpes zoster, shingles
la difteria	diphtheria
la disentería	dysentery
el ébola	ebola
el estafilococo dorado	MRSA, golden staph
la fiebre tifoidea	typhoid fever
el pian, la frambuesa*	yaws
la leptospirosis	leptospirosis
la meningitis	meningitis
la mononucleosis	mononucleosis
la paperas	mumps
la rubéola	rubella (German measles)
el sarampión	rubeola, measles
el tétano, el tétanos	tetanus
la tos ferina	pertussis, whooping cough
la varicela, las viruelas locas	chicken pox

Los flavivirus

el chikungunya	chikungunya
el dengue (clásico, hemorrágico)	dengue (classic, hemorrhagic)
la fiebre amarilla	yellow fever
el zika	zika

Los parásitos

la enfermedad de Chaga	Chaga's disease
la infección por giardias	giaradiasis
las lombrices	(intestinal) worms
el paludismo, la malaria	malaria
la teniasis, la infección por tenia	tapeworm
la toxoplasmosis	toxoplasmosis

*Yaws is a non-venereal form of syphilis that is present in the Americas and can cause a VDRL test to be positive, although more specific tests result in less false positives.

HACIA PRECISIÓN

 10.4 Ejercicio _____

Usar el vocabulario en varios contextos le ayuda con la memorización. Use el vocabulario nuevo de enfermedades infecciosas y tropicales para contestar las siguientes preguntas.

A. ¿Cuáles son algunas enfermedades que están causadas por un virus?
B. ¿Cuáles son algunas enfermedades bacterianas?
C. ¿Para cuáles enfermedades hay vacuna?
D. ¿Cuáles se mejoran con los antibióticos?
E. ¿Cuáles están causadas por comida infectada?
F. ¿Cuáles enfermedades afectan el sistema neurológico?
G. ¿Cuáles son las enfermedades más comunes en el área donde usted trabaja?
H. ¿Cuáles eran más frecuentes en los niños que nacieron antes del 1956?
I. ¿Cuáles pueden ser transmitidas por vectores, como los mosquitos?
J. ¿Cuál puede ser transmitida por las heces de un gato (*cat*) infectado?
K. ¿Cuál es una bacteria anaeróbica que se puede prevenir con una vacuna cada diez años?

Lectura: El estafilococo dorado (*MRSA*)

Muchas personas saludables tienen la bacteria estafilococo dorado en la piel. En algunos casos la bacteria entra en el cuerpo y causa una infección en la sangre o una pulmonía. La meticilina es un antibiótico muy efectivo contra el estafilococo, pero algunos estafilococos son resistentes a la meticilina. Estos se llaman *estafilococo dorado* o *estafilococo resistente a la meticilina*. También se llama *MRSA* por su nombre en inglés.

Estas infecciones son más comunes en los hospitales que en la comunidad. Una infección adquirida (*acquired*) en el hospital se llama *una infección nosocomial*. Para prevenir la infección es importante lavarse las manos. También es importante practicar las precauciones universales, no compartir toallas, lavar bien las sábanas y siempre cubrir las cortadas con un vendaje o una tirita (*bandage*).

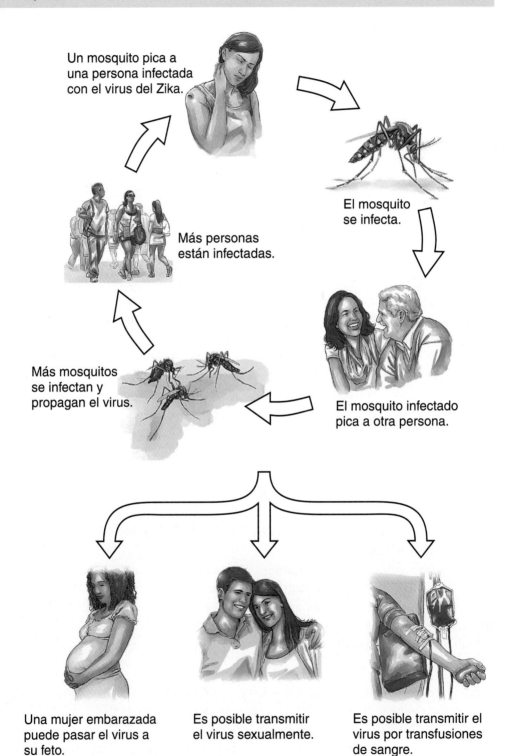

Un mosquito pica a una persona infectada con el virus del Zika.

El mosquito se infecta.

Más personas están infectadas.

Más mosquitos se infectan y propagan el virus.

El mosquito infectado pica a otra persona.

Una mujer embarazada puede pasar el virus a su feto.

Es posible transmitir el virus sexualmente.

Es posible transmitir el virus por transfusiones de sangre.

Lectura: El zika, el dengue y el chikungunya

Hay tres virus que son problemas importantes de salud pública en Latinoamérica. Son el dengue, el chikungunya y el zika. Son de la misma familia del virus de la fiebre amarilla (el género *Flavivirus*). Son originalmente de África y periódicamente provocan brotes, o epidemias, en otras regiones tropicales.

brote	outbreak
picadura	bite
sarpullido	rash
plaqueta	platelet

Estos tres virus se transmiten por vectores, principalmente la especie *Aedes* de mosquitos. Los virus se transmiten de persona infectada a mosquito y de mosquito infectado a persona. Los síntomas empiezan de dos a siete días después de la picadura del mosquito y pueden durar hasta diez días. Una de cada cuatro personas infectadas con el zika no tiene síntomas.

Los síntomas más frecuentes de las tres enfermedades incluyen fiebre, dolores de cabeza y dolores en los huesos, los músculos y las articulaciones. Otros síntomas incluyen nauseas, conjuntivitis y sarpullido. Las fiebres del zika y del dengue son más leves que la fiebre del chikungunya pero pueden durar más tiempo. Los síntomas hemorrágicos como la conjuntivitis son mas comunes en el dengue y el zika. (Típicamente las plaquetas solo bajan con el dengue.) El intenso dolor de las articulaciones es un síntoma más típico del chikungunya. En las personas mayores de edad los dolores en las articulaciones pueden durar más tiempo y pueden ser crónicos.

El zika presenta menos hospitalizaciones que el dengue y el chikungunya. El peligro principal del zika es para las mujeres embarazadas. Una mujer embarazada que tiene zika puede tener un aborto espontáneo o puede transmitir el virus al feto a través de la placenta. Los bebés de madres infectadas con zika pueden nacer con microcefalia. El zika también puede provocar el síndrome de Guillain-Barré si el virus coloniza los nervios. Es poco frecuente, pero el zika puede ser transmitido por vía sanguínea, y una persona infectada puede infectar con virus a otra persona a través del sexo vaginal, anal u oral.

Hasta el momento no hay medicamento para prevenir o curar estos virus. Se puede tomar acetaminofén para la fiebre y el dolor, pero el tratamiento con aspirina y otros antiinflamatorios no esteroideos está contraindicado por el riesgo del síndrome hemorrágico. Se puede aliviar las erupciones con antihistamínicos. También el paciente debe descansar y consumir líquidos.

criadero	breeding area
estancado	stagnant
llanta	tire
permetrina	permethrin
manga	sleeve

Sin vacuna la única prevención es controlar los criaderos de mosquitos y prevenir sus picaduras. Para controlar los criaderos de mosquitos, se debe evitar el agua estancada en objetos como tanques, llantas y otros recipientes. Para prevenir las picaduras se debe aplicar permetrina a la ropa, usar mosquiteros, usar camisas con mangas largas y pantalones largos y ponerse un repelente en la piel.

Lectura: La leptospirosis

La leptospirosis es una infección grave y contagiosa causada por la bacteria *leptospira.* No es muy común en los Estados Unidos, aunque hay casos recientes de perros (*dogs*) infectados y trasmisión de perro a persona. Hay más casos en lugares tropicales. Ocurre cuando el agua o la comida está contaminada con orina o heces de ratas, ratones u

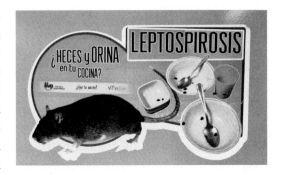

otros animales. Los síntomas incluyen fiebre, fotofobia, dolor de cabeza, de abdomen y de las piernas y los ojos amarillentos. El tratamiento normalmente incluye tomar penicilinas, tetraciclinas, cloramfenicol o eritromicina. Las medidas de prevención incluyen:

- Vacunar a los animales domésticos.
- Eliminar las ratas y los lugares donde se reproducen.
- Lavar los platos, vasos y otros utensilios de cocina antes de usarlos.
- Lavar las latas (*cans*) de comida antes de abrirlas o consumir la comida.

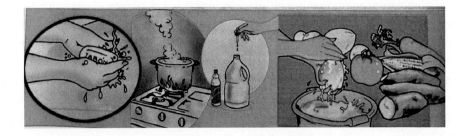

Lectura: El cólera

El cólera es una enfermedad intestinal infecciosa causada por una bacteria. Se transmite cuando se toma agua o comida contaminada con heces fecales. El síntoma principal del cólera es diarrea aguda. Otros síntomas incluyen vómito y calambres severos en el estómago. El cólera normalmente tiene una tasa de mortalidad (*mortality rate*) de un 1 por ciento. Para prevenir el cólera debe lavarse bien las manos con agua y jabón después de evacuar y orinar y antes de preparar comida y comer. Debe cocinar bien los alimentos y no comer los vegetales crudos. Es importante lavar las verduras y las frutas en agua purificada. Para purificar el agua debe

hervir   to boil
hervida   boiled

hervirla por un minuto. Si no es posible hervir el agua, media cucharadita de cloro (Clorox) descontamina cinco galones de agua en treinta minutos.

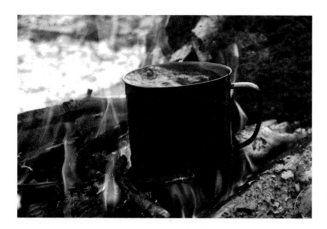

Para purificar el agua, hiérvala por un minuto.

Algunos antibióticos ayudan. Estos incluyen tetraciclina, eritromicina, trimeto-prima, doxiciclina y ciprofloxacina. El tratamiento más importante es la rehidratación por vía oral. Cuando una persona tiene diarrea o vómitos, es urgente beber muchos líquidos para evitar la deshidratación. Tome las bebidas que normalmente toma. También las farmacias venden bebidas de rehidratación.

Para hacer una bebida de rehidratación donde no la puede comprar, use un litro de agua purificada y agregue una cucharadita—o menos—de sal (sal de mesa) y ocho cucharaditas de azúcar. Esta sal de rehidratación oral (SRO) reduce la necesidad de administrar líquidos intravenosos. Es importante no usar más de una cucharadita de sal por litro, porque cuando se incrementa la osmolaridad de la solución también incrementa los efectos adversos de la hipernatremia, como vómitos.

El jugo de fruta y la banana contienen potasio, un mineral que ayuda a combatir la deshidratación. Los adultos deben tomar tres o más litros de líquido diario. Los niños deben tomar un litro o más diario.

HACIA FLUIDEZ

 Actividad 10.5 _____

Con un/a compañero/a, conteste las siguientes preguntas sobre el zika, el dengue y el chikungunya.

    A. ¿Son efectivos los antibióticos en casos de leptospirosis?
    B. ¿Cómo se llaman las infecciones adquiridas en un hospital o una clínica?
    C. ¿Cómo se puede prevenir una infección?
    D. Si el zika resulta en menos hospitalizaciones, ¿cuál es su peligro principal?
    E. ¿Cuál es la tasa de mortalidad del cólera?
    F. ¿Qué podemos hacer para evitar las enfermedades transmitidas por mosquitos?

G. ¿Por qué no debe tomar antiinflamatorios no esteroideos para aliviar el dolor del dengue?

H. ¿Qué puede resultar si el virus de zika coloniza los nervios?

I. ¿Cuál de los virus baja las plaquetas?

J. Dicen que una onza de prevención vale más de una libra de cura. ¿Por qué es verdad en el caso de zika?

 Actividad 10.6

Usted tiene un/a amigo/a que va de voluntario a un país donde hay un brote de cólera. Su amigo/a tiene varias preguntas. Prepare una conversación para presentar a la clase. Algunas preguntas incluyen por ejemplo:

¿Qué es el cólera?
Si me enfermo de cólera, ¿voy a morir?
¿Es posible prevenir el cólera?
¿Cómo se previene el cólera?
¿Cuál es el tratamiento más importante?
¿Qué hago si no hay farmacia o si la farmacia no tiene bebidas de rehidratación?

 ## Educate a Patient about Cancer

Vocabulario: El cáncer

el auto examen	self-exam
benigno/a	benign
la biopsia	biopsy
el cáncer de pulmón	lung cancer
el cansancio	fatigue
la cirugía	surgery
maligno/a	malignant
la metástasis	metastasis
la pérdida de cabello	hair loss
la quimioterapia	chemotherapy
la radioterapia	radiation therapy
el sistema linfático	the lymph system
tumor	tumor

Preguntas útiles

¿Ha tenido cáncer?
¿Hay [historia de] cáncer en la familia?

 ## Lectura: El cáncer

El cuerpo humano es un organismo dinámico. Nuevas **células** forman y células viejas mueren. En algunos casos, el cuerpo forma células nuevas y las células viejas no mueren. Las células adicionales a ve-

> Boldfaced words are new. Find them in the vocabulary list.

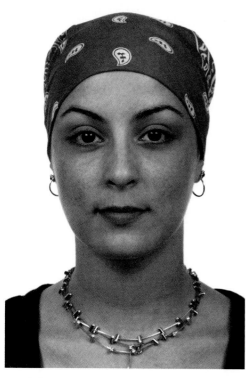

La pérdida de cabello es un posible efecto secundario de la quimioterapia.

ces forman un **tumor**. Cuando hay un tumor, un oncólogo saca unas células para hacer una **biopsia**. Si la biopsia es negativa, el tumor es **benigno** y no es cáncer. Si la biopsia es positiva, el tumor es **maligno** y es cáncer.

Usualmente el nombre de un cáncer específico depende de la parte del cuerpo afectada. Algunos ejemplos son, cáncer del pulmón, cáncer de la próstata y cáncer del cerebro. Si el cáncer de una parte del cuerpo afecta la sangre, el **sistema linfático** u otras partes del cuerpo, se llama la **metástasis**.

Los tratamientos para el cáncer son la **cirugía**, la radioterapia y la quimioterapia. La cirugía es para sacar un tumor maligno. La **radioterapia** usa radiación para destruir células cancerosas. La **quimioterapia** usa medicamentos para destruir células cancerosas. Los tratamientos destruyen células benignas también, pero el cuerpo forma nuevas células. Otros efectos secundarios son **cansancio**, náusea, vómitos, diarrea, estreñimiento y **pérdida de cabello**.

Para prevenir el cáncer, debe decirle a su médico si tiene una historia familiar de cáncer. No fume. No coma carne roja más de dos veces a la semana. Debe comer una dieta balanceada y hacer ejercicio regularmente. Aprenda a hacer el **auto examen** de los senos o los testículos. Dile a su doctor si algo es irregular.

HACIA FLUIDEZ

 10.7 Actividad _____

Con un/a compañero/a, conteste las siguientes preguntas.

A. ¿Cuál es el nombre de la especialidad médica asociada con el cáncer?
B. Cuando hay cáncer en la garganta, ¿cómo se llama el cáncer?
C. ¿Qué es un tumor? ¿Son malignos todos los tumores?
D. ¿Qué hace un oncólogo para saber si un tumor es maligno?
E. ¿Hay tratamientos para el cáncer? ¿Cuáles son?
F. ¿Tienen efectos secundarios los tratamientos para el cáncer?
G. ¿Cómo se previene el cáncer?
H. ¿Cuáles son los cánceres que el uso de tabaco puede causar?
I. ¿Qué es un auto examen de los senos? ¿Quién lo hace y para qué?

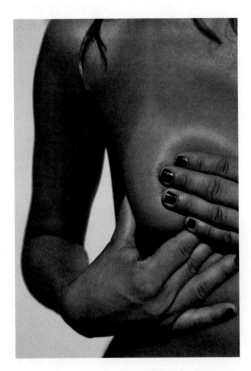

El auto examen de los senos

Ask about Medical History

 ## Estructura: El pretérito perfecto (*The Present Perfect Tense*)

- Use the present perfect tense to speak about a past action that continues to affect the present. As in English, use the auxiliary verb "to have" (*haber*) and the past participle of the verb representing the past experience. To form the past participle of -*ar* verbs, add -*ado* to the stem. To form the participle of -*er* and -*ir* verbs, add -*ido* to the stem.

He consultado con un oncólogo.	I have consulted with an oncologist.
¿Has tenido varicela?	Have you had chicken pox?
¿Ha tenido alguna cirugía?	Have you ever had surgery?
Hemos llamado a la doctora.	We have called the doctor.
¿Han leído la radiografía?	Have they read the x-ray?

- This tense is especially helpful during medical history-taking interviews, both for asking general questions and for asking about specific illnesses.

  ¿De qué enfermedades **ha sufrido** usted?
  ¿Cuáles enfermedades **ha tenido** usted?
  ¿**Ha padecido** usted de paludismo?

- The patient may respond using the present perfect, but it is likely that he or she will use the preterit form of the verb *tener* to specify when something occurred.

He tenido varicela.	I have had chicken pox.
Tuve paperas cuando era niño.	I had mumps when I was a child.

- Recall that in chapter 3 we used the past participle as an adjective with the verb *estar* to say, *El tobillo está hinchado* and *La lengua está hinchada.* When used as an adjective, the past participle must agree with the noun in number and gender. In the present perfect tense (with the verb *haber*), it is not used as an adjective, so it always ends in -*o*.

- The following verbs have irregular past participles. You are already familiar with *muerto* and *roto*.

Infinitivo	*Participio*	*Ejemplo*
decir	dicho	Yo le **he dicho** que sí.
escribir	escrito	¿**Ha escrito** sus medicamentos en un papel?
hacer	hecho	**He hecho** planes para la cirugía.
morir	muerto	Dos de mis tíos **han muerto** del corazón.
ver	visto	No **he visto** a la doctora.
romper	roto	¿Se **ha roto** usted un hueso?
poner	puesto	No me **han puesto** el suero.

Un chiste

Profesor: —¿Se escribe *dormido* o *durmido?*
Estudiante: —Se escribe despierto (*awake*).

HACIA PRECISIÓN

 10.8 Ejercicio _____

Complete las oraciones con el presente perfecto de los verbos entre paréntesis para identificar las acciones o experiencias de las personas indicadas.

A. Mi hermano _____ _____ (tener) piojos.

B. Yo _____ _____ (sufrir) de bronquitis crónica.

C. ¿_____ _____ (poner) tú la vacuna de la hepatitis B?

D. Mis padres _____ _____ (comprar) sus medicamentos.

E. Mi hermano y yo _____ _____ (consultar) con un urólogo.

F. El doctor me _____ _____ (hacer) el examen rectal digital de la próstata.

HACIA FLUIDEZ

 10.9 Actividad _____

Circule en la clase para hacer una encuesta. Pregúnteles a sus compañeros si han tenido las siguientes enfermedades. Por ejemplo, pregunte ¿*Ha tenido la conjuntivitis?* y la otra persona contesta, *Sí, he tenido la conjuntivitis* (o) *No, no he tenido la conjuntivitis.* Anote las respuestas. Después comparta sus resultados con la clase.

Enfermedades	Nombres de compañeros	
conjuntivitis	_____	_____
paludismo	_____	_____
jaquecas	_____	_____
paperas	_____	_____
varicela	_____	_____
amigdalitis	_____	_____
una gripe mala	_____	_____

 10.10 Actividad _____

Con un/a compañero/a, practique una entrevista para tomar la historia médica. Primero, pregúntele al / a la paciente de cuáles enfermedades ha padecido. Después busque más detalles, por ejemplo su edad y dónde vivía cuando se enfermó y si fue hospitalizado.

Modelo: ¿Ha estado hospitalizado alguna vez?
¿De qué enfermedades ha padecido?
¿Ha tenido varicela?
¿Cuántos años tenía cuando tuvo varicela?
¿Dónde vivía en ese tiempo?

> Notice the imperfect tense with *tener* to express age and with *vivir* when not frozen in time.

 10.11 Actividad _____

Con un/a compañero/a prepare una entrevista para exponer a la clase. Usted es pediatra y su compañero/a es madre o padre de un niño que es un paciente nuevo de la clínica. Pregúntele al padre o a la madre sobre la historia médica de su hijo. El padre o madre contesta ad lib.

Modelo: —¿De qué enfermedades ha padecido el niño?
—Tuvo varicela el año pasado.

 10.12 Drama improvisado _____

Play the game "*afortunadamente, desafortunadamente.*" One person suffers from an illness. The next student adds a statement that begins with *afortunadamente* and the following student adds a statement that begins with *desafortunadamente*. See how long you can carry a thread of conversation until you have to change topics.

Modelo: —Padezco de diabetes.
            —Afortunadamente, tengo una receta para la metformina.
            —Desafortunadamente, la farmacia está cerrada.
            —Afortunadamente, tengo metformina en la casa.
            —Desafortunadamente, me gustan los dulces.
            —Afortunadamente, no hay dulces en la casa.
            —Desafortunadamente, hoy es el día de brujas (*Halloween*).

 10.13 Drama improvisado _____

Play the television talk show *Hipocondríaco competitivo* ("Competitive Hypo-chondriac"). You'll need four students to sit in front of the classroom, plus an emcee and a studio audience. As members of the studio audience ask contestants about their medical history and current conditions, things get a little competitive and, dare we say, contagious. Start with minor problems and move up the ladder. Audience members may add sympathetic comments such as, *¡Pobrecito/a!, ¡Qué pena!* and *¡Qué calamidad!* The emcee gives points according to acuity, for example, *Mil puntos para Betty por tener la lengua infectada e hinchada.*

 Estructura: Palabras indefinidas y negativas
(*Indefinite and Negative Words*)

- Indefinite words refer to people and things that we either cannot specify or do not want to specify. Negative words work alone or in conjunction with the word *no* to make a negative statement.

Palabras indefinidas
algo	something
alguien	someone
alguno/a/os/as	some, any
alguna vez	ever
algunas veces	sometimes

Palabras negativas
nada	anything, nothing
nadie	no one
ninguno/a	none, not any

Para completar su léxico
mucho, poco	a lot, a little
siempre	always
nunca, jamás	never
también	also, too
tampoco	neither

- Spanish often uses double negatives. *No necesito nada* means "I don't need anything." The word *no* precedes the verb, and a negative word follows it. The word *no* is omitted when the negative term precedes the verb.

¿Necesita algo para el dolor?	**No necesito nada.**
¿Hay alguien en casa?	**No hay nadie.**
¿Ha tenido cirugía alguna vez?	**Nunca he tenido cirugía.**
¿Algunas veces le duele la mano?	**No me duele nunca / Nunca me duele.**

- *Alguno* and *ninguno* drop their final *-o* when they are used before a masculine, singular noun. Then they become *algún* and *ningún*.

¿Toma usted algún medicamento?	**No tomo ningún medicamento.**
¿Le ayuda algún medicamento?	**Ningún medicamento me ayuda.**

- *Alguno/a/os/as* must agree with its noun with regard to gender and number. *Ninguno/a* isn't used in the plural.

Algunas enfermedades son contagiosas.   **No hay ninguna vacuna.**

HACIA PRECISIÓN

 10.14 Ejercicio _____

Complete la siguiente conversación usando palabras indefinidas y negativas.

Dra. Ávila: ¿Sufre usted de alguna enfermedad?

Doña Rosa: No, no sufro de _____ enfermedad.

Dra. Ávila: ¿Toma usted _____ medicamento?

Doña Rosa: No tomo _____ medicamento.

Dra. Ávila: ¿Es usted alérgica a _____ alimento?

Doña Rosa: No soy alérgica a _____ alimento.

Dra. Ávila: En su familia, ¿_____ ha tenido cáncer?

Doña Rosa: No, en mi familia _____ ha tenido cáncer.

Dra. Ávila: ¿Hay _____ en la casa para ayudarla?

Doña Rosa: Vivo sola. No hay _____ más en casa.

Ask about Symptoms

Vocabulario: Síntomas generales

Síntomas neurológicos

la confusión	confusion
el entumecimiento	numbness, tingling
el problema para hablar	problem speaking
el problema para ver, caminar	problem seeing, walking

Síntomas respiratorios

la dificultad para respirar	difficulty breathing
la falta de aire	shortness of breath
la fatiga*, el cansancio	fatigue
los silbidos	wheezing
los sudores nocturnos	night sweats
la tos, toser	cough, to cough

Síntomas cardíacos

el desmayo	fainting
el dolor del pecho	chest pain
. . . que corre por el brazo	. . . that radiates to the arm
las manos y los pies fríos	cold hands and feet
el mareo	dizziness
la palpitación, temblor del pecho	palpitation
la taquicardia	tachycardia
los tobillos hinchados	swollen ankles (edema)

Síntomas gastrointestinales

el ardor	burning sensation
el gas abdominal	abdominal gas
la náusea	nausea
el vómito	vomiting
el estreñimiento	constipation
la diarrea	diarrhea
los calambres	cramps
la pérdida de peso	weight loss
la pérdida del apetito	loss of appetite

*La fatiga may also refer to shortness of breath.

Síntomas previos a un infarto cerebral

- Entumecimiento o debilidad repentinos de la cara, un brazo o una pierna, especialmente en un lado del cuerpo.

- Confusión o problemas repentinos para hablar, entender, ver o caminar.

- Mareos o dolor de cabeza severo.

**Si tiene alguno de estos síntomas,
llame al 911 de inmediato.**

Síntomas genitourinarios

el flujo de orina débil	weak stream
la incapacidad para orinar	urinary retention
la incontinencia de orina	urinary incontinence
sangre en la orina	hematuria
la urgencia urinaria	urinary urgency
vaciado incompleto de la vejiga	incomplete bladder emptying

Síntomas del reumatismo

la inflamación	inflammation
la hinchazón	swelling
la rigidez	stiffness
el dolor en las articulaciones	joint pain

HACIA FLUIDEZ

 10.15 Actividad

Muchas veces se recetan los medicamentos para aliviar síntomas. Después de estudiar el vocabulario de los síntomas generales, identifique algunas indicaciones comunes de los siguientes medicamentos.

Modelo: Dulcolax
          —Dulcolax es para aliviar el estreñimiento.

A. Mylanta   F. Proventil
B. Compazine   G. Prilosec
C. calamine   H. Afrin
D. Benadryl   I. Robitussin DM
E. la nitroglicerina J. la aspirina

 10.16 Actividad

Identifique algunos de los síntomas de las siguientes enfermedades.

Modelo: la depresión
          —¿Cuáles son algunos de los síntomas de la depresión?
          —Algunos de los síntomas de la depresión son tristeza, pérdida de
          peso y pérdida del apetito.

A. el asma   F. la artritis
B. la úlcera   G. la tuberculosis
C. la gripe   H. el ataque al corazón
D. el hipotiroidismo I. la hipertensión
E. el enfisema   J. la pulmonía

 10.17 Actividad

En grupos pequeños, escriba información para educar a un paciente sobre una de las enfermedades que es común donde un miembro del grupo trabaja. Por ejemplo:

La pulmonía es una inflamación en los pulmones. Es una infección bacteriana o un virus que puede afectar una parte de un pulmón o hasta los dos pulmones. Los síntomas son fiebre, tos, dolor en el pecho y/o dolor cuando respira. El tratamiento es tomar antibióticos o medicamentos antivirales. A veces también el paciente necesita usar un inhalador de alivio rápido o recibir los medicamentos por suero intravenoso y tener terapia respiratoria.

10.18 Actividad _____

Practique el uso del pretérito y el imperfecto. Con un/a compañero/a, observe la receta que escribió el doctor Rey Loza Gómez para ayudar a un americano que viajaba en México y se enfermó de gastroenteritis. Conteste las siguientes preguntas.

A. ¿Cuántos años tenía el paciente?
B. ¿Era el paciente alérgico a algún medicamento?
C. ¿Dónde estaba el paciente cuando se enfermó?
D. ¿Qué síntomas tuvo el paciente?
E. ¿Qué medicamentos recetó el doctor?
F. ¿Cuántas cucharadas de caolín pectina tenía que tomar el paciente en 24 horas?
G. ¿Cuántas tabletas de trimetoprima con sulfa necesitaba el paciente en total para tomar el medicamento en la manera indicada?

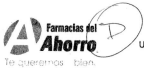

Farmacias del Ahorro
Te queremos bien.

Dr. Rey Loza Gómez
Cedula profesional 2087606
Universidad Autónoma de Guerrero
Real de Cuauhtémoc No. 4

Nombre del paciente: **ROBERT O. CHASE**   Fecha: **30DIC10**
Edad: **55a**   Temperatura:
Peso: Talla:
Presión Arterial: **ALERGIA MED. NO**

     FUROXONA CP.
1.- FURAZOLIDONA CAOLIN PECTINA SUSPEN.
     TOMAR DOS CUCH. C/12 HRS POR 2 DIAS.
2.- BACTRIM F. TAB. 400mg. 80mg. (TRIMETOPRIMA CON SULFA.)
     TOMAR 1 C/8 HRS POR 5 DIAS.
3.- BUSCAPINA COMP. TAB. (BUTILHIOSCINA METAMIZOL SODICO.)
     TOMAR 1 C/ 8 HRS EN CASO DE DOLOR ESTOMACAL

Súrtase esta receta en cualquier Farmacia del Ahorro

 ## Educate a Patient about Tuberculosis

Lectura: La tuberculosis

La tuberculosis es una infección bacteriana. Usualmente afecta los pulmones y es contagiosa. Pasa de una persona a otra por medio del aire, por ejemplo cuando una persona con tuberculosis tose, estornuda o habla. Pero en un 15 por ciento de los casos es una infección que puede ocurrir en otras partes del cuerpo, tal como en el cerebro, los riñones (*kidneys*), los huesos o la espina dorsal.

Hay dos pruebas comunes para la tuberculosis. Una es la prueba cutánea de la tuberculina (el método de Mantoux). Para hacerla, un enfermero pone una inyección intradérmica en el antebrazo usando una jeringuilla pequeña. Dentro de dos o tres días se examina el brazo para ver si hay una reacción. Si hay una reacción suficientemente grande y con hinchazón en el área afectada, el resultado es positivo. La otra prueba es una prueba de sangre para la tuberculosis. Para hacerla, un flebótomo toma una muestra de sangre. Esta prueba se llama la prueba QuantiFERON.

Si la prueba para la tuberculosis es positiva, la persona está infectada con la bacteria, pero la persona no está necesariamente enferma o contagiosa. Para determinar si tiene la enfermedad de tuberculosis de los pulmones hay que hacer una placa del pecho y/o un análisis del esputo. Cuando una persona tiene un resultado positivo, pero la placa del pecho es negativa, la persona no tiene la enfermedad de la tuberculosis, porque en su cuerpo la bacteria está inactiva o no está presente en cantidades suficientes. Esto se llama la tuberculosis latente. La bacteria a veces dura algunas semanas o hasta muchos años sin causar enfermedad. Un doctor a veces receta un medicamento que baja las posibilidades de tener una infección activa. Hay personas que han tenido la vacuna para la tuberculosis (la vacuna BCG, o Bacilo de Calmette-Guerin). La vacuna puede causar un resultado positivo con la prueba cutánea, pero no afecta la prueba de sangre. La vacuna no es común en los Estados Unidos.

Algunos síntomas de la tuberculosis de los pulmones son cansancio, dolor del pecho, tos o tos con sangre, pérdida de peso, una fiebre leve y sudores nocturnos. Hay antibióticos que pueden curar la tuberculosis. Si toma los medicamentos para la tuberculosis es muy importante tomarlos por el tiempo indicado.

HACIA FLUIDEZ

 10.19 Actividad_____

Hágale las siguientes preguntas a un/a compañero/a para reafirmar la comprensión de la lectura de tuberculosis.

A. ¿Es contagiosa la tuberculosis de los pulmones?
B. ¿Cómo pasa la tuberculosis de una persona a otra?
C. ¿Cuáles son los síntomas de la tuberculosis de los pulmones?
D. ¿Cómo se hace la prueba para la tuberculosis?
E. Si el resultado es positivo, ¿tiene tuberculosis el paciente?
F. ¿Cómo se confirma que el paciente tiene tuberculosis de los pulmones?
G. ¿Hay una vacuna para prevenir la tuberculosis?
H. ¿Hay tratamiento para curar la tuberculosis?

Ask about Surgical History

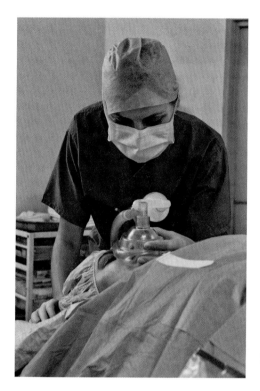

La cirugía (una intervención quirúrgica)

La historia quirúrgica

Like English-speaking lay people, Spanish-speaking lay people may be more likely to describe a surgery or procedure than to know its medical name. The doctor might say, *Usted tiene cálculos en la vesícula* (gall stones). *Hay que operarlo/la,* rather than *Usted necesita una colecistectomía.* Likewise the patient, giving his or her surgical history might say, *Me sacaron la vesícula biliar.*

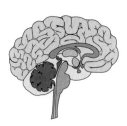

El cerebro

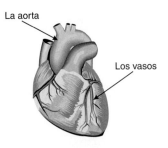

La aorta

Los vasos

El corazón

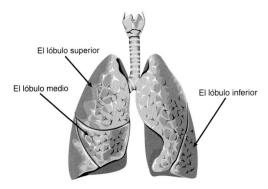

El lóbulo superior

El lóbulo medio

El lóbulo inferior

Los pulmones

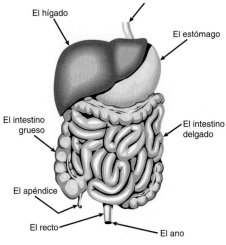

El hígado

El estómago

El intestino grueso

El intestino delgado

El apéndice

El recto

El ano

El sistema digestivo

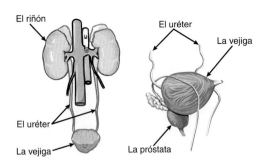

El riñón

El uréter

La vejiga

El uréter

La vejiga

La próstata

El sistema excretor

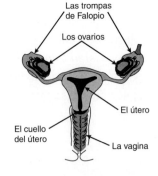

Las trompas de Falopio

Los ovarios

El útero

El cuello del útero

La vagina

El sistema reproductor

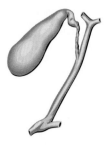

La vesícula biliar

Vocabulario: Los órganos y las glándulas

el cerebro	brain
la amígdala	tonsil
la glándula tiroidea, el tiroides	thyroid
el ganglio linfático	lymph gland
el corazón	heart
el pulmón	lung
el esófago	esophagus
el estómago	stomach
el duodeno	duodenum
el apéndice	appendix
el páncreas	pancreas
la vesícula biliar	gallbladder
el bazo	spleen
el riñón	kidney
el hígado	liver
la vejiga	bladder
el intestino delgado	small intestine
el intestino grueso, el colon	large intestine

Mujeres

la matriz	womb
el útero	uterus
el cuello del útero	cervix
la trompa de Falopio	Fallopian tube
el ovario	ovary
la vagina	vagina

Hombres

el pene	penis
la próstata	prostate gland
el testículo	testicle

HACIA PRECISIÓN

  10.20 Ejercicio _____

Seleccione la opción entre paréntesis que mejor complete las oraciones.

A. Los hombres deben hacerse autoexamen de (la próstata, los testículos).
B. La histerectomía es una cirugía para sacar (el útero, el tiroides).
C. La orina empieza en (los riñones, el hígado) y pasa a (la vesícula, la vejiga).
D. (El duodeno, El pulmón) es el órgano de la respiración.
E. La parte del tubo digestivo que llega al estómago es (el bazo, el esófago).
F. Un óvulo sale de (un ovario, el útero) y entra en la trompa de Falopio.
G. (El corazón, El hígado) es el órgano más grande en el cuerpo.
H. (La amígdala, El bazo) es parte del sistema linfático.
I. La colecistectomía es cuando sacan (el útero, la vesícula biliar).

Vocabulario: Algunas cirugías y procedimientos

el quirófano, la sala de operaciones	operating room
la sala de recuperación	recovery room
la unidad de cuidados intensivos	intensive care unit
la cirugía ambulatoria	ambulatory surgery
la cirugía con hospitalización	inpatient surgery
la artroscopia	arthroscopy
la cirugía láser	laser surgery
la laparoscopia	laparoscopy
el trasplante	transplant

La anestesia

la anestesia local	local anesthesia
la anestesia general	general anesthesia

Los procedimientos

la cirugía a corazón abierto	open-heart surgery
la derivación coronaria	CABG
la revascularización coronaria	CABG
la cirugía de cataratas	cataract surgery
la cirugía de bypass gástrico	gastric bypass surgery
el amarre de las trompas	tubal ligation
la amigdalotomía, la tonsilectomía	tonsillectomy

la apendectomía	appendectomy
la cirugía exploratoria	exploratory surgery
la colecistectomía	cholecystectomy
la colostomía	colostomy
la cirugía de la arteria carótida	carotid artery surgery
la histerectomía	hysterectomy
el marcapasos	pacemaker
la nefrectomía	nephrectomy
la neumonectomía	pneumonectomy
el reemplazo de rodilla, cadera	knee, hip replacement

Pregunta útil

¿Ha tenido alguna cirugía?	Have you ever had surgery?

Expresiones útiles

Enséñeme sus cicatrices.	Show me your scars.
Me sacaron la matriz.	They took out my womb.
Me operaron de la próstata.	They operated on my prostate.

HACIA PRECISIÓN

 10.21 Ejercicio_____

Identifique las siguientes cirugías.

A. _____ Es un procedimiento quirúrgico usado por los cirujanos ortopédicos para visualizar, diagnosticar y tratar problemas en las articulaciones.

B. _____ Es una operación que se hace sin hospitalizar (internar) al paciente.

C. _____ Es un procedimiento quirúrgico para sacar un riñón.

D. _____ El cirujano hace varias incisiones pequeñas para introducir una cámara pequeña que el cirujano usa para observar la cirugía e introducir los instrumentos que el cirujano necesita para hacer la cirugía.

E. _____ Es un procedimiento quirúrgico para diagnosticar una enfermedad abdominal o para saber si la víctima de un trauma tiene heridas internas graves.

HACIA FLUIDEZ

 10.22 Actividad _____

Usted es médico/a de cabecera y su compañero/a es un/a paciente nuevo/a. Prepare para presentar a la clase una entrevista donde le pregunta al / a la paciente
su historia quirúrgica. Identifique el nombre de la cirugía, el año y el nombre del
cirujano.

 10.23 Actividad _____

Usted es cirujano/a y su compañero/a es un/a paciente que necesita cirugía. Prepare para presentar a la clase una entrevista donde le explica al / a la paciente la
cirugía. Aquí hay algunas ideas.

Paciente	*Diagnóstico*	*Cirugía*
Señor Peña	cáncer del pulmón izquierdo	lobectomía
Señora Labredo	apendicitis aguda	apendectomía
Jesusito de la Cruz	amigdalitis frecuente	amigdalotomía
Mariluz Garrido	accidente automovilístico	cirugía exploratoria

 ## Educate a Patient about Vaccinations

Vocabulario: Las vacunas

hepatitis A	hepatitis A (HepA)
hepatitis B	hepatitis B (HepB)
difteria, tétanos y tos ferina	diphtheria, tétanus, and whooping cough (DTaP/Tdap)
poliomielitis	polio
neumocócica conjugada	pneumococcal infection (PCV)
rotavirus	rotavirus (RV)
sarampión, paperas y rubéola	measles, mumps, and rubella (MMR)
varicela	varicela
virus del papiloma humano	human papilloma virus (HPV)
meningocócica conjugada	meningococcal infection (MCV4)
influenza, antigripal	influenza

Estructura: El verbo *ponerse* y las vacunas

- As you have already learned, "I am going to give you an injection," is *Voy a ponerle una inyección.* To ask about vaccination history, you need the preterit of the verb *ponerse* (to put). The verb *ponerse* is irregular in the preterit. Here it is used with indirect object pronouns that indicate to whom the injection was given. If needed, you may review the use of indirect and direct object pronouns in chapter 6.

yo	Le **puse** la vacuna para el tétanos hace un año.
tú	¿Ya me **pusiste** la vacuna para la hepatitis?
él, ella, usted	La enfermera te **puso** una inyección.
nosotros/as	Antes de viajar le **pusimos** dos vacunas.
ellos, ellas, ustedes	Mis padres me **pusieron** la vacuna antigripal.

- Spanish *vacuna* and English "vaccination" are derived from the Latin word for cow (*vacca*), because the vaccine that eradicated smallpox was made from cowpox vesicles obtained from healthy vaccinated bovine animals.

  —¿A usted le pusieron la vacuna para el tétanos?
  —La enfermera me la puso ya.

- A booster vaccine is *una vacuna de refuerzo.*

  Debe tener una vacuna de refuerzo contra el tétanos, la difteria y la tos ferina cada diez años.

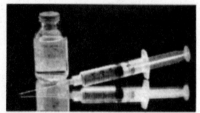

Una vacuna confiable

**Gamma Globulina HUBBER Antitetánica
(Humana) Liofilizada**

Avisamos a todos los Médicos, Centros Médicos, Clínicas, Farmacias y clientes
en general que ya tenemos disponibles en cantidades suficientes.
No necesita refrigeración.

EVITE LOS RIESGOS... UTILICE LO SEGURO.

Distribuye:

CENTRAL DE MEDICAMENTOS, S.A.

Calle Hostos No.105, Sto. Dgo.
Tel. 685-2085 • Y desde el Interior sin cargos al Tel. 1-200-3744

HACIA FLUIDEZ

 10.24 Actividad _____

Pregúntele a su compañero/a si ha tenido las siguientes vacunas.

Modelo: la vacuna para el tétanos
—¿A usted le pusieron la vacuna para el tétanos?
—Sí, me la pusieron.
(o)
—No, no me la pusieron.

> Recall the use of direct and indirect objects together: Me la pusieron is "They gave it to me."

A. la vacuna para la meningitis
B. la vacuna para la difteria
C. la vacuna para la varicela
D. la vacuna para la poliomielitis

E. la vacuna para la pulmonía
F. la vacuna para el sarampión
G. la vacuna para la gripe
H. la vacuna para la hepatitis B

10.25 Actividad

Usted es asociado/a médico/a y su compañero/a es un/a paciente que tiene una cortadura en la mano derecha. Pregúntele al / a la paciente qué pasó y cuándo fue su última vacuna de refuerzo para el tétanos. Explíquele qué necesita hacer, según el plan de tratamiento que está escrito más abajo.

Motivo de la consulta:	«Abrí una lata de sopa y me corté la mano».
Impresión diagnóstica:	Cortadura en la mano derecha
Plan de tratamiento:	Vacuna de refuerzo para el tétanos; cinco puntos; crema antibiótica; vendaje

Después, inventa otro motivo de consulta, impresión diagnóstica y plan de tratamiento para exponer en la clase.

Lectura: La pandemia de gripe

La gripe es una enfermedad de las vías respiratorias. Un virus la causa y la enfermedad es contagiosa. Los síntomas de la gripe incluyen todos los síntomas de un resfriado común, más una fiebre alta, dolores musculares y posibles síntomas gastrointestinales como náusea, vómito y diarrea. Las complicaciones serias de la gripe incluyen la pulmonía, la deshidratación y la insuficiencia cardiaca congestiva.

Muchas personas se enferman con la influenza cada año y muchos de ellos se mejoran sin problema. Pocas personas son hospitalizadas por varios días y de ellas pocas mueren de las complicaciones de la gripe. Hay ciertas personas que no se enferman con la gripe porque sus cuerpos la combaten o porque se han vacunado. La mejor manera para prevenir la gripe es recibir una vacuna contra la gripe todos los años.

La gripe pandémica es una gripe que no tiene vacuna para prevenirla. Para prevenir una pandemia de gripe, debe lavarse las manos frecuentemente y no debe poner las manos cerca de los ojos, la nariz o la boca. Si está enfermo con la gripe o si hay una pandemia de gripe en la comunidad, no debe salir de la casa para ir a lugares públicos como las escuelas o los mercados.

HACIA PRECISIÓN

 10.26 Ejercicio_____

Indique si las siguientes oraciones son verdaderas (*true*) o falsas (*false*).

A. Los antibióticos curan los virus.   V _____   F _____

B. La influenza es contagiosa.   V _____   F _____

C. Hay vacuna para curar la pandemia de gripe.   V _____   F _____

D. La gripe no causa dolores musculares.   V _____   F _____

E. Todos los pacientes se mejoran sin complicación.   V _____   F _____

HACIA FLUIDEZ

  10.27 Reciclaje/Drama improvisado _____

Let's play another game of "Categories." Form a circle, everybody holding one finger up. The first person makes eye contact with a person across the circle and states a word from any vocabulary category that we have covered since chapter 1, for example, a medical specialty, a food, a type of medication, a body part, an infectious disease, or a symptom. That person lowers his or her finger, makes eye contact with another, and states another word from that category. (If the first word belongs to more than one category, then the second or third person's choice determines the category.) Continue until everyone has a word (no duplicates), with the first person being last to receive one. Recall who said what to you and what you said to whom. Next, go through the list in that same order multiple times. Make eye contact with your receiver prior to speaking. When you have perfected this list, a student starts a second list. When you have perfected the second list, do both lists simultaneously.

  10.28 Reciclaje / Drama improvisado_____

As a variation of "Categories," a student leader asks individual students for lists of five items. For example, the leader says, *Kevin, dime cinco enfermedades.* After Kevin says each item, the class counts. Kevin says *zika* and the class energetically says *uno.* Kevin says *chikungunya* and the class says *dos.* After five items, everyone says *cinco enfermedades.* Recycle vocabulary from previous vocabulary lists.

10.29 Reciclaje / Drama improvisado _____

This is a fun improvisation activity in which you'll practice the preterit and the imperfect tenses in the lexical context of symptoms. Two students face each other in front of the classroom. Student three stands a couple of meters behind student two and visible only to student one and the class. Student two asks student one, *¿Por qué llegaste tarde?* Student three mimes a symptom that student one then identifies and uses as an excuse: *Tenía alergia y estornudaba mucho.*

 ## Exposición

 CHAPTER 10 SKILL: DESCRIBING AN ILLNESS

You are going to listen to a recording about cancer and take notes as you listen. Then you will create your own similar description of an illness that is of particular interest or importance to your profession.

1. Listen again to the recording about cancer from this chapter. As you listen, jot down the types of information that are presented. (Look at the categories in the matrix below and use them as a starting point. Does the description contain any additional categories? If so, add them to the matrix.)
2. Following the format of the recording, use the matrix to prepare a brief presentation about a particular illness of your choosing, perhaps one that you see in your current practice or will likely see in your future profession. Write down all the information you will need for your description.

Enfermedad
Pruebas
Síntomas
Tratamientos
Posibles efectos secundarios del tratamiento
Prevención

3. Write your presentation, following the model of the presentation on cancer. Be sure to read it over carefully for completeness of information and errors.
4. Your instructor may either request a copy of your presentation or invite you to share it with the class.

Cultural Note: Feeling at Home Somewhere Else

Mi casa es su casa

Think of another culture you have visited. Suppose you were living there and had to be institutionalized for a long convalescence. Considering your current cultural identity, what would help you to feel "at home?" Even if you were bilingual, would it be important for someone to speak with you in your primary language? What reading materials would you want to have available? Are there certain foods you would crave and others you would want to avoid? What sort of relationship would you want with your caretakers? How comfortable would you feel about being touched or bathed? Would the gender of your caretaker matter? How much of your personal information, treatment plan, and prognosis would you want caretakers to share with your family? Finally, how would you feel about caretakers writing in your medical record, "Patient unable to participate because of language barrier?"

Suppose a well-intentioned staff member were to treat you as a stereotypical person from your culture? For example, you are from the United States, and the dietitian arranges for you to have a special diet of hamburgers and hot dogs while the recreation therapist plays country and western music, but you actually have other preferences. Would the stereotyping cancel the good intentions?

At your current work setting, does a receptionist greet patients and visitors in a familiar language? Do the magazines, newspapers, wall hangings, and dietary choices reflect the cultural diversity of the patients and their families? How diverse is the staff at various levels of the organization? Are health-education pamphlets and discharge instructions available in the languages that patients speak? How long does it usually take to find a qualified interpreter or translator when needed?

Of course Spanish-speakers themselves are culturally diverse to the extent that the large group is considered poly-cultural. They are heterogeneous with regard to cultural origin, religion, ethnicity, geographic origin, education, and socioeconomic position. We may describe North Americans that way, too, and celebrate the way diversity has enriched society. Such diversity challenges health care workers to learn the cultural traditions, worldviews, and practices of their own patient population. However, even when you believe you are knowledgeable about a patient's culture of origin, you cannot safely assume that you are therefore knowledgeable about an individual's personal experience of his or her culture. General cultural knowledge must not promote the stereotyping of individuals.

In health care, there has been a tendency toward standardizing care along clinical pathways. This promotes consistent adherence to empirically proven methods. However, an obstetrician with volunteer experience abroad said about the delivery room, "The problem was that every time we turned our backs, the women would get out of the stirrups and squat in the corners of the room." There was apparent disagreement between care providers and patients about the best position in which to give birth. Health care workers are not necessarily trained to ask the patient his or her belief about treatment. Societies demonstrate varying degrees of expectation with regard to the extent to which newly arriving groups should assimilate.

Aside from the debate about the benefits of gravity-assisted childbirth, there are many areas in which a facility may work to become more "familiar-feeling" to a culturally diverse patient population. One hospital held a meeting between the chief cook, the dietitian, the owner of an ethnic restaurant, and hospital staff members who shared the cultural origins of many of the patients. Staff and patients contributed their favorite recipes from home. Then under the dietitian's guidance about what was nutritionally desirable, the cook was able to translate the recipes to prepare larger quantities of food. The restaurant owners shared information about suppliers of less common foods and spices. As a result, patients felt welcome. Perhaps some were more able to draw upon inner resources of comfort that had been instilled much earlier in life.

Vocabulario del capítulo 10

Padecimientos y la historia abreviada

la epilepsia	epilepsy
la convulsión, el ataque epiléptico	convulsion, seizure
el golpe en la cabeza	closed head injury
la amnesia	amnesia
la concusión	concussion
la pérdida de conocimiento	loss of consciousness
la angina de pecho	angina pectoris
el ataque al corazón	heart attack
el infarto cardíaco	coronary infarction
la trombosis cardíaca	coronary thrombosis
la hipertensión, la presión alta	hypertension
la insuficiencia cardíaca	congestive heart failure
el asma	asthma
el cáncer	cancer
la diabetes	diabetes
la hepatitis	hepatitis
la ictericia, la piel amarillenta	jaundice, yellowish skin
los ojos amarillentos	yellowish eyes
problemas de los riñones	kidney problems
la insuficiencia renal	kidney failure
. . . aguda, crónica	. . . acute, chronic
la fiebre reumática	rheumatic fever
la tuberculosis	tuberculosis

Padecimientos y el repaso de sistemas

la espina bífida	spina bifida
la hemorragia cerebral, el derrame	hemorrhage
el infarto cerebral	cerebral infarct
la jaqueca, la migraña	migraine
la parálisis cerebral	cerebral palsy
el tumor cerebral	brain tumor
la amigdalitis	tonsillitis
la bronquitis crónica	chronic bronchitis
la enfermedad pulmonar obstructiva crónica (EPOC)	COPD
el enfisema	emphysema
la pulmonía, la neumonía	pneumonia
la tuberculosis	tuberculosis

el aneurisma	aneurysm
las hemorroides	hemorrhoids
la hipercolesterolemia	hypercholesterolemia
la hiperlipidemia	hyperlipidemia
la hipertensión, la hipotensión	hypertension, hypotension
el soplo cardíaco	heart murmur
el cálculo biliar (la piedra biliar)	gallstone
la cirrosis hepática	cirrhosis of the liver
el cólico, el empacho	colic, indigestion
el pólipo	polyp
el reflujo esofágico, la acidez	esophageal reflux
la úlcera	ulcer
el agrandamiento de la próstata	BPH
el cálculo (las piedras) en el riñón	renal calculus (stones)
la endometriosis	endometriosis
la infección del aparato urinario	urinary tract infection
la nefritis	nephritis
la hiperglucemia, la hipoglucemia	hyperglycemia, hypoglycemia
el hipertiroidismo, el hipotiroidismo	hyperthyroidism, hypothyroidism
la obesidad	obesity
la artritis reumatoide	rheumatoid arthritis
la distrofia muscular	muscular dystrophy
la esclerosis múltiple	multiple sclerosis
la ciática	sciatica
la osteoporosis	osteoporosis
la catarata	cataract
el eccema	eczema
la irritación del pañal	diaper rash
la melanoma	melanoma
los piojos	head lice
la psoriasis	psoriasis
la sarna	scabies
la anemia	anemia
la hemofilia	hemophilia
la leucemia	leukemia
el linfoma	lymphoma
la anemia drepanocítica	sickle cell anemia

Las enfermedades infecciosas y tropicales

el cólera	cholera
la conjuntivitis	conjunctivitis
la culebrilla	herpes zoster, shingles
la difteria	diphtheria
la disentería	dysentery
el ébola	ebola
el estafilococo dorado	MRSA, golden staph
la fiebre tifoidea	typhoid fever
el pian, la frambuesa	yaws
la leptospirosis	leptospirosis
la meningitis	meningitis
la mononucleosis	mononucleosis
la paperas	mumps
la rubéola	rubella (German measles)
el sarampión	rubeola, measles
el tétano, el tétanos	tetanus
la tos ferina	pertussis, whooping cough
la varicela, las viruelas locas	chicken pox
el chikungunya	chikungunya
el dengue (clásico, hemorrágico)	dengue (classic, hemorrhagic)
la fiebre amarilla	yellow fever
el zika	zika
la enfermedad de Chaga	Chaga's disease
la infección por giardias	giaradiasis
las lombrices	(intestinal) worms
el paludismo, la malaria	malaria
la teniasis, la infección por tenia	tapeworm
la toxoplasmosis	toxoplasmosis

El cáncer

el auto examen	self-exam
benigno/a	benign
la biopsia	biopsy
el cáncer de pulmón	lung cancer
la célula	cell
el cansancio	fatigue
la cirugía	surgery
maligno/a	malignant
la metástasis	metastasis
la pérdida de cabello	hair loss

la quimioterapia	chemotherapy
la radioterapia	radiation therapy
el sistema linfático	the lymph system
tumor	tumor

Síntomas generales

la confusión	confusion
el entumecimiento	numbness, tingling
el problema para hablar	problem speaking
el problema para ver, caminar	problem seeing, walking
la dificultad para respirar	difficulty breathing
la falta de aire	shortness of breath
la fatiga, el cansancio	fatigue
los silbidos	wheezing
los sudores nocturnos	night sweats
la tos, toser	cough, to cough
el desmayo	fainting
el dolor del pecho	chest pain
. . . que corre por el brazo	. . . that radiates to the arm
las manos y los pies fríos	cold hands and feet
el mareo	dizziness
la palpitación	palpitation
la taquicardia	tachycardia
los tobillos hinchados	swollen ankles (edema)
el ardor	burning sensation
el gas abdominal	abdominal gas
la náusea	nausea
el vómito	vomiting
el estreñimiento	constipation
la diarrea	diarrhea
los calambres	cramps
la pérdida de peso	weight loss
la pérdida del apetito	loss of appetite
el flujo de orina débil	weak stream
la incapacidad para orinar	urinary retention
la incontinencia de orina	urinary incontinence
sangre en la orina	hematuria
la urgencia urinaria	urinary urgency
vaciado incompleto de la vejiga	incomplete bladder emptying

la inflamación	inflammation
la hinchazón	swelling
la rigidez	stiffness
el dolor en las articulaciones	joint pain

Los órganos y las glándulas

el cerebro	brain
la amígdala	tonsil
la glándula tiroidea, el tiroides	thyroid
el ganglio linfático	lymph gland
el corazón	heart
el pulmón	lung
el esófago	esophagus
el estómago	stomach
el duodeno	duodenum
el apéndice	appendix
el páncreas	pancreas
la vesícula biliar	gallbladder
el bazo	spleen
el riñón	kidney
el hígado	liver
la vejiga	bladder
el intestino delgado	small intestine
el intestino grueso, el colon	large intestine
la matriz	womb
el útero	uterus
el cuello del útero	cervix
la trompa de Falopio	Fallopian tube
el ovario	ovary
la vagina	vagina
el pene	penis
la próstata	prostate gland
el testículo	testicle

Cirugías y procedimientos

el quirófano, la sala de operaciones	operating room
la sala de recuperación	recovery room
la unidad de cuidados intensivos	intensive care unit
la cirugía ambulatoria	ambulatory surgery
la cirugía con hospitalización	inpatient surgery
la artroscopia	arthroscopy
la cirugía láser	laser surgery

la laparoscopia	laparoscopy
el trasplante	transplant
la anestesia local	local anesthesia
la anestesia general	general anesthesia
la cirugía a corazón abierto	open-heart surgery
la derivación coronaria	CABG
la revascularización coronaria	CABG
la cirugía de cataratas	cataract surgery
la cirugía de bypass gástrico	gastric bypass surgery
el amarre de las trompas	tubal ligation
la amigdalotomía, la tonsilectomía	tonsillectomy
la apendectomía	appendectomy
la cirugía exploratoria	exploratory surgery
la colecistectomía	cholecystectomy
la colostomía	colostomy
la cirugía de la arteria carótida	carotid artery surgery
la histerectomía	hysterectomy
el marcapasos	pacemaker
la nefrectomía	nephrectomy
la neumonectomía	pneumonectomy
el reemplazo de rodilla, cadera	knee, hip replacement

Las vacunas

hepatitis A	hepatitis A (HepA)
hepatitis B	hepatitis B (HepB)
difteria, tétanos y tos ferina	diphtheria, tétanus, and whooping cough (DTaP/Tdap)
poliomielitis	polio
neumocócica conjugada	pneumococcal infection (PCV)
rotavirus	rotavirus (RV)
sarampión, paperas y rubéola	measles, mumps, and rubella (MMR)
varicela	varicela
virus del papiloma humano	human papilloma virus (HPV)
meningocócica conjugada	meningococcal infection (MCV4)
influenza, antigripal	influenza

Palabras indefinidas

algo	something
alguien	someone
alguno/a/os/as	some, any
alguna vez	ever
algunas veces	sometimes

Palabras negativas

nada	anything, nothing
nadie	no one
ninguno/a	none, not any

Para completar su léxico

mucho, poco	a lot, a little
siempre	always
nunca, jamás	never
también	also, too
tampoco	neither

Preguntas útiles

¿Padece del corazón?	Do you have heart problems?
¿Padece de los riñones?	Do you have kidney problems?
¿Ha tenido problemas con el hígado?	Have you had liver problems?
¿Tuvo alguna vez un golpe en la cabeza?	Have you had a head injury?
¿Ha tenido cáncer?	Have you had cancer?
¿Hay [historia de] cáncer en la familia?	Is there [a history of] cancer in your family?
¿Ha tenido alguna cirugía?	Have you ever had surgery?

Expresiones útiles

Enséñeme sus cicatrices.	Show me your scars.
Me sacaron la matriz.	They took out my womb.
Me operaron de la próstata.	They operated on my prostate.

Chapter 11

Internamientos, odontología y la salud mental

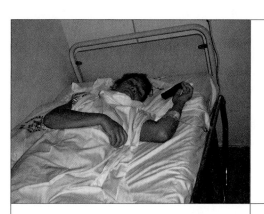

Website   www.yalebooks.com/medicalspanish

Video   *Trama: La laparoscopia; Atracción especial:* At the Drop of a Hat

Audio   *Ejercicio 11.4;* Discharge Planning; *Exposición*

Electronic Workbook

By the end of this chapter you will know additional vocabulary to help you with hospital admissions and discharge planning. You will know the terms associated with dental prophylaxis and treatment. You will learn how to ask about feelings. You will know the vocabulary, questions, and answers related to a neurological examination. You will learn phrases and cultural considerations pertinent to basic mental status exams and substance abuse assessment.

Announce a Hospitalization

Vocabulario: El internamiento

internar, hospitalizar	to admit, to hospitalize
quedarse interno/a	to remain inpatient
la hospitalización	hospitalization
la estadía	stay, length of stay
la habitación privada	private room
la habitación semiprivada	semiprivate room
dar de alta	to discharge from the hospital

Preguntas útiles

¿Ha estado hospitalizado/a?	Have you been hospitalized?
¿Ha estado interno/a?	Have you been inpatient?

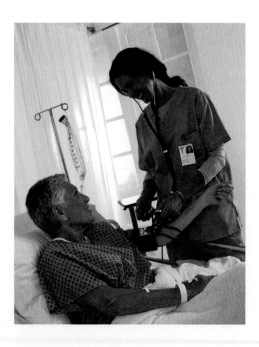

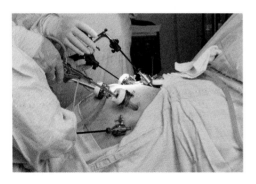

Con la colecistectomía laparoscópica, el
paciente vuelve a su casa el próximo día.

Expresiones útiles

Le damos de alta mañana.   We'll discharge you/him/her tomorrow.

HACIA PRECISIÓN

   11.1 Ejercicio_____

Seleccione las palabras entre paréntesis que mejor completen el párrafo.

Mi madre tiene los tobillos hinchados y dificultad para respirar. El cardiólogo
dice que la va a _____ (dar de alta, internar) para un _____
(ecograma, bazo) y una cateterización cardíaca. Si todo va bien, le va a
_____ (dar de alta, hospitalizar) en dos días. Ella está en la sala
de emergencias y no quiere _____ (quedarse interno, quedarse interna), pero el cardiólogo dice que el corazón es el músculo más importante
del cuerpo y hay que cuidarlo.

HACIA FLUIDEZ

   11.2 Actividad _____

Usted es enfermero/a y su compañero/a es paciente. Explíquele que necesita quedarse interno/a para tener un procedimiento médico y contéstele sus preguntas.
Aquí hay algunas ideas para comenzar.

Nombre	*Diagnóstico*	*Procedimiento*	*Estadía*
doña Olga	colecistitis	colecistectomía	dos días
Juancito	amigdalitis	amigdalotomía	un día
Sra. Méndez	apendicitis	apendectomía	dos días
señor Colón	angina de pecho	angiograma	dos días
Sr. Olivencia	artritis	reemplazo de rodilla	cuatro días

Lectura: Las directivas avanzadas

gravemente enfermo *seriously ill*
derecho a negar *right to refuse*
negarse *to refuse*

Normalmente los hospitales hacen todo lo posible para curar a los pacientes. Cuando un paciente está gravemente enfermo sin posibilidad de recuperación, el paciente tiene derecho de aceptar o negar los tratamientos que no curan su enfermedad pero que lo mantienen con vida por más tiempo, por ejemplo, el ventilador y la reanimación cardiopulmonar. Hay personas que no les gusta la idea de mantenerse con vida con máquinas u otros sistemas artificiales. La directiva avanzada es un documento legal que le permite al paciente dar instrucciones a los doctores con relación al uso de los sistemas artificiales. El documento se llama *directiva* porque el paciente le da instrucción al doctor con respeto a los tratamientos que quiere o que no quiere recibir. Se llama *avanzada* porque es importante firmarlo antes de estar gravemente enfermo, en coma o permanentemente inconsciente. Aunque una persona se niegue (*refuses*) al uso del ventilador o a la reanimación cardiopulmonar, puede aceptar el uso de fluidos intravenosos y/o medicamentos para el dolor que son designados para mantenerlo confortable.

HACIA FLUIDEZ

11.3 Actividad _____

En grupos de tres o cuatro personas, preparen y expongan a la clase una reunión entre un/a doctor/a y una familia donde el/la doctor/a les explica a los familiares una hospitalización (identifique al / a la paciente, el diagnóstico, el procedimiento y la estadía anticipada) y habla de las directivas avanzadas.

 ## Discuss Activities of Daily Living

 ### Estructura: Los verbos reflexivos

- A verb is *reflexive* when it is used with a pronoun that indicates that an action is done to oneself (the subject and object of the verb are the same person) or is done reciprocally (two persons acting on each other). The infinitive form of a reflexive verb appears with the pronoun *se* attached as a suffix. Thus the verb *bañar* means "to bathe," and *bañarse* means "to bathe oneself."

Baño al bebé diario.	I bathe the baby daily.
Me baño por la noche.	I bathe myself at night.
Mi esposa y yo nos bañamos.	My wife and I bathe each other.

- The reflexive pronouns are *me, te, se, nos,* and *se.* Except for *se,* they are the same as the direct and indirect object pronouns. Here they are used with the forms of the verb *lavarse* (*to wash oneself*) in the present indicative tense.

yo	**Me lavo** las manos* antes de examinar a los pacientes.
tú	¿**Te lavas** las manos después de toser o estornudar?
él, ella, usted	La enfermera **se lava** las manos frecuentemente.
nosotros/as	Cuando tenemos sueño **nos lavamos** la cara con agua fría.
ellos, ellas, ustedes	Los niños **se lavan** las manos antes de comer.

- Like the object pronouns, the reflexive pronouns are placed before a conjugated verb or a negative command; they are attached to a verb infinitive, an affirmative command, or the present participle (*lavando, bañando*). When attached to a verb form as a suffix, they may necessitate a written accent to mark the location of the oral stress. (Write the accent when two or more syllables follow the oral stress.)

Tiene que bañarse.	You must take a bath.
Se tiene que bañar.	You must take a bath.
¡Báñese!	Take a bath!
No se bañe mañana.	Don't bathe tomorrow.
El niño está bañándose.	The boy is taking a bath.
El niño se está bañando.	The boy is taking a bath.

- Verbs may be used in their reflexive form—or not—to indicate an individual's level of independence in activities of daily living.

Baño al Sr. Ramírez.	I bathe Sr. Ramírez.
La Sra. Vega se baña.	Sra. Vega bathes herself.

- Following the vocabulary list, below, you'll learn that many of the reflexive verbs that describe activities of daily living have different conjugation patterns. The notations *o–ue, e–ie* and *e–i* signal "stem-changing verbs," in which a vowel in the root of the verb changes in all but the first person plural (*nosotros*). There are those in which an *o* changes to *ue,* those in which an *e* changes to *ie,* and those in which an *e* changes to *i.* In chapter 7 you learned the verb *preferir* (*e–ie*). Stem-changing verbs are treated as regular verbs in the preterit, except for the verbs ending in *-ir,* which change only in the third person singular and plural (as in *vestirse* and *desvestirse,* below).

---

*In Spanish, the reflexive pronoun says whose hands are being washed. English uses the possessive pronoun. To use both would be redundant. Thus, **Me** *lavo las manos* means "I wash **my** hands."

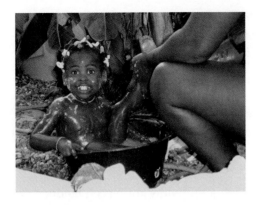

La niña no se baña. Su mamá la baña.

Vocabulario: Actividades de la vida cotidiana

acostarse (o–ue)*	to lie down, to go to bed
afeitarse	to shave oneself
bañarse	to bathe oneself
cepillarse	to brush (one's hair or teeth)
despertarse (e–ie)*	to awaken
ducharse	to shower oneself
levantarse	to get up
peinarse	to comb one's hair
vestirse (e–i) *	to get dressed
ponerse la ropa	to put on one's clothes
desvestirse (e–i)*	to get undressed
quitarse la ropa	to take off one's clothes
virarse	to roll over

*Note the conjugation of these verbs below. *Desvestirse* is conjugated like *vestirse*.

		vestirse (e–i)	
acostarse (o–ue)	*despertarse (e–ie)*	Presente	Pretérito
me ac**ue**sto	me desp**ie**rto	me visto	me vestí
te ac**ue**stas	te desp**ie**rtas	te vistes	te vestiste
se ac**ue**sta	se desp**ie**rta	se viste	**se vistió**
nos acostamos	nos despertamos	nos vestimos	nos vestimos
se ac**ue**stan	se desp**ie**rtan	se visten	**se vistieron**

HACIA PRECISIÓN

11.4 Ejercicio _____

Complete el párrafo con las formas correctas de los verbos entre paréntesis.

Buenos días. Me llamo Juan y mi esposa se llama Melania. Yo ____

_____ (levantarse) a las cinco de la mañana y ____ _____

(bañarse). Melania ____ _____ (levantarse) a las cinco y media y

____ _____ (bañarse). Yo ____ _____ (afeitarse) mientras

Melania ____ _____ (secarse) el cabello. Después, nosotros ____

_____ (vestirse), _____ (desayunarse) y _____ (salir) de

la casa a las siete.

HACIA FLUIDEZ

11.5 Actividad _____

Primero, indique el orden en que usted hace estas actividades en un día típico.
Después describa su día a la clase y añade más detalles sobre cada actividad.

Modelo: *Me despierto muy temprano. Me levanto a las seis y media de la mañana . . .*

_____ desayunar

_____ mirar la televisión y acostarse

_____ cenar

_____ llegar a la casa

_____ despertarse

_____ levantarse

_____ cepillarse los dientes

_____ bañarse y vestirse

_____ salir para trabajar

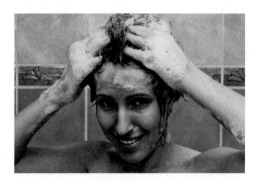

¿Se baña usted por la
mañana o por la noche?

 11.6 Actividad ————————————————————

Haga las siguientes preguntas a un/a compañero/a. Normalmente usamos formas
informales (*tú*) cuando hablamos con un/a compañero/a, pero aquí practicamos
el uso del registro formal (*usted*) para hablar con los pacientes.

Modelo: —¿Se baña usted por la mañana o por la noche?
          —Me baño por la mañana.

A. ¿Se despierta usted antes de las seis de la mañana?
B. ¿A qué hora se levanta por la mañana?
C. ¿Se ducha por la mañana o por la noche?
D. ¿Se afeita todos los días?
E. ¿Se peina o se cepilla el cabello?
F. ¿Se cepilla los dientes antes o después del desayuno?
G. ¿Cuántas veces al día se cepilla los dientes?
H. ¿Se acuesta temprano o tarde los domingos?

 11.7 Actividad ————————————————————

Usamos los verbos reflexivos para hablar de los pacientes independientes, pero
no para hablar de los pacientes dependientes. Con un/a compañero/a observe las
diferencias entre el Sr. Aquino Linares y la Sra. Silva de Palma.

La señora Silva de Palma es independiente. Ella se baña sin ayuda. El Sr. Linares es dependiente. Necesita ayuda y depende completamente de un enfermero para cuidarlo. El enfermero baña y peina al Sr. Linares, pero la Sra. Silva
de Palma se peina sola.

Ahora, identifiquen más diferencias entre los cuidados de los dos pacientes con respeto a sus actividades cotidianas.

El enfermero _____ al Sr. Linares. La Sra. Silva de Palma ____ _____.

El enfermero _____ al Sr. Linares. La Sra. Silva de Palma ____ _____.

El enfermero _____ al Sr. Linares. La Sra. Silva de Palma ____ _____.

 11.8 Actividad _____

Mauricio y Karina son novios pero son muy diferentes. Mauricio es un hombre muy bueno pero tiene malos hábitos de higiene. Karina tiene buenos hábitos de higiene. Observe las fotos de Mauricio y Karina y hable de las diferencias. Agregue (*Add*) otros detalles que no son obvios en las fotos.

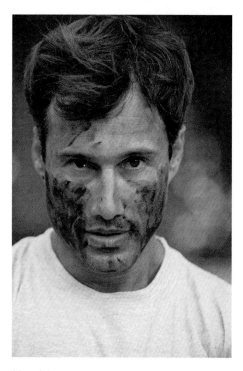
Mauricio

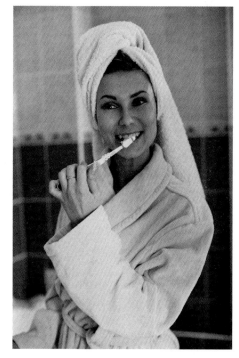
Karina

 11.9 Actividad _____

Observe la imagen de la rutina de Paola (p. 330) y hable de su rutina diaria. Por ejemplo, *Paola se despierta a las seis y diez.* Después, compare la rutina de Paola con la rutina de usted. Por ejemplo, *Paola se despierta a las seis y diez, y yo me levanto a las siete.* O: *Paola se despierta a las seis y diez y yo también me despierto a las seis y diez.*

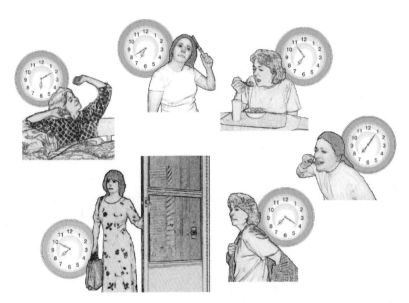

La rutina de Paola

 11.10 Actividad _____

Practique los verbos reflexivos en el pretérito. Use el pretérito para identificar cómo ayer fue diferente a un día normal. Note que en general, los verbos que cambian sus vocales de *o-ue*, de *e-ie* o de *e-i* no cambian en el pretérito. Solamente los que terminan en *-ir* hacen el cambio de vocales en el pretérito, y lo hacen solo en la tercera persona singular y plural (por ejemplo el verbo *vestir*, mas abajo). Consulte *appendix 2* en la pagina 391.

Modelo: Siempre me acuesto temprano, pero ayer fue diferente.
          —Ayer me acosté tarde.

A. Siempre me despierto temprano, pero ayer fue diferente.
B. Siempre me levanto temprano, pero ayer fue diferente.
C. Maribel siempre se viste antes de las ocho pero ayer fue diferente.
D. Mis hijos siempre se cepillan después de desayunar pero ayer fue diferente.
E. Siempre me peino antes de salir pero ayer fue diferente.
F. Juan siempre se afeita antes de la salir pero ayer fue diferente.
G. Siempre me ducho antes de acostarme, pero ayer fue diferente.

11.11 Drama improvisado _____

Play a version of "What's My Line?" Three students volunteer to sit in front of the class and answer questions designed to uncover each one's idiosyncrasies with regard to personal habits. These roles may be secretly assigned, or you may create your own. These ideas will get you started.

A. Una persona que sufre de insomnio.
B. Una persona que tiene buenos hábitos de higiene.
C. Una persona que tiene malos hábitos de higiene.
D. Un hombre que se afeitó ayer por primera vez en diez años.

 11.12 Drama improvisado _____

Play a new version of "Follow the Leader." Recall from chapter 8 that *vamos a* can mean "let's." Everyone walks around the front of the room in no particular pattern. Thinking of the vocabulary of activities of daily living, one student says, *Vamos a afeitarnos.* In unison, the rest of the group says, *Sí, vamos a afeitarnos,* and while walking around, everyone mimes shaving until another student proposes another activity for everyone to do, and so on.

 ## Estructura: *Se* y eventos imprevistos

- The pronoun *se* is used when announcing an unplanned event or one with no specific actor. Use the indirect object pronouns (*me, te, le, nos, les*) to indicate to whom the event happened along with the third person singular or plural of the verb (because the event serves as the subject of the verb). When using *le* or *les,* you may need to further clarify the person to whom the event happened. (You can do this by using *a* + person, as shown in the third example below.) For example,

Se me hinchan los tobillos.	My ankles swell.
Se le fracturó la pierna.	His/her/your leg fractured.
A José se le infectó el corte.	José's cut got infected.

- Perhaps this constitutes a cultural-linguistic pardon that recognizes that some unfortunate events are nobody's fault. *Rompí mi pierna* (I broke my leg) would sound intentional to a Spanish speaker. *Se me rompió la pierna* (My leg broke) was accidental.
- This construction is commonly used with verbs including *olvidar* (to forget), *perder* (*e–ie*) (to lose, to misplace), and *caer* (to drop, to fall); and with verbs related to injuries, including *quemarse, fracturarse,* and *hincharse* among others. For example,

Se me olvidó.	I forgot.
Se me olvidan las cosas.	I forget things.
Se me perdieron las recetas.	The prescriptions got lost.
Se me cayó la botella y se rompió.	The bottle fell and broke.

- Recall that it is the indirect object that changes to show to whom the event has taken place.

Se me olvidó.	I forgot.
Se te olvidó.	You forgot.
A mi mamá se le olvida todo.	My mom forgets everything.

HACIA PRECISIÓN

 11.13 Ejercicio _____

Exprese las siguientes oraciones para enfocar más en el evento que en el actor.

Modelos: Olvidé la cita.
 —Se me olvidó la cita.
 Fracturaste el brazo.
 —Se te fracturó el brazo.

A. Rompíunhueso._____.

B. Olvidé ponerme la insulina._____.

C. Fracturaste el dedo._____.

D. Quemastelamano._____.

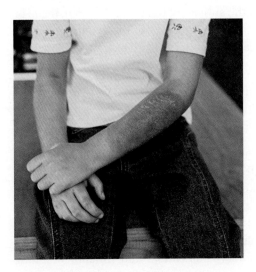

Al niño se le quemó el antebrazo.

E. ¿Perdió usted la receta? _____ _____.

F. Se hincharon mis tobillos._____ _____.

 ## Estructura: Los verbos *dormir* y *poder*

- The verb *dormir* (to sleep) is an *o–ue* stem-changing verb in the present tense. In the preterit it has a stem change only in the third person singular and plural.

	Presente	*Pretérito*
yo	duermo	dormí
tú	duermes	dormiste
él, ella, usted	duerme	**durmió**
nosotros/as	dormimos	dormimos
ellos, ellas, ustedes	duermen	**durmieron**

¿Duerme bien por la noche?	Do you sleep well at night?
¿Durmió bien anoche?	Did you sleep well last night?

- The reflexive form *dormirse* means "to nod off" or "to fall asleep."

Me duermo en la silla.	I fall / I am falling asleep in the chair.
Me dormí tarde anoche.	I fell asleep late last night.

- The verb *poder* (to be able) changes *o–ue* as well. It is often used before another verb in that verb's infinitive form. Its preterit forms are irregular.

	Presente	*Pretérito*
yo	puedo	pude
tú	puedes	pudiste
él, ella, usted	puede	pudo
nosotros/as	podemos	pudimos
ello, ellas, ustedes	pueden	pudieron

Puedo respirar mejor ahora.	I can breathe better now.
No pude respirar bien anoche.	I couldn't breathe well last night.

- After greeting a person, you may want to continue,

¿En qué le puedo ayudar?	How can I help you?

HACIA PRECISIÓN

 11.14 Ejercicio _____

Haga las siguientes preguntas a un/a compañero/a. Use la forma correcta del verbo entre paréntesis. **OJO:** hay dos que usan el pretérito.

A. ¿_____ (poder) usted dormirse sin tomar una pastilla para dormir?

B. ¿Cuánto tiempo hace que usted no _____ (dormir) bien?

C. ¿Cuántas horas _____ (dormir) usted anoche?

D. ¿_____ (poder) usted abrir la botella?

E. ¿_____ (poder) usted tragar (*swallow*) la pastilla grande sin problema?

F. ¿_____ (poder) usted llegar mañana a las siete de la mañana?

G. La enfermera dijo que usted no _____ (dormir) bien anoche. ¿Tiene sueño?

HACIA FLUIDEZ

 11.15 Actividad _____

Usted es psicólogo/a y su compañero/a es un/a paciente que sufre de depresión. Prepare y presente a la clase una entrevista donde ustedes hablan de la dificultad para dormir y la pérdida de apetito (*loss of appetite*). Por ejemplo, en capítulo 7 aprendieron a preguntar ¿Ha bajado de peso?

 # Plan a Hospital Discharge

The phrase *dar de alta* has its origin in military service. When a soldier was injured, he was sent to the hospital with the orders *dar de baja,* because his movement reduced the number of soldiers. He was returned to the ranks with the orders *dar de alta,* because his presence augmented the fighting force. In hospitals, the designation *dar de alta* refers to the doctor's order proclaiming the patient appropriate to return home.

Vocabulario: Planear los cuidados posteriores

dar de alta	to discharge from the hospital
¿Cuándo me dan de alta?	When do they discharge me?
A usted le dan de alta mañana.	They discharge you tomorrow.
¿Necesita ayuda en la casa?	Do you need help at home?
¿Cocina usted para si mismo/a?	Do you cook for yourself?
¿En qué piso vive usted?	On what floor do you live?
¿Hay escalera?	Are there stairs?
¿Hay ascensor?	Is there an elevator?
¿Quién lo/la va a llevar a la casa?	Who is going to take you home?
¿Tiene oxígeno en la casa?	Do you have oxygen at home?

¿Tiene usted familiares o amigos que lo/la ayudan en la casa?
　Do you have family members or friends who help you at home?
¿Tiene o ha tenido un enfermero que lo/la visita en la casa?
　Do you have or have you had a visiting nurse?
¿De qué agencia es/fue el enfermero?
　From what agency is/was the nurse?
¿Cuál es el número de teléfono de la agencia de enfermería?
　What is the telephone number of the visiting nurse agency?

HACIA FLUIDEZ

11.16 Actividad

Usted es un/a enfermero/a que planea los cuidados posteriores para los pacientes hospitalizados. Su compañero/a es paciente. El doctor le va a dar de alta al / a la paciente mañana. El / La paciente sufre de hipertensión y necesita ayuda de una agencia de enfermería para evaluar su presión sanguínea en la casa todos los días por una semana. Explíquele el plan de tratamiento. También pregúntale los datos personales necesarios para inscribirle con la agencia.

A. nombre, dirección, fecha de nacimiento y número de teléfono
B. alergias y los medicamentos que toma actualmente
C. familiares que viven en la casa
D. información del plan médico
E. agencia de enfermería preferida

Teach about Dental Hygiene

Vocabulario: El odontólogo

La boca

el diente	tooth
las encías	gums
los dientes de leche	baby teeth
la muela	molar
la muela del juicio (el cordal)	wisdom tooth
la dentadura postiza	false teeth
la corona	crown
— de oro	gold —
— de porcelana	porcelain —

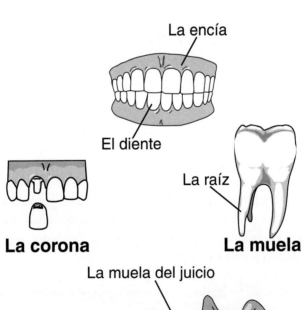

La encía

El diente

La raíz

La corona

La muela

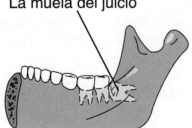

La muela del juicio

Los dientes

La higiene bucal

el/la higienista dental	dental hygienist
la limpieza	cleaning
la crema dental	toothpaste
el hilo dental	dental floss
el fluoruro	fluoride
el enjuague	rinse
el sarro, la placa	plaque
prevenir	to prevent

Los padecimientos y los tratamientos

la caries dental	dental decay, dental cavity
la gingivitis	gingivitis
la periodontitis	periodontitis
el empaste	filling
el sellador (sellante*)	sealant

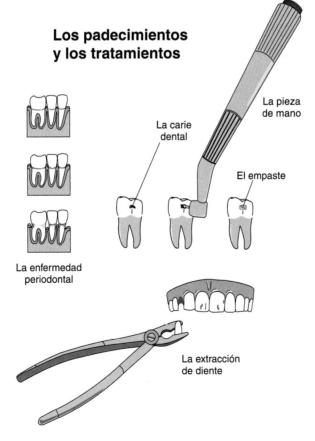

**Los padecimientos
y los tratamientos**

La pieza
de mano

La carie
dental

El empaste

La enfermedad
periodontal

La extracción
de diente

---

*Sellante is not in the official Spanish dictionary but is often heard in this context.

la extracción de diente	tooth extraction
el tratamiento de canal	root canal treatment
enjuagarse la boca	to rinse one's mouth

la caries (s.), **las caries** (pl.)

Lectura: Las caries y las enfermedades de las encías

Las bacterias que normalmente están en la boca pueden causar las caries. Primero, las bacterias forman placa en los dientes. Las bacterias en la placa transforman en ácidos el azúcar que comemos o bebemos. Estos ácidos hacen las caries. Los bebés que duermen con el biberón (*bottle*) pueden tener caries por el azúcar que hay en la leche. Por eso, los bebés no deben dormir con un biberón en la boca. Para prevenir las caries debe comer y beber menos alimentos dulces. También, hay que cepillarse los dientes dos veces al día y usar el hilo dental y una crema dental con fluoruro. El fluoruro protege los dientes. Hay suplementos de fluoruro en forma de tabletas, gotas y enjuagues. Vaya al consultorio del dentista dos veces al año para una limpieza profesional. El dentista puede ponerle selladores (sellantes) en los dientes para prevenir las caries.

La gingivitis es una inflamación de las encías. Algunos de los síntomas de la gingivitis son las encías rojas e hinchadas, dolor cuando toma bebidas o comidas frías, calientes o dulces, y sangre en las encías cuando se cepilla. Sin tratamiento adecuado la gingivitis puede causar la periodontitis. La periodontitis es cuando hay infección entre la encía y el diente. Para evitar las enfermedades de las encías es importante limpiarse la boca diario con hilo dental y cepillo, usar una crema dental con fluoruro y tener exámenes regulares por un dentista o higienista dental.

HACIA FLUIDEZ

 11.17 Actividad _____

Haga las siguientes preguntas a un/a compañero/a para confirmar la comprensión de la lectura.

A. ¿Qué causa las caries?
B. ¿Cómo se previene las caries?
C. ¿Por qué no deben dormir los bebés con un biberón en la boca?
D. Si quiero prevenir las caries, ¿cuál es una buena merienda?
E. ¿Qué es la gingivitis y cuáles son los síntomas?
F. ¿Quién puede explicarme el uso correcto del hilo dental?

La higiene bucal

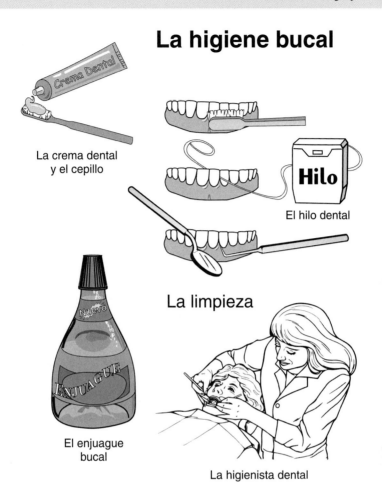

La crema dental
y el cepillo

Hilo

El hilo dental

La limpieza

El enjuague
bucal

La higienista dental

11.18 Actividad

Usted es higienista dental y su compañero/a es paciente. Vamos a usar el registro formal (usted). Use estas preguntas para comenzar una entrevista con su paciente. Después enseñe al paciente cómo evitar las caries y la gingivitis.

A. ¿Con qué frecuencia se cepilla usted los dientes?
B. ¿Con qué frecuencia usa hilo dental?
C. ¿Usa un enjuague con fluoruro?
D. ¿Cuándo fue la última vez que usted vio a un dentista?
E. ¿Cuándo fue la última vez que usted tuvo una limpieza dental?
F. ¿Le duele un diente? ¿Le duele cuando come o toma algo frío o caliente?
G. ¿Hay sangre cuando se cepilla los dientes y las encías?

Conduct a Mental Status Exam

Estructura: El verbo *sentirse*

- Until now we have used the verb *estar* to talk about feelings and the verb *tener* to talk about drive states, such as hunger and thirst.

    —¿Cómo está usted?   —Estoy bien, gracias.
    —¿Tiene usted hambre?   —Sí, tengo hambre.

- *Sentirse* is often used to talk about feelings.

    —¿Cómo se siente usted?   —Estoy cansado pero me siento bien.

- *Sentirse* is a stem-changing reflexive verb like *despertarse* because it goes with reflexive pronouns and the *e* changes to *ie* except in the first person plural (*nosotros*).

    yo   **Me siento** cansado.
    tú   ¿Cómo **te sientes**?
    él, ella, usted   Mi papá **se siente** solo sin mi mamá.
    nosotros/as   **Nos sentimos** bien aquí en México.
    ellos, ellas, ustedes   Los niños **se sienten** mejor hoy.

Vocabulario: Los sentimientos

The following adjectives represent feelings. They must agree with their corresponding nouns in both gender and number. For example *Juan se siente dichoso,* and *Ana y Luisa se sienten contentas.*

Palabras de frecuente uso

agitado	agitated	**enfermo**	ill, sick
agobiado	overwhelmed	**enojado**	angry
agradable	pleasant	**frustrado**	frustrated
agradecido	thankful	**furioso**	furious
alegre	happy	**interesado**	interested
aliviado	relieved	**nervioso**	nervous
ansioso	anxious	**preocupado**	worried
celoso	jealous	**solitario**	lonely
contento	content	**soñoliento**	sleepy
deprimido	depressed	**sorprendido**	surprised
desesperado	desperate	**tímido**	shy
encantado	pleased	**triste**	sad

Palabras para completar su léxico

aborrecido	disgusted	**enfadado**	annoyed
agotado	drained	**enfogonado**	enraged (*slang*)
asustado	frightened	**molesto**	uncomfortable
avergonzado	ashamed	**ofendido**	offended
culpable	guilty	**orgulloso**	proud
descorazonado	disheartened	**rechazado**	rejected
dichoso	lucky	**satisfecho**	satisfied
disgustado	disgusted	**traicionado**	betrayed

These are also used with the verb *estar,* as in *Estoy disgustado,* and *Marisol está ansiosa.* Recall that the choice of *ser* communicates more stable traits.

La niña **es** tímida.   The girl is always shy.
La niña **está** tímida.   The girl is feeling or acting shy right now.

The verb *poner* may be used reflexively when a situation is perceived to cause an emotional response. In this context it can be translated as "I become" / "I get," and is used with reflexive pronouns. For example, *Me pongo nervioso cuando estoy donde el dentista.*

HACIA PRECISIÓN

 11.19 Ejercicio _____

Seleccione las palabras entre paréntesis que mejor completen las oraciones.

   A. Si tomo mucho café me siento (avergonzado, agitado).
   B. Cuando estoy resfriado me siento (molesto, satisfecho).
   C. Cuando trabajo mucho llego a la casa muy (agotado, ofendido).
   D. Estoy (ansioso, dichoso) cuando tengo una cita con el odontólogo.
   E. Me pongo (agobiado, orgulloso) cuando hay mucho trabajo y poco tiempo.
   F. Me siento muy (aliviado, soñoliento) cuando paso la noche sin dormir bien.
   G. Cuando tengo dolor de cabeza y tomo un calmante me siento (celoso, aliviado).

 11.20 Ejercicio_____

Hay mucho vocabulario nuevo. Vamos a organizarlo para recordarlo bien. De la lista de palabras que expresan sentimientos, escriba tres palabras en cada una de las siguientes cinco categorías básicas: alegría (*joy*), tristeza (*sadness*), enojo (*anger*), miedo (*fear*) y vergüenza (*shame*).

la alegría	la tristeza	
_____	_____	
_____	_____	
_____	_____	

el enojo	el miedo	la vergüenza
_____	_____	_____
_____	_____	_____
_____	_____	_____

HACIA FLUIDEZ

 11.21 Actividad _____

Con un/a compañero/a, identifique los sentimientos asociados con las siguientes situaciones. No se olvide que los adjetivos deben concordar (*agree*) con el género del / de la compañero/a que contesta la pregunta.

Modelo: Tengo un trabajo nuevo.
—¿Cómo te sientes?
—Me siento *nervioso/a.*

A.	Tengo cáncer.	F.	Tuve una biopsia ayer.
B.	Me voy a casar.	G.	Voy a tener cirugía.
C.	Hablo español muy bien.	H.	Tengo doscientos dólares.
D.	El paciente está mejor.	I.	Tengo el día libre mañana.
E.	Necesito una inyección.	J.	Mi amiga está muy enferma.

 11.22 Actividad _____

Observe las caras, identifique el sentimiento y exprese en sus propias palabras del por qué de cada expresión. Por ejemplo, *Ella se siente alegre porque su mamá estaba enferma pero ahora está mejor.* Más de un estudiante pueden tener conclusiones diferentes.

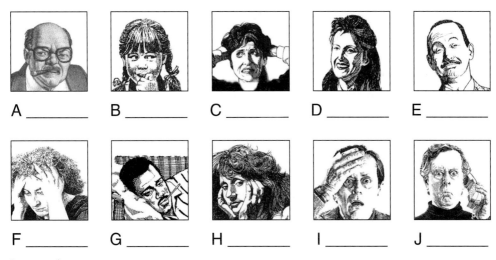

A _____ B _____ C _____ D _____ E _____

F _____ G _____ H _____ I _____ J _____

Las emociones

 11.23 Drama improvisado _____

Play a game of "emo-zones." Write names for emotions or feelings on four or five separate sheets of paper and place them on the floor several feet apart in a circle. At least one student should stand next to each of the papers and make a statement that justifies why he or she feels that way. For example, a student standing next to *celoso* might say, *Estoy celoso/a porque mi novio/a salió anoche con otra persona* or the person standing next to *agobiado* might say, *Me siento agobiado porque tengo doce pacientes esta tarde.* Say it with the appropriate affect. After everyone has a turn, change places and make statements to justify a new emotional state.

 11.24 Drama improvisado _____

Play a few rounds of "At the Drop of a Hat," a game in which you draw an emotion from a hat and then overact a line of script demonstrating that emotion. The instructor will prepare a container with slips of paper identifying emotional states. Students take turns drawing an emotion and reading a line "in character." The "studio audience" then attempts to identify the emotions for points. Here are a few examples of possible lines, but feel free to make up your own.

    A. Tengo que trabajar en el hospital mañana.
    B. El profesor/la profesora va a cocinar esta noche.
    C. Tenemos un examen en la clase de español esta noche.

Vocabulario: Las enfermedades mentales y sus síntomas

la discapacidad intelectual*	intellectual disability
la discapacidad del desarrollo	developmental disability

Los trastornos de ansiedad

la fobia social	social phobia
el trastorno de pánico	panic disorder
el trastorno de estrés postraumático	posttraumatic stress disorder
el trastorno obsesivo compulsivo	obsessive-compulsive disorder

Los trastornos del estado de ánimo

la enfermedad bipolar	bipolar disorder
la depresión	depression
la manía	mania

Los trastornos sicóticos

la sicosis	psychosis
la esquizofrenia	schizophrenia
el trastorno esquizoafectivo	schizoaffective disorder

Los síntomas

las palpitaciones	palpitations
el insomnio	insomnia
la irritabilidad	irritability
la falta de apetito	lack of appetite
la tristeza	sadness
el llanto	weeping, crying jag
el delirio	delusion
la paranoia	paranoia
la alucinación	hallucination
las voces	voices

El suicidio

hacerse daño	to harm oneself
suicidarse, quitarse la vida, matarse	to commit suicide

*Patients may still use *retraso mental* (mental retardation), which was more commonly used prior to Rosa's Law in the United States (S. 2781–111th Congress).

Preguntas útiles

¿Duerme bien?	Do you sleep well?
¿Cómo está su apetito?	How is your appetite?
¿Cómo está su estado de ánimo?	How is your mood?
¿Piensa en suicidarse?	Do you think about suicide?
¿Piensa en quitarse la vida?	Are you planning to commit suicide?
¿Tiene deseo de hacerse daño?	Do you want to hurt yourself?
¿Hay voces que le molestan?	Are there voices that bother you?
¿Oye voces que otra persona no puede oír?	Do you hear voices that others cannot hear?

Oír (*To hear*)
oigo
oyes
oye
oímos
oyen

HACIA FLUIDEZ

 11.25 Actividad _____

Usted es un/a enfermero/a psiquiátrico/a y su compañero/a es su paciente. Practique estas partes de un examen mental abreviado. (Un examen más completo está más abajo en la sección de neurología.)

A. ¿Cómo se llama usted?

B. ¿Qué día es? (¿En qué año estamos? ¿En qué mes estamos? ¿Cuál es la fecha de hoy?)

C. ¿Dónde estamos? (¿En qué país estamos? ¿En qué ciudad estamos? ¿Cómo se llama el lugar donde nosotros estamos?)

D. ¿Cómo se siente usted? ¿Cómo está su estado de ánimo?

E. ¿Duerme bien? (¿Cuánto tiempo hace que no duerme bien?)

F. ¿Come bien? (¿Tiene un apetito normal?)

G. ¿Oye voces que otra persona no puede oír? (¿Qué dicen las voces?)

H. ¿Tiene deseo de hacerse daño?

I. ¿Piensa en suicidarse?

J. Escuche estas tres palabras: *cama, manzana, brazo.* Repítalas.

K. Empezando con cien, reste de siete en siete (reste siete consecutivamente).

L. ¿Cuáles fueron las tres palabras que yo le dije y que usted me repitió hace unos momentos?

M. ¿Cuál es la relación entre una manzana y una pera? (Las dos son . . .)

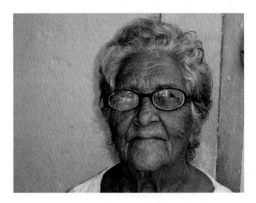

Doña Isabel

 11.26 Actividad _____

En grupos de tres personas preparen para presentar a la clase una entrevista entre un padre, su hijo/a y un/a profesional de salud mental. Invente nombres para las tres personas. La familia vino a la clínica porque hace dos semanas su hijo/a ha estado *hablando solo* (*talking to himself*).

 11.27 Drama improvisado _____

Observe la foto de *doña Isabel.* Ella vivió en Argentina casi toda la vida pero vino a los Estados Unidos para vivir con sus hijos mayores (*grown children*) porque no tenía nadie para cuidarla en Argentina. Ahora tiene síntomas de depresión. Quiere trabajar y sentirse útil (*useful*). Ella no puede comunicarse con sus nietos porque ellos solo hablan inglés y ella no lo habla. En grupos pequeños preparen para exponer a la clase una entrevista entre *doña Isabel,* sus hijos mayores y un/a profesional de salud mental.

 ## Conduct a Neurological Examination

Vocabulario: El examen neurológico

Verbos

arrugar	to wrinkle	**pitar**	to whistle
cubrir	to cover	**resistir**	to resist
empujar	to push	**sonreír**	to smile
frotar	to rub	**soplar**	to blow
fruncir	to frown, to pucker	**tocar**	to touch

Sustantivos y adjetivos

el alfiler	pin	**el ceño**	brow, frown
atento/a	attentive	**orientado/a**	oriented
la bolita de algodón	cotton ball	**el propósito**	purpose
la ceja	eyebrow	**la vigilia**	wakefulness

El neurólogo se especializa en investigar, diagnosticar y tratar problemas del sistema nervioso (el cerebro, la columna vertebral, los nervios y los músculos). Los trastornos que son más común para un neurólogo incluyen la migraña, la enfermedad de Parkinson, la epilepsia, las neuralgias, la esclerosis múltiple, los accidentes circulatorios del cerebro, los problemas de debilidad muscular, el insomnio y la pérdida de memoria (*memory loss*).

El examen neurológico es muy ordenado y tiene el propósito (*purpose*) de descubrir la presencia de un déficit neurológico. Empieza con la vigilia, para observar el nivel de consciencia. Queremos notar si la persona está despierta, atenta y orientada. En casos de trauma, se usa la Escala de Glasgow para personas mayores de cuatro años.

El examen de Glasgow (>4 años)

A. *Apertura ocular* «Abra los ojos».	B. *Respuesta motora* «Enséñeme dos dedos».	C. *Interacción* «¿Cómo se llama usted?»*
Ninguna 1	Ninguna 1	Ninguna 1
Al dolor 2	Extensión 2	Incomprensible 2
Orden verbal 3	Flexión anormal 3	Palabras inapropiadas 3
Espontánea 4	Flexión normal 4	Desorientada, confusa 4
	Localiza el dolor 5	Orientada, conversa 5
	Obedece órdenes 6	

A + B + C = Resultado   Normal = 15, Coma = 3 (mínimo posible)

*Ver "Para observar la orientación", más abajo.

El examen neurológico

Para observar la orientación, pregúntele al paciente,

ciudad
city
vecindario
neighborhood
estado
state
edificio
building

¿Cómo se llama usted?	¿Quién soy yo?
¿Dónde estamos?	¿En qué país estamos?
¿Qué día es?	¿Cuál es la fecha de hoy?
¿En qué año estamos?	¿En qué mes estamos?

Para observar la atención, o la capacidad para mantener la concentración, pregúntele al paciente:

Repita por favor las siguientes tres palabras.
Please repeat the following three words.

Repita por favor los siguientes números: 1—3—9—4.
Please repeat the following numbers: 1—3—9—4.

Ahora repita los siguientes números al revés: 6—2—5—8.
Now repeat the following numbers backwards: 6—2—5—8.

Empezando con cien, reste de siete en siete / reste siete consecutivamente.
Starting with one hundred, subtract sevens consecutively.

¿Cuáles fueron las tres palabras que usted repitió hace unos momentos?
What were the three words that you repeated a few moments ago?

Para evaluar la nominación, muestre al paciente objetos comunes y pregúntele,

¿Cuál es el nombre de esto?
What is the name of this?

Para evaluar la repetición, pregúntele,

Repita por favor, "ni sí, ni no, ni peros".
Repeat, please, "no ands, ifs, or buts."

Para evaluar la comprensión, dele una orden verbal al paciente, por ejemplo,

Tome este papel con la mano derecha, dóblelo en dos y póngalo en el piso.
Take this paper with your right hand, fold it in two, and put it on the floor.

Con la mano derecha tóquese la oreja izquierda.
Touch your left ear with your right hand.

Para evaluar la capacidad lecto-escritura, pídale al paciente,

Favor de leer esta oración en voz alta.	Please read this sentence aloud.
Lea esta oración y haga lo que dice.	Read this sentence and do what it says.
Cierre los ojos.	Close your eyes.
Escriba una oración.	Write a sentence.
Copie este dibujo.	Copy this drawing.

Para evaluar la praxis o descubrir apraxias, pregúntele, por ejemplo,

Saque la lengua.	Stick out your tongue.
Sople.	Blow.
Levante un brazo.	Raise an arm.
Enséñeme cómo se peina el cabello.	Show me how you comb your hair.

Para evaluar la capacidad de abstracción, pregúntele al paciente,

¿En qué son similares la pera y la manzana?	How are a pear and an apple similar?
¿En qué son similares la silla y la mesa?	How are a table and a chair similar?
Las dos son ...	Both are ...

También puede dar un proverbio para interpretar:

¿Qué quiere decir este refrán?	What does this saying mean?
«El día más claro llueve.»	"It rains on the clearest day."
«De tal palo, tal astilla.»	"A chip off the old block."

Examen de los pares craneanos

Cuando quiere que el paciente haga un movimiento específico, puede mostrarle el movimiento y decirle «Haga esto. Así». *(When you want the patient to move in a specific way, you can demostrate the movement and say, "Do this. This way.")*

I	Cubra una fosa nasal y dígame a qué huele esto.	Cover one nostril and tell me what this smells like.
	Ahora cubra la otra fosa nasal y dígame si puede olerlo.	Now cover the other nostril and tell me if you can smell it.
	¿Tiene un buen olor?	Is it a nice scent?
II	Mire la luz.	Look at the light.
	Cubra un ojo y lea esto. ¿Qué dice?	Cover one eye and read this. What does it say?

	Míreme la nariz y dígame cuando puede ver mis dedos.	Look at my nose and tell me when you can see my fingers.
	Tengo que mirarle los ojos para ver los nervios ópticos.	I have to look at your eyes to see the optic nerves.
III, IV y VI	Siga mi dedo con los ojos.	Follow my finger with your eyes.
	Mírese su propia nariz.	Look at your own nose.
	De forma alternativa mire a mi nariz y mi dedo.	Alternate between looking at my nose and my finger.
	Dígame cuando escuches esto.	Tell me when you hear this.
V	Resista cuando le empujo la boca.	Resist when I push on your mouth.
	Dígame si siente esto.	Tell me if you feel this.
	Le voy a tocar con una bolita de algodón.	I am going to touch you with a cotton ball.
	Le voy a tocar con un alfiler.	I am going to touch you with a pin.
VII	Sonría.	Smile.
	Arrugue la frente.	Wrinkle your forehead.
	Frunza el ceño.	Frown.
	Levante sus cejas.	Raise your eyebrows.
	Pite.	Whistle.
	Frunza los labios en un beso.	Pucker your lips into a kiss.
	Abra la boca. Voy a ponerle algo en la boca. Dígame qué es.	Open your mouth. I am going to put something in your mouth. Tell me what it is.
VIII	Dígame cuando puede oír esto.	Tell me when you can hear this.
	Póngase de pie. Cierre los ojos. Camine derecho en una línea imaginaria.	Stand. Close your eyes. Walk straight on an imaginary line.
IX y X	Abra la boca. Diga e-e-e-e-h.	Open your mouth. Say e-e-e-e-h.

XI	Voy a empujar sus hombros. Levántelos y resista mi esfuerzo.	I am going to push your shoulders. Raise them against my force.
	Voy a estabilizar su cabeza. Muévala hacia la derecha (izquierda).	I am going to stabilize your head. Move it to the right (left).
XII	Abra la boca. Saque la lengua. Muéva la lengua a la derecha (a la izquierda).	Open your mouth. Stick out your tongue. Move your tongue to the right (to the left).

Las funciones cerebelosas

Camine en forma habitual.	Walk normally.
Camine con las puntas de los pies.	Walk on your toes.
Póngase de pie con los pies cercanos y los ojos abiertos.	Stand with your feet close together and your eyes open.
Ahora, cierre los ojos.	Now, close your eyes.
Voy a darle golpecitos en la muñeca (el codo, la rodilla). Relájese.	I am going to tap on your wrist (elbow, knee). Relax.
Voy a frotar la planta de su pie.	I am going to rub the bottom of your foot.
Acuéstese boca arriba.	Lie on your back.
Levante las piernas, doblando las caderas y la rodillas.	Raise your legs, bending your hips and knees.

Prueba índice-nariz

Con su dedo índice, toque la punta de su nariz y luego la punta de mi dedo en forma repetida. Primero lentamente, y luego rápidamente.
With your index finger, touch the tip of your nose and then my finger. Do this repeatedly, slowly at first and then quickly.

HACIA FLUIDEZ

 Actividad 11.28 _____

Con un/a compañero/a, practique una evaluación neurológica. Tomen turnos como doctor/a y paciente. Escojan cuáles son las preguntas y pruebas que ustedes usan con más frecuencia en su trabajo.

Address Addictions

Vocabulario: Adicciones

la abstinencia	abstinence
la adicción	addiction
el apoyo	support
dejar de beber/fumar/usar	to quit drinking/smoking/using
la dependencia física	physical dependence
la desintoxicación	detoxification
ebrio/a, borracho/a	intoxicated, drunk
la recaída	relapse
la recuperación	recovery
los síntomas de abstinencia	withdrawal symptoms
sobrio/a	sober
los temblores	tremors, shakes
la tolerancia	tolerance

Preguntas útiles

¿Toma bebidas alcohólicas?

¿Alguien le ha dicho que bebe mucho?

¿Bebe mucho más que antes?

¿A veces toma muy temprano para comenzar el día?

¿Ha tenido problemas en el trabajo por el alcohol?

¿Tiene ansiedad, nauseas, sudor, o temblores cuando no bebe?

¿Ha recibido tratamiento en un centro de desintoxicación?

¿Usa drogas como cocaína, heroína o marihuana?

¿Con qué frecuencia usa la cocaína (la heroína, la marihuana)?

¿Cuándo fue la última vez que usted bebió (usó cocaína)?

Lectura: El alcoholismo y el abuso de drogas

aunque although   Aunque muchas personas no tienen problemas cuando toman bebidas alcohólicas, hay grupos que no deben beber. Los niños, las mujeres embarazadas y las personas que sufren de alcoholismo no deben beber. El consumo de alcohol en exceso puede causar problemas de salud tales como enfermedades del hígado, el corazón y el páncreas. Beber en exceso también puede provocar problemas sociales y familiares tales como accidentes, problemas legales y problemas en el trabajo.

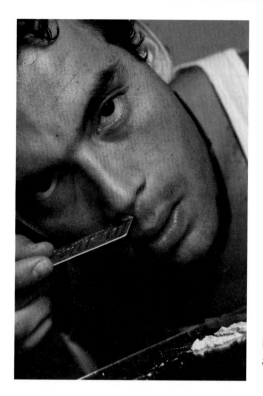

La cocaína es un estimulante que causa una adicción seria.

Los tres síntomas principales del alcoholismo son dificultad para dejar de beber, tolerancia, y dependencia física. La tolerancia es cuando necesita beber más alcohol que antes para sentirse ebrio. Las personas que tienen dependencia física normalmente necesitan tratamiento médico para dejar de beber. Este tratamiento se llama desintoxicación e incluye vitaminas, tranquilizantes y observación para controlar síntomas tales como sudor, náusea, temblores, convulsiones y alucinaciones visuales. Para seguir la recuperación y evitar una recaída es importante tener los servicios de un consejero personal o familiar y de un grupo de apoyo, como Alcohólicos Anónimos.

El abuso de drogas es un problema de salud pública. Las drogas frecuentemente abusadas incluyen cocaína, heroína, marihuana, anfetaminas, esteroides anabólicos y drogas de receta médica, especialmente los opioides. La cocaína es un estimulante que causa una adicción seria. Las personas que usan cocaína la inhalan o la fuman. El abuso de cocaína puede causar una crisis médica como un paro cardíaco o derrame cerebral. La heroína es una droga que proviene de la morfina. El abuso de heroína puede provocar problemas como muertes por sobredosis y enfermedades infecciosas tales como hepatitis y VIH/SIDA transmitidas por jeringuillas compartidas. El consumo habitual de la heroína puede causar tolerancia y dependencia física. Cuando una persona con adicción deja de usar heroína, puede tener síntomas de abstinencia. Estos síntomas incluyen agitación, dolores musculares, diarrea, vómitos y escalofríos.

HACIA FLUIDEZ

 11.29 Actividad_____

Usted es médico/a de cabecera y su compañero/a es un/a paciente que hace poco tiempo estaba ebrio/a y tuvo un accidente automovilístico. Preparen y presenten a la clase una evaluación para descubrir si el/la paciente tiene síntomas de tolerancia y dependencia física y si debe internarse en un centro de desintoxicación.

 ## Exposición

 ### CHAPTER 11 SKILL: REPHRASING INFORMATION

You are going to listen to the recording of a discharge summary and then rephrase what you hear in order to present it to the class.

1. Using the chart below, take note of the specific details while you listen.

Paciente (edad, estado civil, sexo)	
Motivo del internamiento	
Estadía	
Procedimientos	
Diagnóstico	
Medicamentos al ser dado de alta	
Plan de cuidados posteriores	

2. Now create your own discharge summary, using the categories of information included in the chart above. Change the facts so that the summary you create is different from the one you heard. Write clear sentences that summarize the key information without providing a lot of extraneous details. Once you have created a new summary, your instructor may ask you to turn it in or present it to the class.

Cultural Note: *Los nervios*

Cada cabeza es un mundo (Each mind is a world unto itself)

Mental health assessment and treatment are affected by language and by factors beyond language. Clinicians face the danger of mistakenly attributing artifacts of speaking a second language to psychopathology, and also the danger of mistakenly attributing mental health symptoms to linguistic or cultural causes. For example, a marginally bilingual patient who is being interviewed in his or her second language may demonstrate psychomotor retardation and thought blocking that appear similar to depression; or may use neologisms or have word-finding problems that mimic cognitive decline. The same patient may exhibit tangential speech or talk in a circumstantial rather than linear logic that appear similar to hypomania. One patient embarked on a discourse about his situation beginning with seemingly irrelevant history and circumstantial thinking that led his treatment team to suspect dementia. However, despite his apparently tangential thought process, he never lost his train of thought, and he effectively delivered his message.

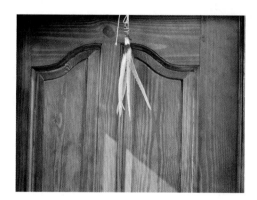

The versatile *sábila* (aloe vera) was hung on this door to keep evil spirits away. Its use for burns is well known, and some studies have shown that drinking aloe juice can produce an additive effect with other antihyperglycemic agents.

Ni soy de aquí ni soy de allá
(I don't belong here and I don't belong there)

Immigrants may have unique psychosocial stressors. For example, more than a few have mortgaged family homesteads for money to pay a "coyote" for passage abroad. This substantially increases the pressure to work and send money home to repay the debt. Others may greatly miss their homeland but not have paperwork that permits round-trip travel. Some feel caught between the desire to return and the embarrassment of not having achieved economic goals they had originally set off to accomplish.

Patients may have limited experience in describing psychiatric problems. When asked about his or her condition, the patient may say, *Padezco de los nervios* or *Sufro de los nervios,* terms related to traditional beliefs that nerves are central to mental distress. When asked what medication he or she takes, the patient may respond, *Tomo una pastilla para los nervios.* Furthermore, while some Latinos may "psychologize" stressors and emotional problems, others may attribute them to physical or spiritual causes. Some patients retain folk explanations for their problems, including a belief in *el espiritismo,* which is related to communication with spirits. Auditory hallucinations may be attributed to *seres* (beings) or to deceased or distant loved ones.

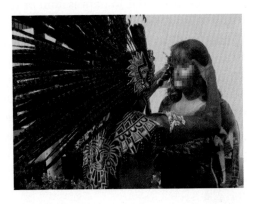

A *chamán* is a folk healer who is believed to have powers to heal illness, tell the future, or invoke or exorcise spirits.

It is important to assess the degree to which a patient has retained original and traditional cultural beliefs and values. Some clues are elicited by asking whom the patient has consulted about the problem: *¿Con quién ha consultado usted?* This may include a doctor, a priest (*sacerdote*), a pastor (*pastor*), or even a folk healer (*espiritista, santero, curandero, chamán*). It is helpful to know what the helpers have said about the problem (*¿Qué le dijo el sacerdote?*) Because of the primacy of family and other community members in a patient's support system, it is beneficial to know how these important people interpret the meaning of the distress and what they believe about taking medications. Clinicians must assess and respect the current values and beliefs of the patient as a starting point before suggesting an alternative approach.

There are aspects of the mental status exam that are not helpful when literally translated from English. Clinicians sometimes assess the patient's general fund of information in order to get a sense of the patient's overall intelligence. It would be unfair to ask a recent immigrant to name the past five United States presidents, the distance from New York to California, or the accomplishments of Samuel Clemens. It may be more appropriate to ask, *¿Cuál es la capital de su país?* or *¿Cuándo se celebra el día de independencia en su país?*

Sometimes the higher mental functions are estimated by assessing the patient's capacity for abstract thinking. Often this is done by asking the patient to interpret proverbs. There is some controversy over whether a proverb should be one with which the patient is expected to be familiar. Even so, it is probably not as helpful to translate "Men who live in glass houses should not throw stones" as it would be to provide a saying that is more commonly known in the patient's community. Here are several common Spanish proverbs:

1. De tal palo, tal astilla (similar to "A chip off the old block").
2. Casa de herrero, cuchillo de palo (The blacksmith's house has a wooden knife).
3. Todo lo que brilla no es oro (All that shines is not gold).
4. Más vale pájaro en mano que cien volando (A bird in hand is worth a hundred flying).
5. No hay rosa sin espinas (There is no rose without thorns).
6. El día más claro llueve (It rains on the clearest day).
7. No hay mal que por bien no venga (similar to "Every cloud has a silver lining").

For an interpretation, ask: *¿Qué significa eso?* (What does that mean?), or *¿Qué quiere decir eso?* (What does that express?).

Ataque de nervios is a culture-bound syndrome that constitutes an accepted—and sometimes expected—behavioral reaction to overwhelming psychosocial distress such as loss or bereavement. It appears in some non-Latino cultures as well. The symptoms resemble those of panic attack, except that unlike panic, *ataque de nervios* has an easily identifiable precipitant. In addition to panic symptoms, sufferers may complain of a sensation of heat rising to the head, may fall to the floor as if having a seizure, or may become aggressive.

Although sometimes sufferers are brought to medical attention, *ataque de nervios* is primarily dealt with in the community and without medical intervention. In some cases, herbal remedies and brief, intensive family support may rival the efficacy of pharmaceuticals. Often, the sufferer will resume his or her premorbid functioning within a day. When the *ataque* takes place outside of the cultural context, medical intervention is more likely. If the practitioner determines that hospitalization is indicated, care should be taken not to isolate the patient from his or her primary support system.

Vocabulario del capítulo 11

El internamiento

internar, hospitalizar	to admit, to hospitalize
quedarse interno/a	to remain inpatient
la hospitalización	hospitalization
la estadía	stay, length of stay
la habitación privada	private room
la habitación semiprivada	semiprivate room
dar de alta	to discharge from the hospital

Actividades de la vida cotidiana

acostarse (o–ue)	to lie down, to go to bed
afeitarse	to shave oneself
bañarse	to bathe oneself
cepillarse	to brush (one's hair or teeth)
despertarse (e–ie)	to awaken
ducharse	to shower oneself
levantarse	to get up
peinarse	to comb oneself
vestirse (e–i)	to get dressed
ponerse la ropa	to put on one's clothes
desvestirse (e–i)	to get undressed
quitarse la ropa	to take off one's clothes
virarse	to roll over

Planear los cuidados posteriores

dar de alta	to discharge from the hospital
¿Cuándo me dan de alta?	When do they discharge me?
A usted le dan de alta mañana.	They discharge you tomorrow.
¿Necesita ayuda en la casa?	Do you need help at home?
¿Cocina usted para si mismo/a?	Do you cook for yourself?
¿En qué piso vive usted?	On what floor do you live?
¿Hay escalera?	Are there stairs?
¿Hay ascensor?	Is there an elevator?
¿Quién lo/la va a llevar a la casa?	Who is going to take you home?
¿Tiene oxígeno en la casa?	Do you have oxygen at home?

¿Tiene usted familiares o amigos que lo/la ayudan en la casa?
 Do you have family members or friends who help you at home?

¿Tiene o ha tenido un enfermero que lo/la visita en la casa?
 Do you have or have you had a visiting nurse?

¿De qué agencia es/fue el enfermero?
 From what agency is/was the nurse?

¿Cuál es el número de teléfono de la agencia de enfermería?
 What is the telephone number of the visiting nurse agency?

El odontólogo

La boca

el diente	tooth
las encías	gums
los dientes de leche	baby teeth
la muela	molar
la muela del juicio (el cordal)	wisdom tooth
la dentadura postiza	false teeth
la corona	crown
—**de oro**	gold—
—**de porcelana**	porcelain—

La higiene bucal

el/la higienista dental	dental hygienist
la limpieza	cleaning
la crema dental	toothpaste
el hilo dental	dental floss
el fluoruro	fluoride
el enjuague	rinse
el sarro, la placa	plaque
prevenir	to prevent

Los padecimientos y los tratamientos

la caries dental	dental decay, dental cavity
la gingivitis	gingivitis
la periodontitis	periodontitis
el empaste	filling
el sellador (sellante)	sealant
la extracción de diente	tooth extraction
el tratamiento de canal	root canal treatment
enjuagarse la boca	to rinse one's mouth

Los sentimientos

agitado	agitated	**deprimido**	depressed
agobiado	overwhelmed	**desesperado**	desperate
agradable	pleasant	**encantado**	pleased
agradecido	thankful	**enfermo**	ill, sick
alegre	happy	**enojado**	angry
aliviado	relieved	**frustrado**	frustrated
ansioso	anxious	**furioso**	furious
celoso	jealous	**interesado**	interested
contento	content	**nervioso**	nervous

preocupado	worried	**sorprendido**	surprised
solitario	lonely	**tímido**	shy
soñoliento	sleepy	**triste**	sad
aborrecido	disgusted	**enfadado**	annoyed
agotado	drained	**enfogonado**	enraged (*slang*)
asustado	frightened	**molesto**	uncomfortable
avergonzado	ashamed	**ofendido**	offended
culpable	guilty	**orgulloso**	proud
descorazonado	disheartened	**rechazado**	rejected
dichoso	lucky	**satisfecho**	satisfied
disgustado	disgusted	**traicionado**	betrayed

Las enfermedades mentales y sus síntomas

la discapacidad intelectual	intellectual disability
la discapacidad del desarrollo	developmental disability

Los trastornos de ansiedad

la fobia social	social phobia
el trastorno de pánico	panic disorder
el trastorno de estrés postraumático	posttraumatic stress disorder
el trastorno obsesivo compulsivo	obsessive-compulsive disorder

Los trastornos del estado de ánimo

la enfermedad bipolar	bipolar disorder
la depresión	depression
la manía	mania

Los trastornos sicóticos

la sicosis	psychosis
la esquizofrenia	schizophrenia
el trastorno esquizoafectivo	schizoaffective disorder

Los síntomas

las palpitaciones	palpitations
el insomnio	insomnia
la irritabilidad	irritability
la falta de apetito	lack of appetite
la tristeza	sadness
el llanto	weeping, crying jag
el delirio	delusion
la paranoia	paranoia
la alucinación	hallucination
las voces	voices

El suicidio

hacerse daño	to harm oneself
suicidarse, quitarse la vida, matarse	to commit suicide

Vocabulario del examen neurológico

arrugar	to wrinkle	**pitar**	to whistle
cubrir	to cover	**resistir**	to resist
empujar	to push	**sonreír**	to smile
frotar	to rub	**soplar**	to blow
fruncir	to frown, to pucker	**tocar**	to touch
el alfiler	pin	**el ceño**	brow, frown
atento/a	attentive	**orientado/a**	oriented
la bolita de algodón	cotton ball	**el propósito**	purpose
la ceja	eyebrow	**la vigilia**	wakefulness

Adicciones

la abstinencia	abstinence
la adicción	addiction
el apoyo	support
dejar de beber/fumar/usar	to quit drinking/smoking/using
la dependencia física	physical dependence
la desintoxicación	detoxification
ebrio/a, borracho/a	intoxicated, drunk
la recaída	relapse
la recuperación	recovery
los síntomas de abstinencia	withdrawal symptoms
sobrio/a	sober
los temblores	tremors, shakes
la tolerancia	tolerance

Preguntas útiles

¿Ha estado hospitalizado/a?	Have you been hospitalized?
¿Ha estado interno/a?	Have you been inpatient?
¿Duerme bien?	Do you sleep well?
¿Cómo está su apetito?	How is your appetite?
¿Cómo está su estado de ánimo?	How is your mood?
¿Piensa en suicidarse?	Do you think about suicide?
¿Piensa en quitarse la vida?	Are you planning to commit suicide?
¿Tiene deseo de hacerse daño?	Do you want to hurt yourself?
¿Hay voces que le molestan?	Are there voices that bother you?
¿Oye voces que otra persona no puede oír?	Do you hear voices that others cannot hear?

¿Toma bebidas alcohólicas?

¿Alguien le ha dicho que bebe mucho?

¿Bebe mucho más que antes?

¿A veces toma muy temprano para comenzar el día?

¿Ha tenido problemas en el trabajo por el alcohol?

¿Tiene ansiedad, nauseas, sudor, o temblores cuando no bebe?

¿Ha recibido tratamiento en un centro de desintoxicación?

¿Usa drogas como cocaína, heroína o marihuana?

¿Con qué frecuencia usa la cocaína (la heroína, la marihuana)?

¿Cuándo fue la última vez que usted bebió (usó cocaína)?

Expresiones útiles

Le damos de alta mañana.   We'll discharge you/him/her tomorrow.

Chapter 12

Maternidad y protección sexual

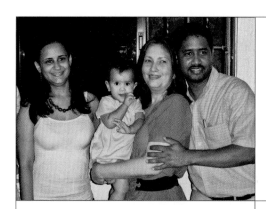

Communication Goals

Vocabulary

Structure

Cultural Note

Website   www.yalebooks.com/medicalspanish
   Video   *Trama: Mi hermano tiene SIDA; Atracción especial:* What's My Line—What's
      Your Temperature?
   Audio   *El embarazo; Ejercicio 12.11; Ejercicio 12.12; Exposición*
   Electronic Workbook

B y the end of this chapter you will know vocabulary that is helpful in labor and delivery and be able to take a patient's history of labor and delivery. You will be able to use informal commands to make direct requests on a more personal basis. You will have had some practice educating patients about safer sex and sexually transmitted diseases.

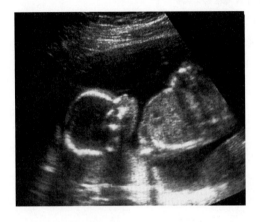

¿Es femenino o masculino? ¿Qué prefieren los padres? Prefieren un bebé saludable.

Confirm a Pregnancy

Vocabulario: El embarazo

La menstruación

menstruar	to menstruate
el período, la regla	period
la ovulación	ovulation
el calambre	cramp
el coágulo	clot
la menopausia, el cambio	menopause, the change

El embarazo

estar embarazada, estar encinta*	to be pregnant
el embarazo ectópico	ectopic pregnancy
el aborto provocado	abortion
el aborto natural, el aborto espontáneo	miscarriage
el parto	delivery
la cesárea	C-section

*Although you may hear the slang *preñada,* it is generally reserved for livestock.

Las pruebas

la prueba del embarazo	pregnancy test
la sonografía, el ultrasonido, el ecograma	ultrasound
la prueba de Pap/Papanicolaou	Pap test

Preguntas útiles

¿Menstrua usted?	Do you menstruate?
¿Menstrua usted todavía?	Do you still menstruate?
¿Cuándo comenzó su último período?	When did your last period start?
¿Son regulares sus períodos?	Are your periods regular?
¿Tiene relaciones sexuales?	Are you sexually active?
¿Sangra más de lo normal?	Do you bleed more than usual?
¿Es su primer embarazo?	Is [this] your first pregnancy?
¿Cuántos embarazos ha tenido?	How many pregnancies have you had?
¿Ha subido de peso?	Have you gained weight?

La prueba de Papanicolaou

Para detectar el cáncer del cuello del útero (*cervical cancer*) todas las mujeres que tienen treinta años de edad o menos y son activas sexualmente deben hacerse la prueba de Pap anualmente. Las mujeres que no son activas sexualmente deben hacerse la prueba de Pap antes de cumplir los veintiún años. Las mujeres mayores de treinta años deben tener la prueba de Pap anualmente o cada dos o tres años dependiendo de sus factores de riesgo.

HACIA PRECISIÓN

12.1 Ejercicio _____

Escriba las preguntas que obtienen (*elicit*) las siguientes respuestas.

A. _____

—Mi ginecóloga es la doctora Hernández Mejía.

B. _____

—Mi último período comenzó el primero de julio.

C. _____

—Mis períodos duran de tres a cuatro días.

D. _____

—Sí, son regulares.

E. _____

—A veces me duelen los períodos.

F. _____

—Tuve una prueba de Pap el año pasado en septiembre.

G. _____

—Me hicieron un ultrasonido el mes pasado.

H. _____

—Hace tres meses que no tengo la menstruación.

I. _____

—Sí. Antes pesaba cincuenta y cinco kilos. Ahora peso como sesenta.

J. _____

—Nunca uso drogas. No fumo tampoco.

HACIA FLUIDEZ

 12.2 Actividad _____

Usted es enfermero/a en una clínica obstétrica y su compañero/a es una paciente que vino para hacerse una prueba de embarazo. La prueba fue positiva y la paciente está embarazada. Hágale las siguientes preguntas a la paciente. La paciente debe contestar ad lib.

A. ¿Cuándo comenzó su último período?
B. ¿Es su primer embarazo? (¿Ha estado embarazada anteriormente?)
C. ¿Cuántos embarazos ha tenido? (¿Cuántas veces ha estado embarazada?)
D. ¿Cuántos hijos tiene?
E. ¿Cuándo fue su último parto?
F. ¿Ha tenido cesárea?
G. ¿Ha tenido abortos espontáneos?
H. ¿Ha tenido abortos provocados?

12.3 Actividad

Entreviste a un/a compañero/a para confirmar los siguientes datos. (Su compañero/a no debe dar información personal actual.) Después presenta a su paciente a la clase.

A. Nombre de paciente: _____

B. Nombre de obstetra: _____

C. Primer día del último período: _____

D. Duración de períodos: _____

E. Aumento de peso durante este embarazo: _____

F. Uso de tabaco, alcohol y drogas: _____

G. Fecha de última prueba de Pap: _____

H. Fecha del último ultrasonido: _____

 12.4 Actividad

Usted es un enfermero/a obstétrico/a y su compañero/a es una paciente que tuvo una prueba de embarazo. La prueba fue positiva. Hable con la paciente para explicar el resultado. Estas preguntas pueden ayudarle a empezar la entrevista.

A. ¿Está sorprendida? ¿Cómo se siente?
B. ¿Cuántos hijos tiene actualmente?
C. ¿Cuántos años tienen sus hijos? ¿Cómo se llaman?
D. ¿Cuándo empezó su último período?
E. [si no tiene hijos] ¿Ha estado embarazada anteriormente?
F. ¿Cuántos embarazos ha tenido?
G. ¿Qué pasó con su primer embarazo?
H. ¿Cuántos años tenía usted entonces?

 12.5 Drama improvisado

Tres estudiantes dramatizan una visita al doctor. Hay un esposo ansioso, su esposa y un/a obstetra. El esposo dice que él ha notado cambios en su esposa que le hace pensar que ella está embarazada. La esposa cree que su esposo está equivocado y dice, *¡No puede ser!*

12.6 Drama improvisado

Grupos de tres estudiantes dramatizan una visita al doctor en la cual la Sra. Peña lleva a su hija Marisol a la clínica después de descubrir que Marisol está embarazada hace seis o siete meses pero ha escondido (*concealed*) el embarazo de su familia hasta hoy.

 ## Teach about Possible Complications

Vocabulario: Posibles complicaciones

los tobillos o pies hinchados	swollen ankles or feet
la cara o manos hinchadas	swollen face or hands
el dolor de cabeza severo	severe headache
los problemas con la vista	vision problems
el vómito persistente	persistent vomiting
el dolor cuando orina	painful urination
diabetes del embarazo	gestational diabetes

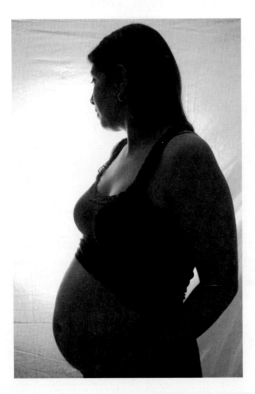

Foto cortesía de Otoniel Acevedo Medina

poco líquido amniótico	insufficient amniotic fluid
la secreción / el flujo vaginal	vaginal secretion
el sangramiento vaginal	vaginal bleeding
la placenta previa	placenta previa
la preeclampsia	preeclampsia

 12.7 Actividad _____

Usted es obstetra en una clínica obstétrica y su compañero/a está embarazada. Asegúrele que gracias a Dios la mayoría de los embarazos no tienen complicaciones. Después, explique a la paciente cuáles son las posibles complicaciones del embarazo y cómo llamar a la clínica para hacer una cita urgente.

 12.8 Actividad _____

Usted es un/a enfermero/a obstétrico/a en una clínica obstétrica y su compañero/a es una paciente embarazada que ha llamado a la clínica para informar que tiene una complicación del embarazo. Pregúntele si tiene o ha tenido otras complicaciones también, por ejemplo si ha tenido o tiene secreciones vaginales, y hágale una cita urgente.

 ## Coach a Delivery

Vocabulario: El parto

nacer	to be born
romper fuente, romper la bolsa de agua	to break water
la presentación de nalgas	breech position
las contracciones del útero	contractions
la dilatación del cuello del útero	dilation of the cervix
el monitoreo fetal	fetal monitor
dar a luz, parir, alumbrar	to deliver
el parto, el alumbramiento	delivery
el parto vaginal, el parto espontáneo	vaginal, spontaneous delivery
el parto prematuro	premature delivery
la cesárea	C-section
los dolores del parto	labor pains
la episiotomía	episiotomy
la placenta	placenta
el medicamento epidural para el dolor	epidural medication for pain

el medicamento para adelantar el parto   medication to advance the delivery

dar el seno, dar el pecho, amamantar*   to breastfeed
la unidad para cuidados intensivos neonatales   neonatal intensive care unit
¡Es un niño! ¡Es una niña!**   It's a boy! It's a girl!
¡Felicidades!   Congratulations!

*For those who feed by bottle, *la mamadera, el biberón, la mamilla,* and *la tetera* are all words for the baby's bottle, depending on the country of origin.

**In the Caribbean region, many say, *¡Es varón!* and *¡Es hembra!* although the use of these terms may offend people from countries where they are used to indicate the gender of non-domesticated animals.

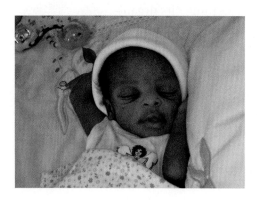

¡Felicidades! ¡Es una niña!

HACIA PRECISIÓN

12.9 Ejercicio _____

Seleccione las palabras entre paréntesis que mejor completen las oraciones.

A. La (operación cesárea, episiotomía) es una incisión en la vulva para facilitar el parto del feto.
B. La (operación cesárea, episiotomía) es necesaria cuando el parto vaginal no es posible.
C. La (placenta, bolsa de agua) es un órgano que está entre la superficie interior del útero y el cordón umbilical.
D. Cuando no hay (dilatación del cuello del útero, placenta previa) se usa medicamento para adelantar el parto.
E. El embarazo (ectópico, inesperado) es un embarazo anormal porque el óvulo fertilizado no está en el útero.
F. El (parto espontáneo, parto prematuro) es un parto antes de treinta y siete semanas de embarazo.

HACIA FLUIDEZ

12.10 Actividad_____

Usted es pediatra y su compañero/a es un padre / una madre nuevo/a. Hagan una entrevista usando el formulario *Historia del parto* para documentar la historia del parto y el primer mes de la vida del bebé.

This form can be downloaded from the website.

Historia del parto

Nombre del niño _____ Fecha de nacimiento _____
Peso al nacer _____ Longitud al nacer _____
Tipo de sangre del niño _____
Puntaje de APGAR: 1 minuto _____ 5 minutos _____
Medicamentos tomados por la madre durante el embarazo:

_____
Uso de alcohol y/o drogas por la madre durante el embarazo:

_____
Padecimientos de la madre durante el embarazo (diabetes, hipertensión, riñones, psiquiatría):

_____
¿Fue embarazo a término (40 semanas)? Sí _____ No _____
Si no fue a término, número de semanas actuales (edad gestacional) _____
¿Está dando leche materna exclusivamente? _____
Número de veces en 24 horas _____
Número de minutos por lado _____
Número de pañales mojados en 24 horas _____
Número de pañales sucios en 24 horas _____ ¿Tiene gases? _____
Tiene vómitos? _____ ¿Tiene problemas de respiración? _____
Antes de salir del hospital, recibió el bebé fototerapia, fluidos por suero, rayos equis, transfusión de sangre u otra intervención? _____
Especifique _____

_____
¿Quiénes viven en la casa?

_____
¿Hay mascotas? _____
¿Duerme en la cuna el bebé? _____
¿A veces se termina la comida antes de tener dinero para comprar más?

_____
¿En la casa hay extintor de incendios / alarma de incendios / detector de monóxido de carbono? _____
Servicio de información toxicológica en los Estados Unidos 1-800-222-1222

Estructura: El imperativo informal

- In chapter 6 you learned formal (*usted*) commands; in chapter 7 you used the verb *deber* to say what a person ought to do. Here you'll learn to make direct requests of persons with whom you may relate on a less formal basis. Use the informal (*tú*) command when addressing children and persons with whom you are on a first-name basis.*

tutear to address informally

- Affirmative (Do it!) commands are formed by using the third person singular.

    tomar   ¡Toma el medicamento!
    comer   ¡Come más vegetales!

- Negative (Don't do it!) commands are formed like the formal (*usted*) commands, and an *s* is added. That is, remove the -*o* from the first person singular form of the present tense and add -*es* for verbs that end in -*ar* and -*as* for verbs that end in -*er* and -*ir*.

    tomar   ¡No tomes el medicamento!
    comer   ¡No comas nada!

- Commands are direct and to the point.

    empujar   ¡Empuja!   ¡No empujes!
    respirar   ¡Respira!   ¡No respires!
    mirar   ¡Mira!   ¡No mires!

- When reflexive or object pronouns are used with commands, the pronouns are added as suffixes to affirmative commands and placed before negative commands as separate words. When the use of a pronoun results in the spoken stress being prior to the penultimate syllable, an accent mark is written.

    acostarse   ¡Acuéstate!   ¡No te acuestes!
                 —boca arriba (*face up*)
                 —boca abajo (*face down*)
    bañarse   ¡Báñate!   ¡No te bañes!
    lavarse   ¡Lávate las manos!   ¡No te laves las manos!
    levantarse   ¡Levántate!   ¡No te levantes!
    moverse   ¡Muévete!   ¡No te muevas!
    virarse   ¡Vírate!   ¡No te vires!

*Note that we have chosen to practice the informal register commands in the context of labor and delivery. You'll still choose to use the formal or informal register with any individual patient. However, frequently in the labor and delivery area the patient is younger and has an existing relationship with the health care provider.

- Here are eight commonly used irregular verbs.*

decir	¡Di!	¡No digas!
hacer	¡Haz!	¡No hagas!
ir	¡Ve!	¡No vayas!
poner	¡Pon!	¡No pongas!
salir	¡Sal!	¡No salgas!
ser	¡Sé!	¡No seas!
tener	¡Ten!	¡No tengas!
venir	¡Ven!	¡No vengas!

*Some students have employed the mnemonic device *Ven di sal haz ten ve pon.*

HACIA PRECISIÓN

12.11 Ejercicio_____

Escriba los imperativos informales que mejor completen las siguientes oraciones afirmativas y negativas.

A. (hacer)   No _____ la cita para hoy. _____ la cita para mañana.

B. (salir)   _____ temprano de la casa. No _____ tarde.

C. (ir)   _____ al consultorio. No _____ al hospital.

D. (bañar)   No _____ al bebé hoy. _____ al bebé mañana.

E. (bañarse)   No _____ hoy. _____ mañana.

F. (ponerse)   _____ la bata del hospital. No _____ ropa interior.

G. (comer)   No _____ nada después de las once. _____ bien mañana.

12.12 Ejercicio_____

Complete los siguientes imperativos informales que son de frecuente uso en el área de partos.

A. ¡No _____ _____ (preocuparse)!

B. ¡_____ (relajarse)!

C. ¡No _____ (comer) nada!

D. Si tienes sed, ¡_____ (comer) pedacitos de hielo (*ice chips*)!

E. ¡_____ (empujar)!

F. ¡No _____ (empujar)!

G. ¡_____ (respirar)!

H. ¡No _____ (respirar)!

 12.13 Ejercicio _____

Complete las dos columnas con los imperativos afirmativos y negativos que faltan.

Imperativo informal afirmativo	*Imperativo informal negativo*
A. ¡_____!	A. ¡No te muevas!
B. ¡Levántate!	B. ¡_____!
C. ¡_____!	C. ¡No te vires!
D. ¡_____ hoy!	D. ¡No te bañes hoy!
E. ¡Come!	E. ¡_____!
F. ¡Acuéstate!	F. ¡_____!
G. ¡_____ el brazo!	G. ¡No levantes el brazo!
H. ¡Respira!	H. ¡_____!

HACIA FLUIDEZ

12.14 Actividad _____

Vamos a jugar *Simon Says*. El profesor va a decir —o no— *Simón dice* antes de dar un imperativo. La clase obedece (*obeys*) —o no— según las instrucciones. Note que ¡Muévete! significa *Move!* (*in general*) pero ¡Mueve el brazo! no es reflexivo porque indica la parte del cuerpo que uno debe mover. Aquí hay algunos imperativos para empezar el juego.

A. ¡Levántate!	E. ¡Abre la boca!
B. ¡No te levantes!	F. ¡Cierra los ojos!
C. ¡Siéntate!	G. ¡No muevas el dedo!
D. ¡Mueve la mano derecha!	H. ¡Levanta el pie izquierdo!

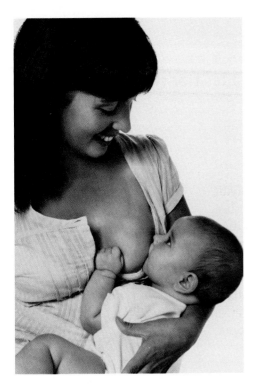

Dar el seno es dar amor.

Lectura: Después del parto—Consejos para las madres

Después del parto es normal sangrar por la vagina por dos o hasta tres semanas y tener una secreción rosada por más tiempo. Si sangra mucho o la
sangre es muy roja, acuéstese con los pies elevados por dos o tres horas. Si
la sangre continua, llame a su médico. No tenga relaciones sexuales por las prime-
ras seis semanas después del parto o hasta que su obstetra, ginecólogo o partera
le dé el permiso. Mientras la superficie del útero se sana del trauma del parto hay
más riesgo de infección.

Note that this is written in the formal register.

    Si amamanta al bebé debe de amamantarlo en el principio de ocho a doce
veces en veinticuatro horas. No se ponga a dieta. Necesita calorías y fluidos para
lactar (producir leche). Coma una dieta balanceada y siga tomando las vitaminas
prenatales.

Promote Safer Sex

Vocabulario: Las enfermedades transmitidas sexualmente

Las enfermedades

la ETS	STD
la clamidia	chlamydia
la gonorrea	gonorrhea
la hepatitis B, C	hepatitis B, C
el herpes	herpes
la enfermedad de VIH	HIV disease
el SIDA	AIDS
la sífilis	syphilis
la verruga venérea	genital wart, papiloma
el virus del papiloma humano	papiloma

Los síntomas

el ardor	burning sensation
las ampollas	blisters
el dolor al orinar	painful urination
el goteo	dripping
las lesiones	lesions
el flujo / la secreción	discharge, secretion
la orina oscura	dark-colored urine

Las prevenciones

abstenerse*	to abstain
el condón de látex**	latex condom
la educación	education
el examen pélvico	pelvic exam

*Conjugate verbs ending in *tener* just like the verb *tener*.

**La abstinencia es la única forma de evitar las enfermedades de transmisión sexual. Si no puede abstenerse, debe tener una relación sexual monógama con un/a compañero/a sano/a. Los condones de látex son efectivos contra el VIH.

Lectura: El SIDA *(AIDS)*

El Síndrome de Inmunodeficiencia Adquirida (SIDA) es una enfermedad muy grave que daña las defensas del cuerpo. Daña la capacidad que tiene el cuerpo para combatir infecciones. Hay un virus llamado VIH (uve-i-hache) que causa el SIDA. Una persona puede tener el virus por muchos años sin estar enferma o tener los síntomas del SIDA. Una persona infectada que no tiene síntomas del SIDA—*un/a portador/a sano/a* del SIDA—puede transmitir el virus a otra persona. Algunos de los síntomas del SIDA son inflamación de los ganglios linfáticos, fiebre persistente sin explicación, sudores nocturnos, una pérdida rápida de peso, fatiga constante, diarrea persistente y manchas blancas en la boca (infección por hongos, o *thrush* en inglés). Hay otras enfermedades que pueden causar estos síntomas y si alguien tiene estos síntomas es posible que no tenga el SIDA. Si usted tiene algunos de estos síntomas sin una buena explicación, hágase una cita con un médico.

dañar
to damage

ganglios linfáticos
lymph glands
sudores nocturnos
night sweats
manchas blancas
white patches

La educación es la mejor defensa contra el SIDA. Es importante saber cómo defenderse. La manera más segura es abstenerse. Si tiene relaciones, es importante tenerlas con una sola persona y saber que esa persona es sana. La comunicación entre parejas es esencial. Hay que hablar con la pareja acerca del SIDA y acerca de su historia sexual. Es muy peligroso tener relaciones sexuales con una persona que se inyecta drogas, o con varias personas. Es importante usar un condón de látex. Debe tener una prueba del VIH antes de planear el embarazo. Una madre infectada puede transmitir el virus al bebé.

abstenerse
to abstain

Es peligroso inyectarse drogas porque las jeringuillas pueden transmitir el SIDA. Para estar saludable, deje de usar las drogas, no use las jeringuillas de otra persona y no comparta las jeringuillas. Si va a usar una jeringuilla más de una vez, lávela con una solución de cloro (Clorox) y agua y después enjuáguela con agua. Hágalo cada vez que la usa.

1. Hable con la pareja sobre el SIDA.
2. Use un condón de látex cada vez que tiene contacto sexual.
3. No use drogas. Si usa drogas, no comparta jeringuillas. Lávelas con una solución de cloro y agua y enjuáguelas con agua.

El SIDA no puede ser transmitido por contacto casual. Compartir comida, usar baños públicos, o abrazarse con una persona infectada no es peligroso.

abrazarse
to hug

Todavía no hay cura para el SIDA pero sí hay tratamiento. Hay drogas antivirales que extienden la vida. Si tiene síntomas del SIDA, es muy importante hablar con el médico o ir a una clínica.

HACIA FLUIDEZ

 12.15 Actividad _____

Con un/a compañero/a confirme su comprensión de la lectura. Contesten las preguntas usando oraciones completas.

    A. ¿Qué es el SIDA, y qué lo causa?
    B. ¿Cuáles son los síntomas del SIDA?
    C. ¿Cuál es la mejor defensa contra el SIDA?
    D. ¿Con quién se debe hablar sobre el SIDA?
    E. ¿Por qué se debe usar un condón de látex?
    F. Si se inyecta drogas, ¿cómo debe lavar la jeringuilla?
    G. ¿Se puede transmitir el SIDA al usar baños públicos?
    H. ¿Hay cura para el SIDA?
    I. ¿Cuándo debe consultarse con un médico?

 12.16 Actividad _____

Con un/a compañero/a haga y conteste las siguientes preguntas y así practique cómo educar a un/a paciente sobre la protección sexual.

    A. ¿Cuál es la manera más segura de evitar las enfermedades de transmisión sexual?
    B. ¿Siempre tienen síntomas las enfermedades transmitidas sexualmente?
    C. ¿Cuáles son algunos de los síntomas de las enfermedades de transmisión sexual?
    D. ¿Qué debe hacer si se tiene algunos de los síntomas?
    E. ¿Quién debe ir al médico o a una clínica regularmente para hacerse un análisis de sangre?
    F. Si tengo relaciones sexuales con varias personas, ¿qué protección debo usar?

 12.17 Actividad _____

Usted es enfermero/a en una clínica del Departamento de Salud Pública. Su compañero/a es un/a paciente que pide una prueba de VIH. Prepare y presente a la clase una entrevista educativa.

12.18 Drama improvisado ⎯⎯⎯⎯⎯⎯⎯⎯⎯⎯⎯⎯⎯⎯⎯⎯

Un/a estudiante dramatiza la vida de Víctor L. Virus, y la clase lo entrevista sobre su vida interesante. Aquí hay algunas posibles preguntas, pero la clase puede inventar sus propias preguntas también. Víctor contesta ad lib.

A. ¿Eres introvertido o extrovertido?
B. ¿Conoces a mi hermano?
C. ¿Tienes una personalidad contagiosa?
D. ¿Qué te gusta hacer?

Victor L. Virus

E. ¿Te gustan las personas que beben? ¿Por qué?
F. ¿Con qué frecuencia te lavas las manos? ¿Debo lavarme las manos frecuentemente?
G. Dicen que tu primera novia no era lo que esperabas. ¿Qué pasó?
H. Si tú y yo salimos una noche, ¿qué debo esperar? ¿Hay algo que no debemos usar?
I. ¿Es verdad que a veces usted duerme por mucho tiempo y al despertarse quiere reproducir?

HACIA FLUIDEZ

 12.19 Reciclaje ⎯⎯⎯⎯⎯⎯⎯⎯⎯⎯⎯⎯⎯⎯⎯⎯⎯⎯⎯

Ahora saben usar los imperativos informales. Haga una lista de expresiones comunes a varios especialidades. Puedes incluir su propia especialidad si no está ya incluida en la lista.

Modelo: El ortopedista: Mantén la pierna elevada. No le hagas peso.

El radiólogo:_____

El nutricionista:_____

El farmacéutico: _____

El higienista dental: _____

El alergólogo: _____

La especialidad de usted: _____

12.20 Reciclaje ⎯⎯⎯⎯⎯⎯⎯⎯⎯⎯⎯⎯⎯⎯⎯⎯⎯⎯⎯⎯⎯⎯⎯⎯⎯⎯

En caso de usar el registro informal con sus pacientes, vamos a practicar los imperativos informales en varios contextos. Use los imperativos informales para dar estas instrucciones.

Modelo: Don't stand up.   ¡No te levantes!

A. Take the medicine every day without fail.

(tomar) ⎯⎯⎯⎯⎯⎯⎯⎯⎯⎯⎯⎯⎯⎯⎯⎯⎯⎯⎯⎯⎯⎯⎯⎯⎯⎯⎯⎯⎯⎯⎯⎯

B. Shake the medicine before using.

(agitar) ⎯⎯⎯⎯⎯⎯⎯⎯⎯⎯⎯⎯⎯⎯⎯⎯⎯⎯⎯⎯⎯⎯⎯⎯⎯⎯⎯⎯⎯⎯⎯

C. Call the clinic tomorrow.

(llamar) ⎯⎯⎯⎯⎯⎯⎯⎯⎯⎯⎯⎯⎯⎯⎯⎯⎯⎯⎯⎯⎯⎯⎯⎯⎯⎯⎯⎯⎯⎯⎯

D. Use the insulin after eating.

(usar) ⎯⎯⎯⎯⎯⎯⎯⎯⎯⎯⎯⎯⎯⎯⎯⎯⎯⎯⎯⎯⎯⎯⎯⎯⎯⎯⎯⎯⎯⎯⎯⎯⎯

E. Make an appointment with the dietitian.

(hacer) ⎯⎯⎯⎯⎯⎯⎯⎯⎯⎯⎯⎯⎯⎯⎯⎯⎯⎯⎯⎯⎯⎯⎯⎯⎯⎯⎯⎯⎯⎯⎯⎯

F. Do not eat anything after midnight.

(comer) ⎯⎯⎯⎯⎯⎯⎯⎯⎯⎯⎯⎯⎯⎯⎯⎯⎯⎯⎯⎯⎯⎯⎯⎯⎯⎯⎯⎯⎯⎯⎯

G. Do not consume fried food.

(consumir) ⎯⎯⎯⎯⎯⎯⎯⎯⎯⎯⎯⎯⎯⎯⎯⎯⎯⎯⎯⎯⎯⎯⎯⎯⎯⎯⎯⎯⎯

H. Follow a low-sodium diet.

(seguir) ⎯⎯⎯⎯⎯⎯⎯⎯⎯⎯⎯⎯⎯⎯⎯⎯⎯⎯⎯⎯⎯⎯⎯⎯⎯⎯⎯⎯⎯⎯⎯

I. Breathe deeply.

(respirar) ⎯⎯⎯⎯⎯⎯⎯⎯⎯⎯⎯⎯⎯⎯⎯⎯⎯⎯⎯⎯⎯⎯⎯⎯⎯⎯⎯⎯⎯⎯

J. Roll over.

(virarse) ⎯⎯⎯⎯⎯⎯⎯⎯⎯⎯⎯⎯⎯⎯⎯⎯⎯⎯⎯⎯⎯⎯⎯⎯⎯⎯⎯⎯⎯⎯⎯

Exposición

CHAPTER 12 SKILL: INTEGRATING AND CONSOLIDATING YOUR WRITING SKILLS

You are going to listen to an obstetrician ask questions and explain activities that are specific to an OB/GYN history and exam. You'll then write a similar interview with a classmate and present it to the class.

1. Listen to the obstetrician ask and answer questions. Take notes on the kinds of information that the doctor requests and provides. Write down at least five different kinds of information.

_____

_____

_____

_____

_____

2. Now, work with a classmate to make a list of the medical history, symptoms, aggravating factors, alleviating factors, physical exam activities, medications, and follow-up tests and procedures that are specific to your current or future area of practice. Together, create an algorithm of questions and instructions that is personalized to you and your partner's practice. Recall that you have learned vocabulary and structures for clarifying the chief complaint, taking a history of illness and treatment, writing medication instructions, and educating a patient about a variety of diagnoses, tests, and procedures. The list below will guide you relative to the location of these topics in the book (chapter numbers appear in parentheses).

¿Qué le pasa? (3)
¿Están vivos sus padres? ¿De qué murieron? (5)
¿Qué enfermedades hay en su familia? (5)
¿Toma algún medicamento o remedio casero todos los días? (6)
¿Es usted alérgico/a a algún medicamento? (6)
¿Con qué frecuencia . . . ? ¿Desde cuándo . . . ? (8)
¿Cuánto tiempo hace que . . . ? ¿Cuánto tiempo dura . . . ? (8)
¿Qué le ayuda? ¿Qué le mejora? ¿Qué le empeora? (8)
¿Qué pasó? ¿Qué ocurría cuando eso pasó? (9)

¿Cuándo fue la última vez que . . . ? (9)
¿De qué enfermedades padece usted? (10)
¿Ha tenido (enfermedad)? ¿Ha tenido cirugía? (10)
¿Ha estado hospitalizado alguna vez? ¿Para qué? (11)
¿Ha estado embarazada? (12)

3. Now write your presentation in the form of an interview. As you write, make use of some of the writing strategies you have learned in previous chapters, such as presenting and organizing information, describing, explaining, and creating and making presentations. Practice this with a classmate "patient," who should make up responses and thereby avoid disclosing personal information.

4. Your instructor may ask to see your final project and invite you to perform it in front of the class.

Cultural Note: Communication about Sexual Matters

El parto es la única cita a ciegas donde conoces el amor de tu vida
(Childbirth is the only blind date where you meet the love of your life)

At times, patients do not easily embrace the goals of health professionals in their teaching about safer sex. Many Latino families do not speak openly about sexual matters. Traditionally, the Catholic Church has disapproved of most forms of contraception. When educating patients about sex, the health care provider should assess and then respect the values of the patient prior to presenting new information in a nonjudgmental manner. Such respect is crucial.

Discussion of gender roles can uncover conflict in the individual and in his or her family. Many adults heard during childhood the refrain, *La mujer es de la casa y el hombre de la calle* (the woman is of the house and the man is of the street). This traditional double standard may pressure women to live at home until marriage, to remain chaste, and to value childbearing more than higher education and a career. The first- or second-generation female immigrant may feel caught between her traditional values and what she perceives to be a different norm in the United States. She may feel guilty over seeking sexual fulfillment as a single woman and insecure about asserting herself in business. She may not speak openly about being sexually active, except when confidentiality is assured. Other required yet sometimes taboo topics in sex education include homosexual behavior, alcoholism, and substance abuse. Raise these in a private setting, and do so only after establishing rapport with the patient.

De padre sano, hijo honrado
(Good fathers make honorable children)

Most hospitals teach childbirth classes to couples using techniques designed by the French physician Fernand Lamaze. These include training the father or a friend to give support to the mother during childbirth. This has practically eradicated the medicated birth, especially the use of twilight and general anesthesia. Latinos are generally eager to participate as couples in this preparation. However, not all do so because the classes are not always available in Spanish when needed and because the practice is not yet as widespread in many of the countries from which the patients have emigrated. In poorer or more densely populated areas, the presence of several deliveries in one room contraindicates the participation of fathers because of modesty.

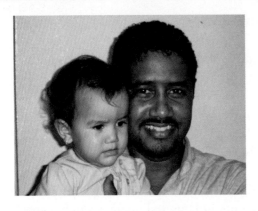

Manuel Franjul Peña cuida a su hija
Ana Camila Franjul Medina.

Some Latinas do not communicate to their partner the expectation that he will take part in the delivery, and some men do not feel comfortable with the idea. Sexual topics are not traditionally discussed in the home. One man standing outside the room in which his wife was in labor admitted that he wanted to be in the room but would not enter because there were female relatives inside who would presumably know more about what to do.

At times the difference in participation between non-Latino and Latino men is not fully understood by health care providers as a difference in tradition. Assessing and understanding the individual family's cultural norms will enable the health care provider to begin the educational process from the perspective of the patient, her partner, and the family. This increases empathy, and may alleviate a father's discomfort in the delivery room.

Vocabulario del capítulo 12

La menstruación

menstruar	to menstruate
el período, la regla	period
la ovulación	ovulation
el calambre	cramp
el coágulo	clot
la menopausia, el cambio	menopause, the change

El embarazo

estar embarazada, estar encinta	to be pregnant
embarazo ectópico	ectopic pregnancy
el aborto provocado	abortion
el aborto natural, el aborto espontáneo	miscarriage
el parto	delivery
la cesárea	C-section

Las pruebas

la prueba del embarazo	pregnancy test
la sonografía, el ultrasonido, el ecograma	ultrasound
la prueba de Pap/Papanicolaou	Pap test

Posibles complicaciones

los tobillos o pies hinchados	swollen ankles or feet
la cara o manos hinchadas	swollen face or hands
el dolor de cabeza severo	severe headache
los problemas con la vista	vision problems
el vómito persistente	persistent vomiting
el dolor cuando orina	painful urination
diabetes del embarazo	gestational diabetes
poco líquido amniótico	insufficient amniotic fluid
la secreción / el flujo vaginal	vaginal secretion
el sangramiento vaginal	vaginal bleeding
la placenta previa	placenta previa
la preeclampsia	preeclampsia

El parto

nacer	to be born
romper fuente, romper la bolsa de agua	to break water
la presentación de nalgas	breech position
las contracciones del útero	contractions
la dilatación del cuello del útero	dilation of the cervix
el monitoreo fetal	fetal monitor

dar a luz, parir, alumbrar   to deliver
el parto, el alumbramiento   delivery
el parto vaginal, el parto espontáneo   vaginal, spontaneous delivery
el parto prematuro   premature delivery
la cesárea   C-section
los dolores del parto   labor pains
la episiotomía   episiotomy
la placenta   placenta
el medicamento epidural para el dolor   epidural medication for pain
el medicamento para adelantar el parto   medication to advance the delivery
dar el seno, dar el pecho, amamantar   to breastfeed
la unidad para cuidados intensivos   neonatal intensive care unit
   neonatales
¡Es un niño! ¡Es una niña!   It's a boy! It's a girl!
¡Felicidades!   Congratulations!

Las enfermedades transmitidas sexualmente
la ETS   STD
la clamidia   chlamydia
la gonorrea   gonorrhea
la hepatitis B, C   hepatitis B, C
el herpes   herpes
la enfermedad de VIH   HIV disease
el SIDA   AIDS
la sífilis   syphilis
la verruga venérea   genital wart, papiloma
el virus del papiloma humano   papiloma

Los síntomas
el ardor   burning sensation
las ampollas   blisters
el dolor al orinar   painful urination
el goteo   dripping
las lesiones   lesions
el flujo / la secreción   discharge, secretion
la orina oscura   dark-colored urine

Las prevenciones
abstenerse   to abstain
el condón de látex   latex condom
la educación   education
el examen pélvico   pelvic exam

Preguntas útiles

¿Menstrua usted?	Do you menstruate?
¿Menstrua usted todavía?	Do you still menstruate?
¿Cuándo comenzó su último período?	When did your last period start?
¿Son regulares sus períodos?	Are your periods regular?
¿Tiene relaciones sexuales?	Are you sexually active?
¿Sangra más que lo normal?	Do you bleed more than usual?
¿Es su primer embarazo?	Is [this] your first pregnancy?
¿Cuántos embarazos ha tenido?	How many pregnancies have you had?
¿Ha subido de peso?	Have you gained weight?

Appendix 1

El abecedario
(The Spanish Alphabet)

Knowing the alphabet in Spanish (also called *el alfabeto*) will help you spell words aloud and conduct vision exams. To ask how the name Baldemira is spelled, use *¿Cómo se escribe Baldemira?* or *¿Cómo se deletrea Baldemira?* Currently there are 27 letters in the Spanish alphabet.

Letra	Nombre	Letra	Nombre	Letra	Nombre
a	a	j	jota	r	ere
b	be	k	ka	s	ese
c	ce	l	ele	t	te
d	de	m	eme	u	u
e	e	n	ene	v	uve
f	efe	ñ	eñe	w	uve doble
g	ge	o	o	x	equis
h	hache	p	pe	y	ye
i	i	q	cu	z	zeta

Some grammars include *rr* in the alphabet. The fourth edition of the *Diccionario académico* (1803) included *ch* and *ll* in the alphabet. Although these letters are digraphs (comprised of two letters each), they are considered letters because each represents a single sound. Words beginning with these two digraphs occupied their own sections in Spanish dictionaries until 1994, when the Asociación de Academias de la Lengua Española reordered those words into their places in the universal Latin alphabet. Now, words beginning with *ch* are found between words that begin with *ce* and those that begin with *ci,* and words beginning with *ll* are placed between words that begin with *li* and those that begin with *lo.* In 2010 the Real Academia Española changed the name of the letter *y* from *i griega* (Greek i) to *ye.* This eliminated the need to call the letter *i* by the name *i latina* (Latin i).

Appendix 2

A Guide to Some Irregular and Stem-Changing Verbs

Most of these verbs and morphologies have been introduced in the text. They are included here as a reference and for further study. The future tense expresses action that will happen in the future, as in *Me acostaré temprano el domingo* (I shall go to bed early on Sunday). Recall that in the text you learned to use the expression *ir + a + infinitivo* to tell the near future, as in *Voy a acostarme temprano esta noche.*

acostarse (o–ue)   to lie down, to go to bed

present	me acuesto, te acuestas, se acuesta, nos acostamos, se acuestan
preterit	me acosté, te acostaste, se acostó, nos acostamos, se acostaron
imperfect	me acostaba, te acostabas, se acostaba, nos acostábamos, se acostaban
future	me acostaré, te acostarás, se acostará, nos acostaremos, se acostarán
usted command	¡Acuéstese! ¡No se acueste!
tú command	¡Acuéstate! ¡No te acuestes!
past participle	acostado

almorzar (o–ue)   to eat lunch

present	almuerzo, almuerzas, almuerza, almorzamos, almuerzan
preterit	almorcé, almorzaste, almorzó, almorzamos, almorzaron
imperfect	almorzaba, almorzabas, almorzaba, almorzábamos, almorzaban
future	almorzaré, almorzarás, almorzará, almorzaremos, almorzarán
usted command	¡Almuerce! ¡No almuerce!
tú command	¡Almuerza! ¡No almuerces!
past participle	almorzado

comenzar (e–ie)   to begin

present	comienzo, comienzas, comienza, comenzamos, comienzan
preterit	comencé, comenzaste, comenzó, comenzamos, comenzaron
imperfect	comenzaba, comenzabas, comenzaba, comenzábamos, comenzaban
future	comenzaré, comenzarás, comenzará, comenzaremos, comenzarán
usted command	¡Comience! ¡No comience!
tú command	¡Comienza! ¡No comiences!
past participle	comenzado

dar   to give

present	doy, das, da, damos, dan
preterit	di, diste, dio, dimos, dieron
imperfect	daba, dabas, daba, dábamos, daban
future	daré, darás, dará, daremos, darán
usted command	¡Dé! ¡No dé!
tú command	¡Da! ¡No dés!
past participle	dado

decir   to say, to tell

present	digo, dices, dice, decimos, dicen
preterit	dije, dijiste, dijo, dijimos, dijeron
future	diré, dirás, dirá, diremos, dirán
imperfect	decía, decías, decía, decíamos, decían
usted command	¡Diga! ¡No diga!
tú command	¡Di ¡No digas!
past participle	dicho

despertarse (e–ie)   to wake up

present	me despierto, te despiertas, se despierta, nos despertamos, se despiertan
preterit	me desperté, te despertaste, se despertó, nos despertamos, se despertaron
imperfect	me despertaba, te despertabas, se despertaba, nos despertábamos, se despertaban
future	me despertaré, te despertarás, se despertará, nos despertaremos, se despertarán
usted command	¡Despiértese! ¡No se despierte!
tú command	¡Despiértate! ¡No te despiertes!
past participle	despierto

dormir (o–ue)   to sleep

present	duermo, duermes, duerme, dormimos, duermen
preterit	dormí, dormiste, durmió, dormimos, durmieron
imperfect	dormía, dormías, dormía, dormíamos, dormían
future	dormiré, dormirás, dormirá, dormiremos, dormirán
usted command	¡Duérmase! ¡No se duerma!
tú command	¡Duérmete! ¡No te duermas!
past participle	dormido

estar   to be

present	estoy, estás, está, estamos, están
preterit	estuve, estuviste, estuvo, estuvimos, estuvieron
imperfect	estaba, estabas, estaba, estábamos, estaban
future	estaré, estarás, estará, estaremos, estarán
usted command	¡Esté! ¡No esté!
tú command	¡Está! ¡No estés!
past participle	estado

hacer   to do, to make

present	hago, haces, hace, hacemos, hacen
preterit	hice, hiciste, hizo, hicimos, hicieron
imperfect	hacía, hacías, hacía, hacíamos, hacían
future	haré, harás, hará, haremos, harán
usted command	¡Haga! ¡No haga!
tú command	¡Haz! ¡No hagas!
past participle	hecho

ir   to go

present	voy, vas, va, vamos, van
preterit	fui, fuiste, fue, fuimos, fueron
imperfect	iba, ibas, iba, íbamos, iban
future	iré, irás, irá, iremos, irán
usted command	¡Vaya! ¡No vaya!
tú command	¡Ve! ¡No vayas!
past participle	ido

poder (o–ue)   to be able

present	puedo, puedes, puede, podemos, pueden
preterit	pude, pudiste, pudo, pudimos, pudieron
imperfect	podía, podías, podía, podíamos, podían
future	podré, podrás, podrá, podremos, podrán
past participle	podido

poner   to put, to place

present	pongo, pones, pone, ponemos, ponen
preterit	puse, pusiste, puso, pusimos, pusieron
imperfect	ponía, ponías, ponía, poníamos, ponían
future	pondré, pondrás, pondrá, pondremos, pondrán
usted command	¡Ponga! ¡No ponga!
tú command	¡Pon! ¡No pongas!
past participle	puesto

preferir (e–ie)   to prefer

present	prefiero, prefieres, prefiere, preferimos, prefieren
preterit	preferí, preferiste, prefirió, preferimos, prefirieron
imperfect	prefería, preferías, prefería, preferíamos, preferían
future	preferiré, preferirás, preferirá, preferiremos, preferirán
usted command	¡Prefiera! ¡No prefiera!
tú command	¡Prefiere! ¡No prefieras!
past participle	preferido

querer (e–ie)   to want, to like

present	quiero, quieres, quiere, queremos, quieren
preterit	quise, quisiste, quiso, quisimos, quisieron
imperfect	quería, querías, quería, queríamos, querían
future	querré, querrás, querrá, querremos, querrán
usted command	¡Quiera! ¡No quiera!
tú command	¡Quiere! ¡No quieras!
past participle	querido

saber   to know

present	sé, sabes, sabe, sabemos, saben
preterit	supe, supiste, supo, supimos, supieron
imperfect	sabía, sabías, sabía, sabíamos, sabían
future	sabré, sabrás, sabrá, sabremos, sabrán
usted command	¡Sepa! ¡No sepa!
tú command	¡Sabe! ¡No sepas!
past participle	sabido

sentarse (e–ie)   to sit down

present	me siento, te sientas, se sienta, nos sentamos, se sientan
preterit	me senté, te sentaste, se sentó, nos sentamos, se sentaron
imperfect	me sentaba, te sentabas, se sentaba, nos sentábamos, se sentaban
future	me sentaré, te sentarás, se sentará, nos sentaremos, se sentarán
usted command	¡Siéntese! ¡No se siente!
tú command	¡Siéntate! ¡No te sientes!
past participle	sentado

sentirse (e–ie)   to feel

present	me siento, te sientes, se siente, nos sentimos, se sienten
preterit	me sentí, te sentiste, se sintió, nos sentimos, se sintieron
imperfect	me sentía, te sentías, se sentía, nos sentíamos, se sentían
future	me sentiré, te sentirás, se sentirá, nos sentiremos, se sentirán
usted command	¡Siéntase! ¡No se sienta!
tú command	¡Siéntete! ¡No te sientas!
past participle	sentido

ser   to be

present	soy, eres, es, somos, son
preterit	fui, fuiste, fue, fuimos, fueron
imperfect	era, eras, era, éramos, eran
future	seré, serás, será, seremos, serán
usted command	¡Sea! ¡No sea!
tú command	¡Sé! ¡No seas!
past participle	sido

tener   to have

present	tengo, tienes, tiene, tenemos, tienen
preterit	tuve, tuviste, tuvo, tuvimos, tuvieron
imperfect	tenía, tenías, tenía, teníamos, tenían
future	tendré, tendrás, tendrá, tendremos, tendrán
usted command	¡Tenga! ¡No tenga!
tú command	¡Ten! ¡No tengas!
past participle	tenido

venir   to come

present	vengo, vienes, viene, venimos, vienen
preterit	vine, viniste, vino, vinimos, vinieron
imperfect	venía, venías, venía, veníamos, venían
future	vendré, vendrás, vendrá, vendremos, vendrán
usted command	¡Venga! ¡No venga!
tú command	¡Ven! ¡No vengas!
past participle	venido

vestirse (e–i)   to dress oneself

present	me visto, te vistes, se viste, nos vestimos, se visten
preterit	me vestí, te vestiste, se vistió, nos vestimos, se vistieron
imperfect	me vestía, te vestías, se vestía, nos vestíamos, se vestían
future	me vestiré, te vestirás, se vestirá, nos vestiremos, se vestirán
usted command	¡Vístase! ¡No se vista!
tú command	¡Vístete! ¡No te vistas!
past participle	vestido

English to Spanish Glossary

The translations in this glossary are generally limited to the context in which the words are used in the book. The abbreviation (*v*) indicates a verb, and (*f*) indicates feminine.

a

abdomen **el abdomen**
able (to be able) (*v*) **poder** (o–ue)
abortion **el aborto (provocado, espontáneo)**
about **sobre**
abrasion **la abrasión**
abstain (*v*) **abstener** (conjugate like *tener*)
abstinence **la abstinencia**
accident **el accidente**
accuracy **la precisión**
acetaminophen **el acetaminofén**
ache **el dolor sordo**
ache (*v*) **doler** (o–ue)
active **activo/a**
acute **agudo/a**
addict **el/la adicto/a**
addiction **la adicción**
address **la dirección**
admission (hospital) **el internamiento, la estadía**
admit (*v*) **internar, hospitalizar, dar de baja**
adrenaline **la adrenalina**
advance (*v*) **adelantar**
aerosol **el aerosol**
after **después de**
afternoon **la tarde**
afterward **después**

age **la edad**
agitated **agitado/a**
AIDS **el SIDA**
ailment **el padecimiento, la enfermedad**
air **el aire**
— pollution **la contaminación del aire**
alcohol **el alcohol**
alcoholism **el alcoholismo**
alive **vivo/a**
allergen **el alérgeno**
allergic **alérgico/a**
allergy **la alergia**
aloe vera **la sábila**
also **también**
always **siempre**
Alzheimer's disease **la enfermedad de Alzheimer**
ambulance **la ambulancia**
ambulatory **ambulatorio/a**
American **americano/a**
Americanized **americanizado/a**
amnesia **la amnesia**
amniotic fluid **el líquido amniótico**
amount **la cantidad**
analgesic **analgésico/a**
analysis **el análisis**
anaphylactic shock **el shock anafiláctico**
anaphylaxis **la anafilaxis**
and **y**
anemia **la anemia**

anesthesia **la anestesia**
anesthesiologist **el/la anestesiólogo/a**
aneurysm **el aneurisma**
anger **el enojo, el enfado**
anger (*v*) **enojar(se), enfadar(se)**
angina pectoris **la angina de pecho**
angiogram **el angiograma**
angry **enojado/a, enfadado/a**
animal **el animal**
   — dander **la caspa de animal**
anise **el anís**
ankle **el tobillo**
annoy (*v*) **molestar**
annoyance **la molestia**
annoyed **enfadado/a**
answer (*v*) **contestar**
antacid **el antiácido**
antibiotic **el antibiótico**
antibody **el anticuerpo**
anticholinergic **el anticolinérgico**
anticoagulant **el anticoagulante**
anticonvulsant **el anticonvulsivo**
antidepressant **el antidepresivo**
antidiarrheal **el antidiarreico**
antihistamine **el antihistamínico**
antihyperglycemic **el antihiperglucémico**
antiinflammatory **el antiinflamatorio**
antipyretic **el antipirético**
antispasmodic **el antiespasmódico**
anus **el ano**
anxiety **la ansiedad**
anxious **ansioso/a, nervioso/a**
anyone **alguien**
apoplexy **la apoplejía**
appendectomy **la apendectomía**
appendicitis **la apendicitis**
appendix **el apéndice**
appetite **el apetito**
apple **la manzana**
apply (*v*) **aplicar**
appointment **la cita**
April **abril**
area **el área** (*f*)
argue (*v*) **discutir, pelear**
arise (*v*) **levantar(se)**
arm **el brazo**
arrhythmia **la arritmia**
arrive (*v*) **llegar**
arthritis **la artritis**
arthroscopy **la artroscopia**

as, like **como**
ashamed **avergonzado/a**
ask (a question) (*v*) **preguntar**
ask (for something) (*v*) **pedir** (e–i)
asphyxia **la asfixia**
aspirin **la aspirina**
asthma **el asma** (*f*)
atomizer **el atomizador**
atrial fibrillation **la fibrilación auricular**
attack **el ataque**
   heart — **el ataque al corazón**
attentive **atento/a**
audiologist **el/la audiólogo/a**
audiology **audiología**
August **agosto**
aunt **la tía**
avocado **el aguacate**
avoid (*v*) **evitar**
awake **despierto/a**
awaken (*v*) **despertar(se)** (e–ie)

b

baby **el/la bebé**
   — teeth **los dientes de leche**
back **la espalda**
bacterial **bacteriano/a**
bacterium **la bacteria**
bad **malo/a**
badly **mal**
banana **la banana, el plátano, el guineo**
bandage **el vendaje, la tirita, la curita**
barbiturate **el barbitúrico**
bath **el baño**
bathe (*v*) **bañar(se)**
bathroom **el baño, el cuarto de baño**
be (*v*) **ser** (*irregular*), **estar** (*irregular*)
bean **el frijol, la habichuela, la judía**
because **porque**
bed **la cama**
bedpan **la silleta, el pato de cama**
beef **la carne de res**
beer **la cerveza**
before **antes de**
behind **detrás de**
believe (*v*) **creer**
benefit **el beneficio**
benign **benigno/a**
betrayed **traicionado/a**
better **mejor**

better (to get better) (v) **mejorar**
beverage **la bebida**
biceps **el bíceps braquial, el bíceps femoral**
bilingual **bilingüe**
biopsy **la biopsia**
birth **el nacimiento, el parto, el alumbramiento**
bite (of insect) **la picadura**
black **negro/a**
blackboard **la pizarra**
bladder **la vejiga**
blanket **la frazada**
bleed (v) **sangrar**
blind **ciego/a**
blister **la ampolla**
blond **rubio/a**
blood **la sangre**
  — pressure **la tensión arterial, la presión arterial, la presión sanguínea, la presión de la sangre**
blow **el golpe**
blow (v) **soplar**
board **la tabla**
body **el cuerpo**
boil (v) **hervir** (e–ie)
bone **el hueso**
bore (v) **aburrir**
bottle **la botella, el frasco**
  baby's — **el biberón, la tetera**
brain **el cerebro**
bread **el pan**
break (v) **quebrar, romper**
break water (v) **romper fuente**
breakfast **el desayuno**
breakfast (v) **desayunar**
breast **el seno**
breastfeed (v) **amamantar, dar el seno, dar el pecho**
breathe (v) **respirar**
breathing **la respiración**
breech position **la presentación de nalgas**
breeding area **el criadero**
broccoli **el brócoli**
bronchia **el bronquio**
bronchial **bronquial**
bronchoscopy **la broncoscopia**
broth **el caldo**
brother **el hermano**
brother-in-law **el cuñado**

brow **el ceño**
bruise **el moretón**
bruit **el soplo**
brunette **moreno/a**
brush **el cepillo**
brush (v) **cepillar(se)**
bump **el golpe**
bump (v) **golpear(se)**
burn **la quemadura**
burn (v) **quemar(se)**
burned **quemado/a**
burning sensation **el ardor**
butter **la mantequilla**
buttock **el glúteo, la nalga, el pompis**
buy (v) **comprar**
bypass **la desviación, la revascularización**

C

CABG (coronary artery bypass graft) **la desviación coronaria, la revascularización coronaria**
cake **la torta, el pastel, el bizcocho** (Carib.)
calcium **el calcio**
calf **la pantorrilla** (anat.)
call **la llamada**
call (v) **llamar**
calm (v), to calm down **calmar(se)**
calorie **la caloría**
can **la lata**
can (to be able) (v) **poder** (o–ue)
cancer **el cáncer**
candy **el dulce**
canned **enlatado/a**
capsule **la cápsula, la gragea**
car **el coche, el carro, el automóvil**
carbohydrate **el carbohidrato**
card **la tarjeta**
cardiac **cardíaco/a**
cardiologist **el/la cardiólogo/a**
cardiology **la cardiología**
cardiovascular disease **la enfermedad cardiovascular**
care **el cuidado**
care for (v) **cuidar**
carpal **carpiano/a**
carpet **la alfombra**

carpus **el carpo**
carrier (asymptomatic) **el portador (sano)**
carrot **la zanahoria**
carry (v) **llevar**
cast **el yeso**
cataract **la catarata**
catheter **la sonda, el catéter**
catheter (urinary) **la algalia, la sonda**
cavity **la caries, la caries dental**
cell **la célula**
cereal **el cereal**
cerebral **cerebral**
cerebral palsy **la parálisis cerebral**
cerebrovascular accident (CVA) **el ac-cidente cerebrovascular**
cervix **el cuello del útero, el cuello de la matriz**
cesarean, C-section **la cesárea**
Chaga's disease **el mal de Chaga**
chair **la silla**
cheek **la mejilla, el cachete**
cheekbone **el pómulo**
cheese **el queso**
chemotherapy **la quimioterapia**
chest **el pecho**
chest pain **el dolor del pecho**
chew (v) **masticar**
chewable **masticable**
chicken **el pollo**
    — pox **la varicela, la viruela loca**
chikungunya **el chikungunya**
child **el/la niño/a, el/la muchacho/a**
chills **los escalofríos**
chin **la barbilla**
Chinese **el chino** (*lang.*)
chlamydia **la clamidia**
chocolate **el chocolate**
cholecystectomy **la colecistectomía**
cholera **el cólera**
chronic **crónico/a**
cigarette **el cigarillo**
cinnamon **la canela**
cirrhosis **la cirrosis, la cirrosis hepática**
city **la ciudad**
clarify (v) **clarificar**
class **la clase**
classic **clásico/a**
clavicle **la clavícula**
clean **limpio/a**
clean (v) **limpiar**

cleaning **la limpieza**
clear **claro/a**
clinic **la clínica**
clinical **clínico/a**
close (v) **cerrar** (e–ie)
closed **cerrado/a**
clot **el coágulo, el émbolo**
clothes **la ropa**
clothing **la ropa**
cocaine **la cocaína**
coccyx **el cóccix**
cockroach **la cucaracha, el bicho**
coconut **el coco**
codeine **la codeína**
cold **frío/a**
cold (common cold) **el resfriado, el res-frío, el catarro, la monga** (*slang*)
colesterol **el colesterol**
colic **el cólico, los cólicos**
collide (v) **chocar**
collision **el choque**
colon **el colon**
colonoscopy **la colonoscopia**
color **el color**
colostomy **la colostomía**
comb **el peine**
comb (v) **peinar(se)**
come (v) **venir** (*irregular*)
comfortable **cómodo/a, confortable**
common **común**
complicated **complicado/a**
complication **la complicación**
concussion **la concusión**
condom **el condón, el preservativo**
confirm (v) **confirmar**
congestion **la congestión, el catarro**
congestive heart failure **la insuficiencia cardíaca**
congratulations **felicidades**
conjunctivitis **la conjuntivitis**
conscious **consciente**
constant **constante, continuo/a**
constipation **el estreñimiento**
consult **la consulta**
consult (v) **consultar**
content **contento/a**
contraceptive **el contraceptivo, el anticonceptivo**
contraction **la contracción**
convulsion **la convulsión**

cook **el/la cocinero/a**
cook (*v*) **cocinar**
COPD **la enfermedad pulmonar obstructiva crónica, el enfisema**
cope (*v*) **lidiar**
cotton ball **la bolita de algodón**
cough **la tos**
cough (*v*) **toser**
cough suppressant **el antitusígeno**
counselor **el/la consejero/a**
cover (*v*) **cubrir**
CPR **la reanimación cardiopulmonar**
cramp **el calambre**
cranium **el cráneo**
crash **el choque**
crash (*v*) **chocar**
crazy **loco/a**
cream **la crema, el ungüento**
crisis **la crisis**
crown **la corona**
crush (*v*) **polvorizar**
crushing **pesado/a**
crutch **la muleta**
cry (*v*) **llorar**
crying jag, weeping **el llanto**
CT scan **la tomografía computarizada**
culture (laboratory) **el cultivo**
curious **curioso/a**
current **actual**
custodian (legal) **el/la tutor/a**
custody **la custodia**
custom **la costumbre**
cut **el corte, la cortada, la cortadura, el tajo**
cut (*v*) **cortar(se)**
cyst **el quiste**

d

damage (*v*) **dañar**
dangerous **peligroso/a**
dark **oscuro/a**
date **la fecha**
daughter **la hija**
daughter-in-law **la nuera, la yerna**
day **el día**
day before yesterday **anteayer**
dead **muerto/a**
deaf **sordo/a**
deafness **la sordera**

death **la muerte**
decaffeinated **descafeinado/a**
December **diciembre**
decongestant **el descongestionante**
deep **profundo/a**
dehydration **la deshidratación**
deliver (a baby) (*v*) **dar a luz, parir, alumbrar**
delivery (birth) **el parto, el alumbramiento**
   premature — **el parto prematuro**
deltoid **deltoides**
delusion **el delirio**
demonstrate (*v*) **demostrar**
dengue **el dengue**
dental floss **el hilo dental**
dental hygienist **el/la higienista dental**
dentist **el/la dentista, el/la odontólogo/a**
dentistry **la odontología**
denture **la dentadura postiza**
dependence **la dependencia**
depressed **deprimido/a**
depression **la depresión**
dermatologist **el/la dermatólogo/a**
dermatology **la dermatología**
description **la descripción**
desk **el escritorio**
desperate **desesperado/a**
dessert **el postre**
diabetes **la diabetes**
   gestational — **la diabetes del embarazo**
diagnosis **el diagnóstico**
dialysis **la diálisis**
diarrhea **la diarrea**
die (*v*) **morir** (o–ue)
diet **la dieta, el plan de alimentación**
dietician **el/la dietista**
dilation **la dilación**
dilute (*v*) **deluir**
dine (*v*) **cenar**
dinner **la comida, la cena**
diphtheria **la difteria**
disabled **incapacitado/a, el/la inválido/a, con capacidades diferentes**
discover (*v*) **descubrir**
disease **la enfermedad**
disgusted **disgustado/a**
disheartened **descorazonado/a**
dislocation **la dislocación**

— of a bone **la luxación**
disorder **el trastorno**
distressed **angustiado/a**
diuretic **el diurético**
divorce **el divorcio**
divorce (*v*) **divorciarse**
divorced **divorciado/a**
dizziness **el mareo**
dizzy **mareado/a**
do, make (*v*) **hacer** (*irregular*)
doctor **el/la doctor/a, el/la médico/a**
doctor's office **el consultorio**
doll **la muñeca**
door **la puerta**
Down syndrome **el síndrome de Down**
dorsal **dorsal**
drain (surgical) **el drenaje**
drain (*v*) **drenar**
drained **agotado/a**
draw blood (*v*) **sacar sangre**
drill (dental) **la fresa dental, la pieza de mano**
drink **la bebida**
drink (*v*) **beber**
drip (*v*) **gotear**
dripping **el goteo**
drive (*v*) **manejar**
drop **la gota**
drug **la droga**
drunk **ebrio/a, borracho/a**
dry (*v*) **secar(se)**
dryness **la sequedad**
dust **el polvo**
dust mite **el ácaro del polvo**
dysentery **la disentería**

e

each, every **cada**
ear **el oído** (*inner*), **la oreja** (*outer*)
early **temprano**
eat (*v*) **comer**
ebola **el ébola**
echogram **el ecograma**
ectopic pregnancy **el embarazo ectópico**
eczema **el eccema**
egg **el huevo**
eighth **el/la octavo/a**
elbow **el codo**
elderly **mayor, anciano/a**

electrocardiogram **el electrocardiograma**
electroencephalogram **el electroencefalograma**
elevator **el ascensor**
eliminate (*v*) **eliminar**
elixir **el elixir**
embolism **la embolia, el émbolo**
emergency **la emergencia, la urgencia**
emergency room **la sala de urgencias**
emphysema **el enfisema**
enchanted **encantado/a**
end **el fin**
end (*v*) **terminar**
endocrinologist **el/la endocrinólogo/a**
endometriosis **la endometriosis**
endoscopy **la endoscopía**
English **el inglés** (*lang.*)
enrage (*v*) **enojar(se), enfogonar(se)** (*slang*)
enraged **enojado/a, enfogonado/a** (*slang*)
ENT doctor **el/la otorrinolaringólogo/a**
epilepsy **la epilepsia**
epinephrine **la epinefrina**
episiotomy **la episiotomía**
esophageal reflux **el reflujo esofágico**
esophagus **el esófago**
eucalyptus **el eucalipto**
ever **alguna vez**
every **cada**
exam **el examen**
examination **la examinación**
examine (*v*) **examinar**
exhale (*v*) **exhalar**
expectorant **el expectorante**
explain (*v*) **explicar**
exploratory **exploratorio/a**
extraction **la extracción**
eye **el ojo**
eyebrow **la ceja**
eyeglasses **los lentes, los anteojos**

f

face **la cara**
faint (*v*) **desmayar(se)**
fall (*v*) **caer(se)**
Fallopian tube **la trompa de Falopio**
false teeth **los dientes postizos, la dentadura, la caja de dientes, el puente** (*bridge*)

fan **el ventilador, el abanico** (Carib.)
far **lejos**
fascinate (*v*) **fascinar**
fast **rápido/a**
fast (*v*) **ayunar**
fat **gordo/a**
fat **la grasa**
fat-free **descremado/a**
father **el padre**
father-in-law **el suegro**
fatigue **el cansancio, la fatiga**
fear **el miedo**
February **febrero**
feces **la materia fecal, las heces, el excremento**
feed (*v*) **alimentar, dar de comer**
feel (*v*) **sentir(se)** (e–ie)
female **femenino/a, hembra**
femur **el fémur**
fetus **el feto**
fever **la fiebre**
fiber **la fibra**
fibula **el peroné**
fifth **el/la quinto/a**
fight (*v*) **luchar, pelear**
filling (dental) **el empaste**
film **la placa**
find (*v*) **encontrar** (o–ue)
fine **bien**
finger **el dedo**
fingernail **la uña**
first **el/la primero/a**
fish **el pescado**
fish (*v*) **pescar**
floor **el piso**
flow **el flujo**
flu **la gripe, la influenza**
fluid **el fluido**
fluoride **el fluoruro**
foam **la espuma**
folk healer **el/la espiritista, el/la curandero/a, el/la chamán**
follow (*v*) **seguir** (e–i)
food **el alimento, la comida**
foot **el pie**
forearm **el antebrazo**
forehead **la frente**
forget (*v*) **olvidar**
formula (baby) **la fórmula**
foster child **el/la hijo/a de crianza**

fourth **el/la cuarto/a**
fracture **la fractura**
   comminuted — **la fractura conminuta**
   compound — **la fractura compuesta**
   multiple — **la fractura múltiple**
   open — **la fractura abierta**
   simple — **la fractura simple**
   spiral — **la fractura espiral**
   transverse — **la fractura oblicua**
French **el francés** (*lang.*)
french fries **las papas fritas**
frequency **la frecuencia**
frequent **frecuente**
frequently **frecuentemente**
Friday **el viernes**
fried **frito/a**
fried food **la fritura**
friend **el/la amigo/a**
fright **el susto**
frighten (*v*) **asustar**
frightened **asustado/a**
from **de**
(in) front of **delante de, enfrente de**
frown (*v*) **fruncir**
frozen **helado/a**
fruit **la fruta**
frustrated **frustrado/a**
furious **furioso/a**

g

gallbladder **la vesícula biliar**
gallstone **el cálculo en la vesícula**
gasp (*v*) **jadear**
gasping **el jadeo**
gastritis **la gastritis**
gel **el gel**
gelatin **la gelatina**
generalist **el/la médico/a general, el/la generalista, el/la médico/a de cabecera**
generous **generoso/a**
genital wart **la verruga venérea**
geriatric **geriátrico/a**
geriatrician **el/la geriatra**
geriatrics **la geriatría**
German **el alemán** (*lang.*)
giardiasis **la infección por giardias**
ginger **el jengibre**
gingivitis **la gingivitis**
give (*v*) **dar** (*irregular*)

gland **la glándula**
glass **el vaso**
glaucoma **la glaucoma**
glove **el guante**
gluteus maximus **el glúteo mayor**
go (*v*) **ir** (*irregular*)
go to bed (*v*) **acostarse** (o–ue)
God **Dios**
godchild, godson, goddaughter **el/la ahijado/a**
godfather **el padrino**
godmother **la madrina**
gold **el oro**
golden **dorado/a**
gonorrhea **la gonorrea**
good **bueno/a**
good-bye **adiós**
gout **la gota**
grain **el grano**
grandchild **el/la nieto/a**
grandparent **el/la abuelo/a**
grape **la uva**
grapefruit **la toronja**
grease **la grasa**
great-aunt **la tía abuela**
great-grandchild **el/la bisnieto/a**
great-grandfather **el bisabuelo**
great-grandmother **la bisabuela**
great-uncle **el tío abuelo**
green **verde**
greenish **verdoso/a**
grind (*v*) **moler** (o–ue)
ground **molido/a, majado/a**
gum (anat.) **la encía**
gunshot wound **la herida de bala**
gynecologist **el/la ginecólogo/a**
gynecology **la ginecología**

h

hair **el pelo, el cabello**
half-brother **el medio hermano, el hermano de madre / de padre**
half-sister **la media hermana, la hermana de madre / de padre**
hallucination **la alucinación**
hallway **el pasillo**
hand **la mano**
handsome **guapo/a**
happen (*v*) **pasar**

happiness **la felicidad, la alegría**
happy **feliz, contento/a, alegre**
hard **duro/a**
hardworking **trabajador/a**
harm **el daño**
harm (*v*) **dañar**
have (*v*) **tener** (*irregular*)
he **él**
head **la cabeza**
head injury **la herida en la cabeza**
headache **el dolor de cabeza**
health **la salud**
hear (*v*) **oír**
hearing **el oído**
heart **el corazón**
   — attack **el ataque al corazón**
   — murmur **el soplo en el corazón**
height **la altura**
helicopter **el helicóptero**
hello **hola**
help **la ayuda**
help (*v*) **ayudar**
hemoglobinopathy **la hemoglobinopatía**
hemophilia **la hemofilia**
hemorrhage **la hemorragia**
hemorrhagic **hemorrágico/a**
hemorrhoids **las hemorroides**
hepatitis **la hepatitis**
here **aquí**
hernia **la hernia**
heroin **la heroína, la manteca** (*slang*)
herpes **el herpes**
herpes zoster **la culebrilla**
hip **la cadera**
history **la historia**
HIV **el VIH**
hives **las ronchas, el sarpullido, la urticaria**
Holter monitor **la supervisión Holter**
honey **la miel de abeja**
hope **la esperanza**
hope (*v*) **esperar**
   I hope so! **¡Ojalá!**
hopeless **desesperado/a**
hopelessness **la desesperación**
hospital **el hospital**
hospitalization **la hospitalización, el internamiento**
hour **la hora**
how? **¿cómo?**

how many? **¿cuántos/as?**
how much? **¿cuánto/a?**
humerus **el húmero**
hunger **el hambre**
hurt (*v*) **doler** (o–ue)
hypercholesterolemia **la hipercolesterolemia**
hyperglycemia **la hiperglucemia**
hypertension **la hipertensión, la presión alta**
hyperthyroidism **el hipertiroidismo**
hypoglycemia **la hipoglucemia**
hypotension **la hipotensión, la presión baja**
hypothyroidism **el hipotiroidismo**
hysterectomy **la histerectomía**

i

I **yo**
ibuprofen **el ibuprofeno**
ice **el hielo**
ice cream **el helado, el mantecado**
ilium **el íleon**
ill **enfermo/a**
illness **la enfermedad, el padecimiento**
implant **el implante**
implant (*v*) **implantar**
in front of **delante de, enfrente de**
inch **la pulgada**
incontinence **la incontinencia**
infarct **el infarto**
infarction **el infarto**
   miocardial — **el infarto de miocardio**
infect (*v*) **infectar**
infection **la infección**
inflame (*v*) **inflamar**
inflammation **la inflamación**
influenza **la influenza**
inhalation **la inhalación**
inhale (*v*) **inhalar**
inhaler **el inhalador, la pompa** (*slang*)
inject (*v*) **inyectar**
injection **la inyección**
injure (*v*) **lastimar, herir**
injury **la herida**
   traumatic — **la herida traumática, el traumatismo**
insomnia **el insomnio**
insufficiency **la insuficiencia**

insurance **el seguro**
   medical — **el plan médico**
intelligent **inteligente, listo/a**
intensive care **el cuidado intensivo**
intensive care unit **la unidad de cuidados intensivos**
interest (*v*) **interesar**
interested **interesado/a**
interesting **interesante**
internist **el/la médico/a internista**
intestinal **intestinal**
   — worm **la lombriz intestinal**
   — bug **el bicho intestinal**
intestine **el intestino**
   large — **el intestino grueso**
   small — **el intestino delgado**
intradermic **intradérmico/a**
intramuscular **intramuscular**
intravenous **intravenoso/a**
iron (Fe) **el hierro**
irritability **la irritabilidad**
ischemic heart disease **la cardiopatía isquémica**
Italian **el italiano** (*lang.*)
itch **la picazón, la comezón, el prurito**
itch (*v*) **picar, sentir comezón, sentir picazón**
IV fluid **el suero**

j

January **enero**
Japanese **el japonés** (*lang.*)
jaundice **la ictericia**
jaundiced **amarillento/a**
jaw **la mandíbula**
jealous **celoso/a**
job **el trabajo**
joint **la articulación, la coyuntura**
juice **el jugo, el zumo**
July **julio**
June **junio**

k

kidney **el riñón**
kidney stone **el cálculo en el riñón, la piedra en el riñón**
kill (*v*) **matar**
kilogram **el kilogramo**

kind **amable, simpático/a**
kitchen **la cocina**
knee **la rodilla**
kneecap **la patela, la rótula**
know (*v*) **saber** (*irregular*), **conocer**
　(*irregular*)
knuckle **el nudillo**

l

labor **el parto**
　— pain **el dolor del parto**
　to be in — **estar de parto**
laboratory **el laboratorio**
laceration **la laceración, la cortadura**
lactation **la lactancia**
language **el idioma, la lengua, el lenguaje**
laparoscopy **la laparoscopia**
lard **la manteca**
large **grande**
large intestine **el intestino grueso**
laser **el láser**
late **tarde**
later **luego**
latex **el látex**
laxative **el laxante**
learn (*v*) **aprender**
left **el/la izquierdo/a**
leg **la pierna**
lemon **el limón**
length of stay **la estadía**
leptospirosis **la leptospirosis**
leukemia **la leucemia**
lice **los piojos**
like (*v*) **gustar, querer** (e–ie)
like, as **como**
like this **así**
lime **el limón**
lip **el labio**
liquid **el líquido**
listen (*v*) **escuchar**
listen with a stethoscope (*v*) **auscultar**
lithium **el litio**
live (*v*) **vivir**
liver **el hígado**
lonely **solitario/a**
long **largo/a**
look (*v*) **mirar**
loose **flojo/a**
lose (*v*) **perder** (e–ie)

loss **la pérdida**
　— of consciousness **la pérdida de**
　　conocimiento
luck **la suerte**
　good — **la buena suerte**
lucky **dichoso/a**
lukewarm **tibio/a**
lump **la bolita, la pelotita**
lumpectomy **la lumpectomía**
lunch **el almuerzo**
lunch (*v*) **almorzar** (o–ue)
lung **el pulmón**
lymph gland **el ganglio linfático**

m

machine **la máquina**
make, do (*v*) **hacer** (*irregular*)
malaise **el malestar general**
malaria **el paludismo**
male **masculino/a, el varón**
malignant **maligno/a**
man **el hombre**
mango **el mango**
mania **la manía**
manic-depressive **el/la**
　maníacodepresivo/a
manner **la manera**
March **marzo**
married **casado/a**
marry (*v*) **casar(se)**
masseter **masetero**
mash (*v*) **majar**
maternal **materno/a**
matter (*v*) **importar**
May **el mayo**
meal **la comida**
measles **el sarampión**
　German — **la rubéola**
meat **la carne**
medical record **el expediente médico, la**
　historia médica
medication **el medicamento, la medicina**
medicine **la medicina**
meningitis **la meningitis**
menopause **la menopausia, el cambio de**
　vida
menstruate (*v*) **menstruar**
menstruation **la menstruación, la regla,**
　el período

mental illness **la enfermedad mental**

mental retardation **la discapacidad intelectual, la discapacidad del desarrollo**

metabolism **el metabolismo**

metacarpal **metacarpiano/a**

metacarpus **el metacarpo**

metastasis **la metástasis**

metatarsus **el metatarso**

midday **el mediodía**

midnight **la medianoche**

midwife **la comadrona, la partera**

migraine **la jaqueca, la migraña**

milk **la leche**

milligram **el miligramo**

millilitre **el mililitro**

mine **mío/a/os/as**

miocarditis **la miocarditis**

miscarriage **el aborto natural, la pérdida**

miss (*v*) **hacer falta** (*irregular*)

molar **la muela**

mold **el moho**

mole **el lunar**

Monday **el lunes**

money **el dinero, la plata**

monitor **el monitor**

monitor (*v*) **monitorear**

mononucleosis **la mononucleosis**

month **el mes**

monthly **mensual, mensualmente**

more **más**

   — or less **más o menos**

morning **la mañana**

mother **la madre**

mother-in-law **la suegra**

mouth **la boca**

move (*v*) **mover** (o–ue)

move up (*v*) **adelantar**

MRI **las imágenes por resonancia magnética**

MRSA **el estafilococo resistente a la meticilina, el estafilococo dorado**

mucolytic **el mucolítico**

mucus **el moco**

multiple sclerosis **la esclerosis múltiple**

mumps **la paperas**

muscle **el músculo**

muscular dystrophy **la distrofia muscular**

my **mi, mis**

n

name **el nombre**

   first — **el nombre de pila**

   surname **el apellido**

nap **la siesta**

narrow **estrecho/a**

natural **natural**

nausea **la náusea**

nebulize (*v*) **nebulizar**

nebulizer **el nebulizador**

neck **el cuello**

need **la necesidad**

need (*v*) **necesitar**

needle **la jeringuilla, la aguja**

negative **negativo/a**

neither **tampoco**

neonatal intensive care **el cuidado intensivo neonatal**

nephrectomy **la nefrectomía**

nephritis **la nefritis**

nerve **el nervio**

nervous **nervioso/a**

neurologist **el/la neurólogo/a**

neurology **la neurología**

never **nunca, jamás**

newborn **el/la recién nacido/a**

next **próximo/a**

night **la noche**

   — sweats **los sudores nocturnos**

ninth **el/la noveno/a**

nitroglycerine **la nitroglicerina**

nobody, no one **nadie**

noon **el mediodía**

normally **normalmente**

nose **la nariz**

nosocomial **nosocomial**

nothing **nada**

noun **el sustantivo**

November **noviembre**

now **ahora**

numbness **el entumecimiento**

nurse **el/la enfermero/a**

nurse practitioner **enfermero/a con licencia para diagnosticar y tratar padecimientos y recetar medicamentos**

nurse's aide **el/la ayudante de enfermero**

nursing **la enfermería**

nutritionist **el/la nutricionista**

o

oatmeal **la avena**
obese **obeso/a**
obesity **la obesidad**
obstetrician **el/la obstetra**
obstetrics **la obstetricia**
October **octubre**
odor **el olor**
offend (*v*) **ofender**
offended **ofendido/a**
offer (*v*) **ofrecer** (*irregular*)
offering **la ofrenda**
office **la oficina**
    doctor's — **el consultorio**
oil **el aceite**
ointment **el ungüento, la crema**
old **viejo/a, anciano/a**
on (top of) **encima de**
oncologist **el/la oncólogo/a**
oncology **la oncología**
open **abierto/a**
open (*v*) **abrir**
operating room **la sala de operaciones, el quirófano**
ophthalmologist **el/la oftalmólogo/a**
ophthalmology **la oftalmología**
or **o**
oral **oral**
orange **la naranja, la china** (Carib.)
oregano **el orégano**
oriented **orientado/a**
orthopedic **ortopédico/a**
orthopedic surgeon **el/la cirujano ortopédico/a**
orthopedics **la ortopedia**
orthopedist **el/la ortopedista**
osteoporosis **la osteoporosis**
otorhinolaryngologist (ENT) **el/la otorrinolaringólogo/a**
otorhinolaryngology **la otorrinolaringología**
ought (*v*) **deber**
ounce **la onza**
our **nuestro/a**
outbreak (of a disease) **el brote**
outpatient **ambulatorio/a**
ovary **el ovario**
overdose **la sobredosis**
overweight **sobrepeso/a**
overwhelmed **agobiado/a**

ovulate (*v*) **ovular**
ovulation **la ovulación**
owe (*v*) **deber**
oxygen **el oxígeno**

p

pacemaker **el marcapasos**
pain **el dolor**
    burning pain — **quemante**
    dull pain — **latente, sordo**
    sharp pain — **agudo, punzante**
labor pain **el dolor del parto**
pain (*v*) **doler** (o–ue)
pale **pálido/a**
palpate (*v*) **palpar, tocar**
palpitation **la palpitación**
palsy **la parálisis**
pancreas **el páncreas**
pandemic **la pandemia**
pandemic **pandémico/a**
pant (*v*) **jadear**
panting **el jadeo**
Pap test **la prueba de Papanicolaou, el examen de Papanicolaou**
paper **el papel**
papilloma **el papiloma**
paralysis **la parálisis**
paramedic **el/la paramédico/a**
paranoia **la paranoia**
paranoid **paranoico/a**
parents **los padres**
patch **el parche**
paternal **paterno/a**
paternity **la paternidad**
patient **el/la paciente**
peanut butter **la manteca de cacahuate, la mantequilla de maní** (Carib.)
pectoralis major **pectoral mayor**
pediatric **pediátrico/a**
pediatrician **el/la pediatra**
pediatrics **la pediatría**
pen **el bolígrafo, la pluma, el lapicero**
penis **el pene**
pepper **el ají, el pimiento**
percuss (*v*) **percutir, dar golpecitos**
period **el período, el periodo, la regla, la menstruación**
periodontitis **la periodontitis**

permethrin **la permetrina**
permission **el permiso**
persistent **persistente**
personal **personal**
pertussis **la tos ferina**
phalange **la falange**
pharmacist **el/la farmacéutico/a**
pharmacy **la farmacia**
phlegm **la flema**
phobia **la fobia**
physical exam **el examen físico**
physical therapist **el/la terapeuta físico/a**
physician **el/la médico/a, el/la doctor/a**
physician's assistant **el/la asociado/a médico/a**
piece **el pedazo**
pill **la pastilla, la píldora, la tableta, el comprimido**
pillow **la almohada**
pin **el alfiler**
place **el lugar**
placenta **la placenta**
— previa **la placenta previa**
plain **sencillo/a**
platelet **la plaqueta**
plaque (dental) **el sarro**
plastic surgeon **el/la cirujano/a plástico/a**
pleasant **agradable**
please **por favor**
please (v) **gustar, encantar**
pleasure **el placer**
pneumonectomy **la neumonectomía, la pulmonectomía**
pneumonia **la pulmonía, la neumonía**
podiatrist **el/la podólogo/a**
podiatry **la podiología**
pole **el palo**
policy **la póliza**
polio **la polio, la poliomelitis**
pollen **el polen**
polyp **el pólipo**
poor **pobre**
porcelain **la porcelana**
portion **la porción**
Portuguese **el portugués** (*lang.*)
positive **positivo/a**
potato **la papa**
pound **la libra**
practice (v) **practicar**
precaution **la precaución**

preeclampsia **la preeclampsia**
pregnancy **el embarazo**
pregnant **embarazada, encinta**
prescribe (v) **recetar**
prescription **la receta**
press (v) **palpar, presionar, oprimir**
pressure **la presión, la tensión**
prevent (v) **prevenir** (*irregular*)
preventative **preventivo/a**
prevention **prevención**
prickly pear cactus **el nopal**
private **privado/a**
procedure **el procedimiento**
process **el proceso**
prognosis **el pronóstico**
prolapse **el prolapso**
prostate **la próstata**
prostatitis **la prostatitis**
prosthesis **la prótesis**
protein **la proteína**
proud **orgulloso/a**
provoke (v) **provocar**
prune **la ciruela**
psoriasis **la psoriasis**
psychiatric **psiquiátrico/a**
psychiatrist **el/la psiquiatra**
psychiatry **la psiquiatría**
psychologist **el/la psicólogo/a**
psychology **la psicología**
psychosis **la psicosis**
psychotic **psicótico/a**
pucker (v) **fruncir**
puff **la inhalación**
pulmonologist **el/la neumonólogo/a**
pulsating **latente**
pulse **el pulso**
punctual **puntual**
purée **puré**
purpose **el propósito**
push (v) **empujar**
put (v) **poner** (*irregular*)
pyramid **la pirámide**

q

quadriceps **el cuádriceps**
quarter **cuarto/a**
question **la pregunta**
question (v) **preguntar** (*to ask*), **cuestionar** (*to doubt, wonder*)

quick **rápido/a**
quinine **la quinina**

r

radiation therapy **la radioterapia**
radio **el radio**
radiologist **el/la radiólogo/a**
radiology **la radiología**
rash **la erupción, la irritación, el sarpullido**
reach **el alcance**
reaction **la reacción**
read (*v*) **leer**
receive (*v*) **recibir**
receptionist **el/la recepcionista**
record (*v*) **grabar**
recorder **la grabadora**
recovery room **la sala de recuperación, la sala de restablecimiento**
rectum **el recto**
rectus abdominis **el recto abdominal**
rectus femoris **el recto femoral**
red **rojo/a, colorado/a**
refrigerator **el refrigerador, la nevera**
regular **regular**
reject (*v*) **rechazar**
rejected **rechazado/a**
rejection **el rechazo**
relieved **aliviado/a**
remain (*v*) **quedar(se)**
remedy **el remedio**
    home — **el remedio casero**
remember (*v*) **recordar** (o–ue)
remove (*v*) **sacar, quitar(se)**
renal calculus **el cálculo en el riñón, las piedras en el riñón**
renal failure **la insuficiencia renal**
replacement **el reemplazo**
resist (*v*) **resistir**
resistant **resistente**
respiratory therapist **el/la terapeuta respiratorio/a**
rest **el descanso**
rest (*v*) **descansar**
result **el resultado**
resuscitate (*v*) **resucitar**
resuscitation **la resucitación**
return (*v*) **volver** (o–ue), **regresar**
rheumatic fever **la fiebre reumática**

rheumatologist **el/la reumatólogo/a**
rheumatology **la reumatología**
rib **la costilla**
rice **el arroz**
rich **rico/a**
right **el/la derecho/a**
rinse **el enjuague**
rinse (*v*) **enjuagar**
risk **el riesgo**
robe **la bata**
roll over (*v*) **virar(se)**
room **el cuarto, la habitación**
root canal **el tratamiento de canal**
rosemary **el romero**
rub (*v*) **frotar**
rubella **la rubéola**
rum **el ron**
run (*v*) **correr**

s

sacrum **el sacro**
sad **triste**
sadness **la tristeza**
salad **la ensalada**
salmon **el salmón**
salt **la sal**
same **igual**
sample **la muestra**
sandwich **el emparedado, el sándwich**
sartorius **el sartorio**
satisfied **satisfecho/a**
Saturday **el sábado**
sausage **la salchicha, el chorizo**
say (*v*) **decir** (*irregular*)
scabies **la sarna**
scapula **el omóplato**
scare **el susto**
scare (*v*) **asustar**
scared **asustado/a**
schizophrenia **la esquizofrenia**
school **la escuela**
sciatic **ciático/a**
sciatica **la ciática**
scrotum **el escroto**
sealant **el sellador, el sellante**
seat belt **el cinturón de seguridad**
second **segundo/a**
secretary **el/la secretario/a**
secretion **la secreción**

sedative **el sedante, el calmante**

see (*v*) **ver** (*irregular*)

self exam **el autoexamen**

sensation **la sensación**

September **septiembre**

serratus **el serrato**

seventh **el/la séptimo/a**

severe **severo/a**

sew (*v*) **coser**

sexually transmitted disease **la enferme-dad transmitida sexualmente**

shake (*v*) **agitar**

shakes **los temblores**

shame **la vergüenza**

share (*v*) **compartir**

shave (*v*) **afeitar(se)**

she **ella**

sheet **la sábana**

shine (*v*) **brillar**

shingles **la culebrilla**

shoe **el zapato**

shop (*v*) **hacer compras** (*irregular*)

short **bajo/a** (*height*), **corto/a** (*length*)

shortness of breath **la dificultad para respirar, la falta de aire, la fatiga**

should (*v*) **deber**

shoulder **el hombro**

shy **tímido/a**

sick **enfermo/a**

sickle cell anemia **la anemia drepa-nocítica de células falciformes**

sickness **la enfermedad**

side **el lado**

side effect **el efecto secundario**

sight **la vista**

single **soltero/a**

sister **la hermana**

sister-in-law **la cuñada**

sit (*v*) **sentar(se)** (e–ie)

sixth **el/la sexto/a**

skeleton **el esqueleto**

skin **la piel**

skinny **flaco/a**

sleep (*v*) **dormir** (o–ue)

sleeping pill **la pastilla para dormir**

sleeve **la manga**

slow **despacio, lento/a**

small **pequeño/a**

small intestine **el intestino delgado**

smallpox **la viruela**

smell **el olor**

smell **el olfato** (*sense of*)

smell (*v*) **oler** (*irregular*)

smile (*v*) **sonreír**

smoke **el humo**

— detector **el detector de humo**

smoke (*v*) **fumar**

smoker **el/la fumador/a**

snack **la merienda**

sneeze **el estornudo**

sneeze (*v*) **estornudar**

sober **sobrio/a**

social **social**

social work **el trabajo social**

social worker **el/la trabajador/a social**

soda pop **el refresco, la gaseosa**

soft **blando/a**

soft drink **la gaseosa, el refresco**

some **alguno/a**

someone **alguien**

something **algo**

sometimes **a veces**

son **el hijo**

son-in-law **el yerno**

sonogram **el sonograma, el ecograma**

sonograph **la sonografía, el ecograma**

soup **la sopa**

soybean **la soja**

Spaniard **el/la español/a**

Spanish **el español** (*lang.*)

speak (*v*) **hablar**

specialty **la especialidad**

speech therapist **el/la terapeuta de len-guaje, el/la terapeuta del habla**

spend (money) (*v*) **gastar**

spend (time) (*v*) **pasar**

spice **la especia**

spina bifida **la espina bífida**

spine **la espina dorsal, la columna**

spirit **el ánimo, el espíritu**

spirometry **la espirometría**

spit (*v*) **escupir**

spleen **el bazo**

spontaneous **espontáneo/a**

sprain **la torcedura, el esguince**

sprain (*v*) **torcer(se)** (o–ue)

sprained **torcido/a**

spray **el aerosol**

spray (*v*) **rociar**

sputum **el esputo**

squash **la calabaza**
stab wound **la puñalada**
stagnant **estancado/a**
stain **la mancha**
stain (*v*) **manchar**
staphylococcus **el estafilococo**
starch **el almidón**
start **el principio, el comienzo**
start (*v*) **empezar** (e–ie)
stepbrother **el hermanastro**
stepfather **el padrastro**
stepmother **la madrastra**
stepsister **la hermanastra**
sternocleideomastoid
    esternocleidomastoideo/a
sternum **el esternón**
steroid **el esteroide**
stethoscope **el estetoscopio**
stiffness **la rigidez**
stitch **el punto**
stitch (*v*) **coser**
stomach **el estómago**
straight **derecho/a**
street **la calle**
stress **el estrés**
stretcher **la camilla**
stroke **la apoplejía, la embolia cerebral,**
    la hemorragia cerebrovascular, el
    accidente cerebrovascular
strong **fuerte**
student **el/la estudiante**
study (*v*) **estudiar**
subcutaneous **subcutáneo/a**
sudden **repentino/a, de repente**
    — death **la muerte súbita**
suffer (*v*) **sufrir**
    — from an illness (*v*) **padecer**
sugar **el azúcar, la azúcar** (ambiguous
    gender)
suicide **el suicidio**
suicide (*v*) **suicidarse, matarse, quitarse**
    la vida
Sunday **el domingo**
supper **la cena**
supplementary **complimentario/a**
suppository **el supositorio**
surgeon **el/la cirujano/a**
surgery **la cirugía**
surname **el apellido**
suspension **la suspensión**

swallow **el trago**
swallow (*v*) **tragar**
sweat **el sudor**
sweat (*v*) **sudar**
sweet **dulce**
swell (*v*) **hinchar**
swelling **la hinchazón**
swollen **hinchado/a**
symptom **el síntoma**
syndrome **el síndrome**
syphilis **la sífilis**
syringe **la jeringa, la jeringuilla**
syrup **el jarabe** (*medicine*), **el almíbar**
system **el sistema**

t

tablespoon **la cuchara**
tablespoonful **la cucharada**
tachycardia **la taquicardia**
take (*v*) **tomar**
take out (*v*) **sacar**
talk (*v*) **hablar**
tall **alto/a**
tapeworm **la teniasis**
tarsus **el tarso**
taste **el gusto, el sabor**
taste (*v*) **probar** (o–ue)
tea **el té, la infusión, la tisana**
tear (secretion) **la lágrima**
teaspoon **la cucharita**
teaspoonful **la cucharadita**
technician **el/la técnico/a**
telephone **el teléfono**
tell (*v*) **decir** (*irregular*)
temperature **la temperatura**
tenth **el/la décimo/a**
test **la prueba**
testicle **el testículo**
tetanus **el tétano, el tétanos**
thalasemia **la talasemia**
thank you **gracias**
thankful **agradecido/a**
that **ese, esa, aquel, aquella**
the **el, la**
then **entonces**
therapist **el/la terapeuta**
there **allí, allá**
thermometer **el termómetro**
they **ellos, ellas**

thigh **el muslo**
thin **delgado/a**
third **el/la tercero/a**
thirst **la sed**
this **este, esta**
those **esos, esas, aquellos, aquellas**
throat **la garganta**
thrombosis **la trombosis**
thrush **una infección oral producida por hongos**
Thursday **el jueves**
thus **así**
thyroid **el tiroides, la glándula tiroidea**
time **el tiempo, la hora**
tibia **la tibia**
tibialis anterior **tibial anterior**
tire (v) **cansar**
tired **cansado/a**
toast **la tostada, el pan tostado**
toast (v) **tostar**
today **hoy**
toe **el dedo del pie**
tolerance **la tolerancia**
tomato **el tomate, el jitomate**
tomorrow **mañana**
tongue **la lengua**
tongue-twister **el trabalengua**
tonsil **la amígdala**
tonsillectomy **la tonsilectomía, la tonsilotomía, la amigdalectomía**
tonsillitis **la amigdalitis**
too **también**
tooth **el diente**
toothpaste **la crema dental**
(on) top of **encima de**
topical **tópico/a**
tormented **mortificado/a**
touch (sense of) **el tacto**
touch (v) **tocar**
toward **hacia**
towel **la toalla**
toxoplasmosis **la toxoplasmosis**
tradition **la tradición**
tranquilizer **el calmante**
transplant **el trasplante**
transplant (v) **trasplantar**
trapezius **el trapecio**
traumatic **traumático/a**
   — injury **el traumatismo, la herida traumática, el politraumatismo**

treat (v) **tratar**
treatment **el tratamiento**
tremors **los temblores**
triceps **el tríceps braquial, femoral**
triglyceride **el triglicérido**
true **verdadero, cierto**
truth **la verdad**
try (v) **intentar, tratar de**
tuberculosis **la tuberculosis**
Tuesday **el martes**
tumor **el tumor**
tuna **el atún**
typhoid fever **la tifoidea**

U

ulcer **la úlcera**
ulna **el cúbito**
ultrasound **la sonografía, el ecograma**
umbilical cord **el cordón umbilical**
uncle **el tío**
under **debajo de**
understand (v) **comprender, entender**
unit **la unidad**
United States **los Estados Unidos**
until **hasta**
urgency **la urgencia**
urinate (v) **orinar**
urine **la orina**
   — sample **la muestra de orina**
urologist **el/la urólogo/a**
urology **la urología**
us **nosotros, nosotras**
useful **útil**
useless **inútil**
uterus **el útero, la matriz**

V

vaccinate (v) **vacunar**
vaccination **la vacuna**
vagina **la vagina**
vaginal **vaginal**
valve disease **la valvulopatía**
varicela **la varicela**
vegetable **el vegetal, la verdura, la legumbre**
vehicular **automovilístico/a**
vein **la vena**
vertebra **la vértebra**

very **muy**
victim **la víctima**
virus **el virus**
visit **la visita**
visit (*v*) **visitar**
visitor **el/la visitante**
vitamin **la vitamina**
voice **la voz**
vomit **el vómito**
vomit (*v*) **vomitar**

W

wait (*v*) **esperar**
waiting room **la sala de espera**
wakefulness **la vigilia**
walk (*v*) **caminar**
walker **el andador**
want (*v*) **querer** (e–ie)
wash (*v*) **lavar(se)**
we **nosotros, nosotras**
weak **débil**
weakness **la debilidad**
wear (*v*) **llevar**
Wednesday **el miércoles**
week **la semana**
weekend **el fin de semana**
weekly **semanal, semanalmente**
weeping, crying **el llanto**
weigh (*v*) **pesar**
weight **el peso**
well **bien, sano/a**
what? **¿qué?, ¿cuál?**
wheelchair **la silla de ruedas**
wheeze **el silbido**
where? **¿dónde?**
from where? **¿de dónde?**
to where? **¿adónde?**
which? **¿cuál?**
whistle (*v*) **pitar**
white **blanco/a**
withdrawal symptom **el síntoma de abstinencia**
who **quien**
who? whom? **¿quién?**
whole **entero/a**
    — grain **integral**
whooping cough **la tos ferina**
why? **¿por qué?**
widow **la viuda**

widower **el viudo**
wife **la esposa, la mujer**
wig **la peluca**
window **la ventana**
wine **el vino**
wisdom **la sabiduría**
wisdom tooth **el cordal, la muela del juicio**
withdraw (*v*) **retirar**
woman **la mujer**
womb **la matriz**
word **la palabra**
work (*v*) **trabajar**
worse **peor**
worsen (*v*) **empeorar**
wound **la herida**
wrinkle (*v*) **arrugar**
wrist **la muñeca**
write (*v*) **escribir**
written **escrito/a**

X

x-ray **la radiografía, los rayos equis, la placa**
x-ray technician **el/la técnico/a de radiografía**

Y

yaws **el pian, la frambuesa**
year **el año**
yellow **amarillo/a**
yellowish **amarillento/a**
yesterday **ayer**
yogurt **el yogur**
you **tú, usted, ustedes**
young **joven**
your **tu, su**
yours **tuyo/a, suyo/a**
yucca **la yuca**

Z

zero **el cero**
zika **el zika**

Spanish to English Glossary

The translations in this glossary are generally limited to the context in which the words are used in the book.

a

el abanico fan
el abdomen abdomen
aborrecido/a disgusted
el aborto espontáneo miscarriage
el aborto natural miscarriage
el aborto provocado abortion
la abrasión abrasion
abril April
abrir to open
abstener to abstain
la abstenencia abstinence
la abuela grandmother
el abuelo grandfather
aburrido/a bored, boring
aburrir to bore
el ácaro del polvo dust mite
el accidente accident
 — **cerebrovascular** cerebrovascular accident
el aceite oil
el acetaminofén acetaminophen
acostar(se) (o–ue) to lie down, to go to bed
activo/a active
actual current
adelantar to advance, to move up
la adicción addiction
el/la adicto/a addict
adiós good-bye

¿adónde? to where?
la adrenalina adrenaline
el aerosol aerosol
afeitar(se) to shave
agitado/a agitated
agitar to agitate
agobiado/a overwhelmed
agosto August
agotado/a drained
agradable pleasant
agradecido/a thankful
el agua (f) water
el aguacate avocado
aguantar to bear, to endure
agudo/a acute
la aguja needle
el/la ahijado/a godson, goddaughter, godchild
ahora now
el aire air
el alcance reach
el alcohol alcohol
el alcoholismo alcoholism
alegre happy
la alegría happiness
el alemán German (lang.)
el alérgeno allergen
la alergia allergy
alérgico/a allergic
el alfiler pin

la **alfombra** rug, carpet
la **algalia** urinary catheter
algo something
alguien someone, anyone
algún, alguno/a some
alguna vez ever
algunas veces sometimes
alimentar to feed
el **alimento** food
aliviado/a relieved
el **alivio** relief
allá there
allí there
el **almíbar** syrup
el **almidón** starch
la **almohada** pillow
almorzar (o–ue) to eat/have lunch
el **almuerzo** lunch
alto/a tall
la **alucinación** hallucination
el **alumbramiento** birth
alumbrar to give birth
amable kind, nice
amamantar to breastfeed
amarillento/a yellowish, jaundiced
amarillo/a yellow
la **ambulancia** ambulance
ambulatorio/a ambulatory, outpatient
la **amígdala** tonsil
la **amigdalitis** tonsillitis
la **amigdalotomía** tonsilectomy
el/la **amigo/a** friend
la **amnesia** amnesia
la **ampolla** blister
la **anafilaxis** anaphylaxis, anaphylactic
   shock
analgésico/a analgesic
el **análisis** analysis
anciano/a elderly
el **andador** walker
la **anemia** anemia
   — **drepanocítica de células falci-**
      formes sickle cell anemia
la **anestesia** anesthesia
la **anestesiología** anesthesiology
el/la **anestesiólogo/a** anesthesiologist
la **aneurisma** aneurysm
la **angina de pecho** angina pectoris
el **angiograma** angiogram
angustiado/a distressed

el **animal** animal
el **ánimo** spirit
el **anís** anise
el **ano** anus
anoche last night
la **ansiedad** anxiety
ansioso/a anxious
anteayer day before yesterday
el **antebrazo** forearm
antes de before
el **antiácido** antacid
el **antibiótico** antibiotic
el **anticoagulante** anticoagulant
el **anticonvulsivo** anticonvulsant
el **anticuerpo** antibody
el **antidepresivo** antidepressant
el **antidiarreico** antidiarrheal
el **antiespasmódico** antispasmodic
el **antihiperglucémico** antihyperglycemic
el **antihistamínico** antihistamine
el **antiinflamatorio** antiinflammatory
el **antipirético** antipyretic
el **antitusígeno** antitussive
el **año** year
el **apellido** surname
la **apendectomía** appendectomy
el **apéndice** appendix
la **apendicitis** appendicitis
el **apetito** appetite
aplicar to apply
la **apoplejía** apoplexy, stroke
aprender to learn
aquel, aquella that
aquellos, aquellas those
aquí here
el **ardor** burning sensation
la **área** área
la **arritmia** arrhythmia
el **arroz** rice
arrugar to wrinkle
la **articulación** joint
la **artritis** arthritis
la **artroscopía** arthroscopy
el **ascensor** elevator
la **asfixia** asphyxia
así thus, in this way, like this
asilo asylum, nursing home
el **asma** (*f*) asthma
el/la **asociado/a médico/a** physician's
   assistant

la **aspirina** aspirin
asustado/a scared, frightened
asustar to scare, to frighten
atacar to attack
el **ataque** attack
   — **al corazón** heart attack
atento/a attentive
el **atomizador** atomizer
el **atún** tuna
la **audiología** audiology
el/la **audiólogo/a** audiologist
auscultar to listen with a stethoscope
automovilístico/a vehicular
la **avena** oatmeal
avergonzado/a ashamed
ayer yesterday
la **ayuda** help
el/la **ayudante** assistant, helper
ayudar to help
ayunar to fast
el/la **azúcar** sugar
azucarado/a sugar-added

b

la **bacteria** bacterium
bacteriano/a bacterial
bajo/a short (height)
bañar(se) to bathe
el **baño** bath, bathroom
la **barbilla** chin
el **barbitúrico** barbiturate
la **bata** robe, hospital gown
el **bazo** spleen
el/la **bebé** baby
beber to drink
la **bebida** beverage
el **beneficio** benefit
benigno/a benign
el **biberón** baby's bottle
el **bíceps braquial, bíceps femoral** biceps
bien well
bilingüe bilingual
la **biopsia** biopsy
el/la **bisabuelo/a** great-grandfather,
   great-grandmother
el/la **bisnieto/a** great-grandson,
   great-granddaughter
el **bizcocho** cake (Carib.)
blando/a soft

la **boca** mouth
el **bolígrafo** pen
la **bolita** lump
   — **de algodón** cotton ball
borracho/a drunk
la **botella** bottle
el **brazo** arm
el **brócoli** broccoli
la **broncoscopia** bronchoscopy
bronquial bronchial
el **bronquio** bronchial tube
el **brote** outbreak (of a disease)
buenmozo handsome
bueno/a good

c

el **cabello** hair
la **cabeza** head
cada each, every
la **cadera** hip
caer (*irregular*) to fall
la **calabaza** squash
el **calambre** cramp
el **calcio** calcium
el **cálculo en el riñón** kidney stone
el **caldo** broth
la **calle** street
el **calmante** tranquilizer, sedative,
   analgesic
calmar(se) to calm, to calm down
el **calor** heat
la **caloría** calorie
la **cama** bed
la **camilla** stretcher, gurney
caminar to walk
el **cáncer** cancer
la **canela** cinnamon
cansado/a tired
el **cansancio** fatigue
cansar to tire, to grow tired
la **cantidad** amount
la **cápsula** capsule
la **cara** face
cardíaco/a cardiac
la **cardiología** cardiology
el/la **cardiólogo/a** cardiologist
la **cardiopatía isquémica** ischemic heart
   disease
la **caries, la caries dental** cavity

la **carne** meat
— **de res** beef
casado/a married
casar(se) to marry
la **caspa** dandruff
— **de animal** animal dander
la **catarata** cataract
el **catarro** congestion, common cold
el **catéter** catheter
la **ceja**   eyebrow
celoso/a jealous
la **célula** cell
la **cena** supper, dinner
cenar to eat/have supper, dinner
el **ceño** brow
cepillar(se) to brush
el **cereal** cereal
— **cocido** cooked cereal
— **seco** dry cereal
cerebral cerebral
el **cerebro** brain
cero zero
la **cerveza** beer
la **cesárea** C-section, cesarean
el/la **chamán** folk healer
el **chino** Chinese
chiquito/a small
chocar to collide, to crash
el **chocolate** chocolate
el **choque** collision, crash
la **ciática** sciatica
ciático/a sciatic
la **cicatriz** scar
ciego/a blind
el **cinturón de seguridad** seat belt
la **cirrosis** cirrhosis
la **ciruela** plum, prune
la **cirugía** surgery
el/la **cirujano/a** surgeon
— **ortopédico/a** orthopedic surgeon
— **plástico/a** plastic surgeon
la **cita** appointment
la **ciudad** city
la **clamidia** chlamydia
clarificar to clarify
la **clase** class
clásico/a classic
la **clavícula** clavicle
la **clínica** clinic
clínico/a clinical

el **coágulo** clot
la **cocaína** cocaine
el **cóccix** coccyx
el **coche** car
la **cocina** kitchen
cocinar to cook
el/la **cocinero/a** cook
el **coco** coconut
la **codeína** codeine
el **codo** elbow
la **colecistectomía** cholecystectomy
la **colecistitis** cholecystitis
el **cólera** cholera
el **colesterol** colesterol
el **cólico, los cólicos** colic
el **colon** colon
la **colonoscopia** colonoscopy
el **color** color
colorado/a red
la **colostomía** colostomy
la **comadrona** midwife
combatir to fight
comer to eat
la **comezón** itch, itching
la **comida** meal
¿**cómo?** how?
como like, as
cómodo/a comfortable
compartir to share
complementario/a supplemental
la **complicación** complication
complicado/a complicated
comprar to buy
comprender to understand
el **comprimido** pill
común common
la **concusión** concussion
el **condón** condom
confirmar to confirm
la **congestión** congestion
congestionado/a congested
la **conjuntivitis** conjunctivitis
consciente conscious
el/la **consejero/a** counselor
constante constant
consultar to consult
el **consultorio** doctor's office
la **contaminación** contamination
— **del aire** air pollution
contento/a happy, contented

contestar to answer
la contracción contraction
el contraceptivo contraceptive
la convulsión convulsion
el corazón heart
el cordal wisdom tooth
el cordón umbilical umbilical cord
la corona crown
   — **de oro** gold crown
   — **de porcelana** porcelain crown
correr to run
corriente regular, everyday
la cortadura cut
cortar(se) to cut
el corte cut
cortés polite
la cortesía politeness
corto/a short (length)
coser to sew
la costilla rib
la costumbre custom
la coyuntura joint
el cráneo cranium
creer to believe
la crema cream, ointment
   — **dental** toothpaste
el criadero breeding area
la crisis crisis
crónico/a chronic
el cuádriceps quadriceps
¿cuál? which?
¿cuándo? when?
¿cuánto/a? how much?
¿cuántos/as? how many?
cuarto/a quarter, fourth
el cuarto room
el cúbito ulna
cubrir to cover
la cuchara tablespoon
la cucharada tablespoonful
la cucharadita teaspoonful
la cucharita teaspoon
el cuello neck
   — **del útero,** — **de la matriz** cervix
el cuerpo body
el cuidado intensivo intensive care
   — **neonatal** neonatal intensive care
cuidar to care for
la culebrilla herpes zoster, shingles
la culpa guilt

culpable guilty
el cultivo culture (laboratory)
el/la cuñado/a brother-in-law,
   sister-in-law
curioso/a curious
la curita small bandage
la custodia custody

d

dañar to damage, to harm
el daño damage, harm
dar (*irregular*) to give
   — **a luz** to give birth
   — **de alta** to discharge
   — **de baja** to admit
de of, from
¿de dónde? from where?
debajo de under
deber ought, should, to owe
débil weak
la debilidad weakness
el/la décimo/a tenth
decir (*irregular*) to say, to tell
el dedo finger
   — **del pie** toe
defecar to move one's bowels
dejar to leave behind
delante de (in) front of
delgado/a thin
el delirio delusion
deltoides deltoid
demasiado/a too much
demostrar (o–ue) to demonstrate
el dengue dengue
la dentadura teeth, set of teeth
   — **postiza** dentures, false teeth
el/la dentista dentist
la dependencia dependence
la depresión depression
deprimido/a depressed
derecho/a right, straight
la derivación coronaria CABG, coronary
   artery bypass graft
el/la dermatólogo/a dermatologist
la dermatología dermatology
el derrame leak, spill, hemorrhage
desayunar to eat/have breakfast
el desayuno breakfast
descafeinado/a decaffeinated

descansar to rest
el descanso rest
el descongestionante decongestant
descorazonado/a disheartened
descremado/a fat-free
la descripción description
descubrir to discover
desesperado/a hopeless, desperate
la deshidratación dehydration
desmayar(se) to faint
despacio/a slow, slowly
despertar(se) (e–ie) to awaken
despierto/a awake
después afterward
después de after
detrás de behind
el día day
la diabetes diabetes
   — **del embarazo** gestational diabetes
el diagnóstico diagnosis
la diálisis dialysis
la diarrea diarrhea
dichoso/a lucky
diciembre December
el diente tooth
   — **de leche** baby tooth
la dieta diet
el/la dietista dietician
la difteria diphtheria
la dilatación dilation
diluir to dilute
el dinero money
la dirección address
la discapacidad disability
   — **del desarrollo** developmental
     disability
   — **intelectual** intellectual disability
discapacitado/a disabled
la disentería dysentery
disgustado/a disgusted
la dislocación dislocation
la distrofia muscular muscular dystrophy
el diurético/a diuretic
divorciado/a divorced
divorciar(se) to divorce, to get divorced
el divorcio divorce
el/la doctor/a doctor
doler (o–ue) to ache, to hurt
el dolor pain
   — **agudo, punzante** sharp pain

   — **del parto** labor pain
   — **latente, sordo** dull pain
   — **quemante** burning pain
el domicilio domicile, residence
el domingo Sunday
¿dónde? where?
dorado/a golden
   el estafilococo — MRSA
dormir (o–ue) to sleep
dorsal dorsal
el drenaje drain, drainage
drenar to drain
la droga drug
duchar(se) to shower
dulce sweet
el dulce candy
durar to last, endure
duro/a hard

e

el ébola ebola
ebrio/a drunk
la eccema eczema
el ecograma sonogram, sonograph
ectópico/a ectopic
la edad age
el efecto secundario side effect
el the
él he
el electrocardiograma electrocardiogram
el electroencefalograma
   electroencephalogram
eliminar to eliminate
el elixir elixir
ella she
ellos/as they
embarazada pregnant
el embarazo pregnancy
la embolia embolism
   — **cerebral** stroke
la emergencia emergency
el empacho indigestion
el emparedado sandwich
el empaste filling (dental)
empeorar to worsen
empezar (e–ie) to start, begin
empujar to push
encantado/a pleased
encima de on top of

encinta pregnant
encontrar (o–ue) to find
la endocrinología endocrinology
el/la endocrinólogo/a endocrinologist
la endometriosis endometriosis
la endoscopía endoscopy
enero January
enfadado/a annoyed
enfadar(se) to become annoyed
la enfermedad sickness, illness
  — **arterial coronaria** coronary artery disease
  — **cardiovascular** cardiovascular disease
  — **de Chaga** Chaga's disease
  — **pulmonar obstructiva crónica** COPD
  — **transmitida sexualmente** sexually transmitted disease
la enfermería nursing, nurses station
el/la enfermero/a nurse
enfermo/a sick, ill
la enfisema emphysema
enfogonado/a enraged (*slang*)
enfogonar(se) to enrage (*slang*)
enjuagar to rinse
el enjuague rinse
enlatado/a canned
enojado/a angry
enojar to anger
enojar(se) to get angry
el enojo anger
la ensalada salad
enseñar to teach, to show
entero/a whole
el entumecimiento numbness
la epilepsia epilepsy
la epinefrina epinephrine
la episiotomía episiotomy
la erupción rash
esa that
los escalofríos chills
la esclerosis múltiple multiple sclerosis
escribir to write
escrito/a written
el escritorio desk
el escroto scrotum
escuchar to listen
la escuela school
escupir to spit

ese that
el esguince sprain
el esófago esophagus
la espalda back
el español Spanish (*lang.*)
el/la español/a Spaniard
la especia spice
la especialidad specialty
la esperanza hope
esperar to wait, to hope
la espina bífida spina bifida
la espina dorsal spine
el espíritu spirit
la espirometría spirometry
espontáneo/a spontaneous
la espuma foam
el esputo sputum
el esqueleto skeleton
la esquizofrenia schizophrenia
esta this
la estadía length of stay
los Estados Unidos the United States
el estafilococo staphylococcus
el estafilococo dorado MRSA
estancado/a stagnant
estar (*irregular*) to be
la estatura height
este this
esternocleidomastoideo/a sternocleideomastoid
el esternón sternum
el esteroide steroid
el estetescopio stethoscope
el estómago stomach
estornudar to sneeze
el estornudo sneeze
estrecho/a narrow
el estreñimiento constipation
el estrés stress
el/la estudiante student
estudiar to study
el eucalipto eucalyptus
evacuar to move one's bowels
evitar to avoid
el examen exam
la examinación examination
examinar to examine
exhalar to exhale
el expectorante expectorant
el expediente médico medical record

explicar to explain
exploratorio/a exploratory
la extracción extraction

f

la falange phalange
la falta de aire shortness of breath
el/la farmacéutico/a pharmacist
la farmacia pharmacy
fascinar to fascinate
la fatiga fatigue, shortness of breath
febrero February
la fecha date
las felicidades congratulations
feliz happy
el fémur femur
el feto fetus
la fibra fiber
la fibrilación auricular atrial fibrillation
la fiebre fever
    — **reumática** rheumatic fever
    — **tifoidea** typhoid fever
el fin de semana weekend
firmar to sign
flaco/a skinny
la flema phlegm
flojo/a loose
el fluido fluid
el flujo flow
el fluoruro fluoride
la fobia phobia
la fórmula formula
la fractura fracture
    — **abierta** open fracture
    — **compuesta** compound fracture
    — **conminuta** conminuted fracture
    — **espiral** spiral fracture
    — **oblicua** transverse fracture
    — **simple** simple fracture
la frambuesa yaws
el francés French (*lang.*)
el frasco bottle
la frazada blanket
la frecuencia frequency
frecuente frequent
frecuentemente frequently
la frente forehead
la fresa dental drill tip
el frío cold

frío/a cold
frito/a fried
la fritura fried food
frotar to rub
fruncir to frown, to pucker
frustrado/a frustrated
la fruta fruit
fuerte strong
el/la fumador/a smoker
fumar to smoke
furioso/a furious

g

el ganglio linfático lymph gland
la garganta throat
la gaseosa soft drink
gastar to spend money
la gastritis gastritis
el gel gel
la gelatina gelatin
generoso/a generous
el/la geriatra geriatrist
la geriatría geriatrics
geriátrico/a geriatric
la ginecología gynecology
ginecológico/a gynecologic
el/la ginecólogo/a gynecologist
la gingivitis gingivitis
la glándula gland
    — **tiroide** thyroid gland
la glaucoma glaucoma
el glúteo buttock
el glúteo mayor gluteus maximus
el golpe bump, blow
golpear(se) to bump, hit
el golpecito tap
la gonorrea gonorrhea
gordo/a fat
la gota drop, gout
gotear to drip
el goteo dripping
la grabadora recorder
grabar to record
gracias thank you
la gragea capsule
el grano grain
la grasa fat, grease
la gripa (Colombia) common cold
la gripe flu, common cold

el guante glove
guapo/a handsome (with *ser*), angry (with
   estar, Carib.)
el guinco banana
gustar to please
el gusto taste

h

la haba, la habichuela bean
la habitación room
hablar to talk, to speak
hacer (*irregular*) to do, to make
hacer falta to miss
hacia toward
el hambre hunger
hambriento/a hungry
hasta until
hay there is, there are
las heces fecales feces
helado/a frozen
el helado ice cream
el helicóptero helicopter
la hembra female
la hemofilia hemophilia
la hemoglobina hemoglobin
la hemoglobinopatía hemoglobinopathy
la hemorragia hemorrhage
hemorrágico/a hemorrhagic
las hemorroides hemorrhoids
la hepatitis hepatitis
la herida wound, injury
   — de bala gunshot wound
herir (e–ie) to injure
el/la hermanastro/a brother-in-law,
   sister-in-law
el/la hermano/a brother, sister
el/la hermano/a de madre / de padre half-
   brother, half-sister
la hernia hernia
la heroína heroin
el herpes herpes
hervir (e–ie) to boil
el hielo ice
el hierro iron (Fe)
el hígado liver
higiénico/a hygienic
el/la higienista dental dental hygienist
el/la hijastro/a stepson, stepdaughter
el/la hijo/a son, daughter

el/la hijo/a de crianza foster child
el hilo dental dental floss
hinchado/a swollen
hinchar to swell
la hinchazón swelling
la hipercolesterolemia
   hypercolesterolemia
la hiperglucemia hyperglycemia
la hipertensión hypertension
el hipertiroidismo hyperthyroidism
la hipoglucemia hypoglycemia
la hipotensión hypotension
el hipotiroidismo hypothyroidism
la histerectomía hysterectomy
la historia history
hola hello
el hombre man
el hombro shoulder
la hora hour
el hospital hospital
la hospitalización hospitalization
hospitalizar hospitalize
hoy today
el hueso bone
el huevo egg
el húmero humerus
el humo smoke

i

el ibuprofeno ibuprofen
la ictericia jaundice
el idioma language
igual equal, same
igualmente equally, same here, same to
   you
el íleon ilium
implantar to implant
el implante implant
importar to matter
incluir (*irregular*) to include
la incontinencia incontinence
el infarto infarct, infarction
   — de miocardio miocardial
     infarction
la infección infection
   — por giardias giardiasis
   — por tenia tapeworm
infectar to infect
la inflamación inflammation

inflamado/a inflamed
inflamar to inflame
la influenza influenza
la infusión infusion, tea
el inglés English (*lang.*)
la inhalación puff, inhalation
el inhalador inhaler
el insomnio insomnia
la insuficiencia insufficiency
   — **cardíaca** congestive heart
    failure
   — **renal** renal failure
integral whole-grain
inteligente intelligent
intentar to try
interesado/a interested
interesante interesting
interesar to interest
el internamiento hospitalization
internar to admit (to an institution)
el intestino intestine
   — **delgado** small intestine
   — **grueso** large intestine
intradérmico/a intradermic
intramuscular intramuscular
inútil useless
inválido/a disabled
la inyección injection
ir (*irregular*) to go
la irritabilidad irritability
la irritación rash
el italiano Italian (*lang.*)
izquierdo/a left

j

jadear to gasp, to pant
el jadeo gasping, panting
jamás never
el japonés Japanese (*lang.*)
la jaqueca migraine, headache
el jarabe syrup (medicine)
el jengibre ginger
la jeringa, la jeringuilla syringe
el jitomate tomato
joven young
el jueves Thursday
el jugo juice
julio July
junio June

k

el kilogramo kilogram

l

la the
el labio lip
la laceración laceration
la lactancia lactation
el lado side
la lágrima tear (secretion)
la laparoscopia laparoscopy
largo/a long
el láser laser
lastimar to injure, to wound
latente pulsating
el látex latex
lavar(se) to wash (oneself)
el laxante laxative
la leche milk
   — **artificial** formula
   — **materna** mother's milk
leer to read
lejos far
la lengua tongue, language
el lenguaje language
los lentes eyeglasses
lento/a slow
la leptospirosis leptospirosis
la leucemia leukemia
levantar(se) to get up, to arise, to raise
leve light, slight
la libra pound
el libro book
lidiar to cope
el limón lemon, lime
la limpieza cleaning
limpio/a clean
el líquido liquid
   — **amniótico** amniotic fluid
el litio lithium
la llamada call
llamar to call
llamar(se) to call oneself
el llanto weeping, crying jag
la llegada arrival
llegar to arrive
llevar to carry, to wear
llorar to cry

loco/a crazy
la lombriz intestinal intestinal worm
luego later
el lugar place
la lumpectomía lumpectomy
el lunar mole
el lunes Monday
la luxación dislocation of a bone
la luz light

m

la madrastra stepmother
la madre mother
la madrina godmother
majado/a mashed
majar to mash
mal badly
el malestar general malaise
maligno/a malignant
malo/a bad
la mancha stain
manchar to stain
la mandíbula jaw
manejar to drive, to manage
la manera manner
la manga sleeve
la manía mania
el/la maníacodepresivo/a
  manic-depressive
la mano hand
la manteca lard, heroin (*slang*)
la manteca de cacahuate, la mantequilla
  de maní peanut butter
la mantequilla butter
la manzana apple
la mañana morning
mañana tomorrow
la máquina machine
el marcapasos pacemaker
mareado/a dizzy
el mareo dizziness
la marihuana marijuana
el martes Tuesday
marzo March
más more
más o menos more or less
masetero masseter
masticable chewable
matar(se) to kill, to commit suicide

la matriz womb
mayo May
mayor older, elderly
la medianoche midnight
el medicamento medication
la medicina medicine
el/la médico/a doctor
  — de cabecera, — generalista general
    practitioner
  — internista internist
el mediodía midday, noon
la mejilla cheek
mejor better
mejorar to get better
la meningitis meningitis
la menopausia menopause
la menstruación menstruation
menstruar to menstruate
mensual, mensualmente monthly
la merienda snack
el mes month
la metástasis metastasis
el miedo fear
la miel de abeja honey
el miembro member, penis
el miércoles Wednesday
la migraña migraine
el miligramo milligram
el mililitro millilitre
la miocarditis miocarditis
mirar to look
el moco mucus
el moho mold
moler (o–ue) to grind
molestar to bother, to annoy
la molestia bother, annoyance
molesto/a uncomfortable, annoyed
molido/a ground
la monga common cold (*slang*)
el monitor monitor
la mononucleosis mononucleosis
moreno/a dark, brunette
el moretón bruise
morir (o–ue) to die
mortificado/a tormented
mover(se) (o–ue) to move
el/la muchacho/a child
el mucolítico mucolytic
la muela molar
  — del juicio wisdom tooth

la muerte death
　— **súbita** sudden death
la muestra sample
la mujer woman
la muleta crutch
la muñeca wrist, doll
el músculo muscle
el muslo thigh
muy very

n

nacer (*irregular*) to be born
el nacimiento birth
nada nothing
nadie nobody, no one
la nalga buttock
la nariz nose
natural natural
la náusea nausea
el nebulizador nebulizer
nebulizar to nebulize
la necesidad need
necesitar to need
la nefrectomía nephrectomy
la nefritis nephritis
negativo/a negative
el nervio nerve
nervioso/a nervous
la neumonectomía pneumonectomy
la neumonía pneumonia
el/la neumonólogo/a pulmonologist
la neurología neurology
el/la neurólogo/a neurologist
la nevera refrigerator
ningún, ninguno/a none, not any
el/la niño/a child
la nitroglicerina nitroglycerine
la noche night
el nombre name
　— **de pila** first name
el nopal prickly pear cactus
normalmente normally
nosocomial nosocomial
nosotros/as we, us
noveno/a ninth
noviembre November
el nudillo knuckle
la nuera daughter-in-law
nuestro/a our, ours

nunca never
el/la nutricionista nutritionist

o

o or
la obesidad obesity
obeso/a obese
el/la obstetra obstetrician
la obstetricia obstetrics
obstétrico/a obstetric
octavo/a eighth
octubre October
la odontología dentistry
el/la odontólogo/a dentist
ofender to offend
ofendido/a offended
ofrecer to offer
la ofrenda offering
la oftalmología ophthalmology
el/la oftalmólogo/a ophthalmologist
el oído ear (inner), hearing
oír to hear
¡Ojalá! I hope so!
ojalá que . . . I wish that . . .
el ojo eye
oler (*irregular*) to smell
el olfato smell
el olor odor, smell
olvidar to forget
el omóplato scapula
la oncología oncology
el/la oncólogo/a oncologist
la onza ounce
oprimir to press
oral oral
el orégano oregano
la oreja ear (outer)
orgulloso/a proud
orientado/a oriented
la orina urine
orinar to urinate
el oro gold
la ortopedia orthopedics
ortopédico/a orthopedic
el/la ortopedista orthopedist
oscuro/a dark
la osteoporosis osteoporosis
la otorrinolaringología ENT
el otorrinolaringólogo ENT doctor

el ovario ovary
la ovulación ovulation
ovular to ovulate
el oxígeno oxygen

p

el/la paciente patient
padecer (*irregular*) to suffer (from an
   illness)
el padecimiento malady, illness, chronic
   condition
el padrastro stepfather
el padre father
los padres parents
el padrino godfather
la palabra word
pálido/a pale
el palo pole, stick
palpar to palpate
la palpitación palpitation
el paludismo malaria
el pan bread
   — **integral** whole-grain bread
   — **tostado** toast
el páncreas pancreas
la pandemia pandemic
pandémico/a pandemic
la pantorrilla calf (anat.)
la papa potato
las papas fritas french fries
la paperas mumps
el papiloma papilloma
la parálisis paralysis, palsy
   — **cerebral** cerebral palsy
el/la paramédico/a paramedic
la paranoia paranoia
paranoico/a paranoid
el parche patch
la pareja partner, couple
parir to give birth
el/la partero/a midwife
el parto birth
   — **prematuro** premature birth
pasar to happen, to pass
el pasillo hallway
el pastel cake
la pastilla pill
la patela kneecap
la paternidad paternity

paterno/a paternal
el pato de cama bedpan
el pecho chest
pectoral mayor pectoralis major
el pedazo piece
el/la pediatra pediatrician
la pediatría pediatrics
pediátrico/a pediatric
pedir (e–i) to ask for, to beg
peinar(se) to comb
el peine comb
pelear to argue, to fight
el peligro danger
peligroso/a dangerous
el pelo hair
la pelotita lump
la peluca wig
el pene penis
peor worse
pequeño/a small
percutir to percuss
perder (e–ie) to lose
la pérdida loss
   — **de conocimiento** loss of
      consciousness
el perico cocaine (*slang*)
el período, el periodo period
la periodontitis periodontitis
la permetrina permethrin
el permiso permission
el peroné fibula
persistente persistent
persistir to persist
personal personal
pesado/a crushing, heavy
pesar to weigh
el pescado fish
pescar to fish
el peso weight
el pian yaws
la picadura bite
picar to itch
la picazón itch, itching
el pie foot
la piel skin
la pierna leg
la píldora pill
el pimiento bell pepper
los piojos lice
la pirámide pyramid

el **piso** floor
pitar to whistle
la **pizarra** blackboard
la **placa** film, plaque, x-ray
la **placenta** placenta
— **previa** placenta previa
el **placer** pleasure
el **plan de alimentación** diet
el **plan médico** health insurance
la **plaqueta** platelet
la **plata** silver, money
pobre poor
poder (o–ue) to be able
la **podiología** podiatry
el/la **podólogo/a** podiatrist
el **polen** pollen
la **polio, la poliomielitis** polio
el **pólipo** polyp
el **politraumatismo** traumatic injury
la **póliza** policy
el **pollo** chicken
el **polvo** dust
el **ácaro del** — dust mite
polvorizar to crush
la **pompa** inhaler (*slang*)
el **pompis** buttock
el **pómulo** cheekbone
poner (*irregular*) to put
¿**por qué?** why?
la **porcelana** porcelain
la **porción** portion
porque because
el **portador** carrier
— **sano** asymptomatic carrier
el **portugués** Portuguese (*lang.*)
positivo/a positive
el **postre** dessert
practice practicar
la **precaución** precaution
la **precisión** accuracy, precision
la **preeclampsia** preeclampsia
la **pregunta** question
preguntar to ask a question
la **presentación de nalgas** breech position
la **presión** pressure
— **arterial** blood pressure
— **de la sangre** blood pressure
— **sanguínea** blood pressure
presionar to press
la **prevención** prevention

prevenir (conj. like *venir*) to prevent
preventivo/a preventive
primero/a first
el/la **primo/a** cousin
privado/a private
probar (o–ue) to test, taste, try
el **procedimiento** procedure
el **proceso** process
profundo/a deep
el **prolapso** prolapse
el **pronóstico** prognosis
el **propósito** purpose
la **próstata** prostate
la **prostatitis** prostatitis
prostético/a prosthetic
la **proteína** protein
la **prótesis** prosthesis
provocar to provoke
el/la **próximo/a** next
la **prueba** test
— **de Papanicolaou** Pap test
el **prurito** itch
la **psicología** psychology
el/la **psicólogo/a** psychologist
la **psicosis** psychosis
psicótico/a psychotic
el/la **psiquiatra** psychiatrist
la **psiquiatría** psychiatry
psiquiátrico/a psychiatric
la **psoriasis** psoriasis
el **pueblo** town
la **puerta** door
la **pulgada** inch
el **pulmón** lung
la **pulmonía** pneumonia
el/la **pulmonólogo/a** pulmonologist
el **pulso** pulse
el **punto** stitch, period, dot, point
puntual punctual
punzante stabbing
la **puñalada** stab wound
puré purée

q

que that
¿**qué?** what?, how?
quebrado/a broken
quedar(se) to remain
quemado/a burned

la **quemadura** burn
quemar(se) to burn
querer (e–ie) to want, to like
el **queso** cheese
¿**quién?** who?, whom?
la **quimioterapia** chemotherapy
la **quinina** quinine
quinto/a fifth
el **quirófano** operating room
el **quiste** cyst
quitar(se) to remove

r

el **radio** radio, radius (bone)
la **radiografía** x-ray
la **radiología** radiology
el/la **radiólogo/a** radiologist
la **radioterapia** radiation therapy
rápido/a quick
la **raquiña** itch, itching (*slang*)
la **reacción** reaction
la **reanimación cardiopulmonar** CPR
el/la **recepcionista** receptionist
la **receta** prescription
recetar to prescribe
rechazado/a rejected
rechazar to reject
el **rechazo** rejection
recibir to receive
el **recibo** receipt
el/la **recién nacido/a** newborn
recordar (o–ue) to remind, to remember
el **recto** rectum
el **recto abdominal** rectus abdominis
el **recto femoral** rectus femoris
el **reemplazo** replacement
el **reflujo esofágico** esophageal reflux
el **refresco** soda pop
el **refrigerador** refrigerator
la **regla** period, menstruation
regresar to return
regular regular, O.K.
el **remedio** cure
    — **casero** home remedy
repentino/a, de repente sudden
la **res, la carne de res** beef
el **resfriado** common cold
el **resfrío** common cold
resistente resistant

resistir to resist
la **respiración** respiration
respirar to breathe
la **resucitación** resuscitation
resucitar to resuscitate
el **resultado** result
retirar to withdraw
el **retraso mental** mental retardation
la **reumatología** rheumatology
el/la **reumatólogo/a** rheumatologist
la **revascularización coronaria** CABG,
    coronary artery bypass graft
rico/a rich
el **riesgo** risk
la **rigidez** stiffness
el **riñón** kidney
rociar to spray
la **rodilla** knee
el **romero** rosemary
romper(se) to break
    — **fuente** to break water
el **ron** rum
las **ronchas** hives
la **ropa** clothes, clothing
la **rubéola** rubella, German measles
rubio/a blond, fair

s

el **sábado** Saturday
la **sábana** sheet
saber (*irregular*) to know
la **sábila** aloe vera
sacar to take out
el **sacro** sacrum
la **sal** salt
la **sala de**
    — **emergencia** emergency room
    — **espera** waiting room
    — **operaciones** operating room
    — **recuperación** recovery room
    — **urgencias** emergency room
la **salchicha** sausage
la **salud** health
sanar to heal
sangrar to bleed
la **sangre** blood
sano/a healthy, healed
el **sarampión** measles
la **sarna** scabies

el sarpullido hives
el sarro plaque (dental)
el sartorio sartorius
satisfecho/a satisfied
secar(se) to dry
la secreción secretion
el/la secretario/a secretary
la sed thirst
el sedante sedative
seguir (e–i) to follow
segundo/a second
el seguro insurance
seguro/a safe, sure
el sellador sealant
el sellante sealant
la semana week
sencillo/a plain, easy
el seno breast, sinus
    — **frontal** frontal sinus
    — **paranasal** paranasal sinus
la sensación sensation
sentar(se) (e–ie) to sit
sentir(se) (e–ie) to feel
septiembre September
séptimo/a seventh
la sequedad dryness
ser (*irregular*) to be
el serrato serratus
severo/a severe
sexto/a sixth
el shock anafiláctico anaphylactic shock
la sicosis psychosis
sicótico/a psychotic
el SIDA AIDS
siempre always
la siesta nap
la sífilis syphilis
el silbido wheeze
la silla chair
    — **de ruedas** wheelchair
la silleta bedpan
simpático/a kind
el síndrome syndrome
    — **de Down** Down syndrome
el síntoma symptom
    — **de abstinencia** withdrawal
      symptom
el sistema system
sobre on, about, around
la sobredosis overdose

sobrepeso/a overweight
sobrio sober
la soja soybean
solitario/a alone
la sonda catheter
la sonografía ultrasound
sonreír to smile
la sopa soup
soplar to blow
el soplo bruit
    — **cardíaco** heart murmur
la sordera deafness
sordo/a deaf
sorprendido/a surprised
su your, his, her, their
subcutáneo/a subcutaneous
sudar to sweat
el sudor sweat
los sudores nocturnos night sweats
la suegra mother-in-law
el suegro father-in-law
el sueño dream, sleep
el suero IV fluid
la suerte luck
suicidarse to commit suicide
el suicidio suicide
el supositorio suppository
la suspensión suspension
el susto fright
suyo/a/os/as yours, his, hers, theirs

t

la tabla board
el tacto touch
el tajo cut
la talasemia thalassemia
también also, too
tampoco neither
la taquicardia tachycardia
tarde late
la tarde afternoon
la tarjeta card
el té tea
el/la técnico/a technician
el teléfono telephone
los temblores tremors, shakes
la temperatura temperature
temprano early
tener (*irregular*) to have

la **teniasis** tapeworm
la **tensión arterial** blood pressure
el/la **terapeuta** therapist
— **de lenguaje** speech therapist
— **del habla** speech therapist
— **físico/a** physical therapist
— **respiratorio/a** respiratory therapist
tercero/a third
el **termómetro** thermometer
el **testículo** testicle
el **tétano, el tétanos** tetanus
la **tía** aunt
la **tía abuela** great-aunt
la **tibia** tibia
tibial anterior tibialis anterior
tibio/a lukewarm
el **tiempo** time, weather
tímido/a shy
el **tío** uncle
el **tío abuelo** great-uncle
la **tirita** small bandage
el **tiroides** thyroid
la **tisana** infusion (drink), tea
la **toalla** towel
el **tobillo** ankle
tocar to touch
la **tolerancia** tolerance
tomar to take
el **tomate** tomato
la **tomografía computarizada** CT scan
la **tonsilectomía** tonsilectomy
la **tonsilotomía** tonsilotomy
tópico/a topical
la **torcedura** sprain
torcer(se) (o–ue) to sprain
torcido/a sprained
la **toronja** grapefruit
la **torta** cake
la **tos** cough
— **ferina** pertussis, whooping cough
toser to cough
la **tostada** toast
la **toxoplasmosis** toxoplasmosis
el/la **trabajador/a social** social worker
trabajar to work
el **trabajo** job
— **social** social work
el **trabalengua** tongue-twister
la **tradición** tradition
tragar to swallow

traicionado/a betrayed
trasnochar to stay up all night
el **trapecio** trapezius
trasplantar to transplant
el **trasplante** transplant
el **trastorno** disorder
— **bipolar** bipolar disorder
— **de ansiedad** anxiety disorder
el **tratamiento** treatment
— **de canal** root canal
tratar to treat
traumático/a traumatic
el **traumatismo** traumatic injury
el **tríceps braquial, femoral** triceps
los **triglicéridos** triglycerides
triste sad
la **tristeza** sadness
la **trombosis** thrombosis
la **trompa de Falopio** Fallopian tube
tu your
tú you
la **tuberculosis** tuberculosis
el **tumor** tumor
tutear to address informally
el/la **tutor/a** custodian (legal)
tuyo/a/os/as yours

u

la **úlcera** ulcer
el **ungüento** ointment
la **unidad** unit
la **uña** fingernail
la **urgencia** urgency, emergency
la **urología** urology
el/la **urólogo/a** urologist
la **urticaria** urticaria
usted you
el **útero** uterus
útil useful
la **uva** grape

v

la **vacuna** vaccination
vacunar to vaccinate
la **vagina** vagina
la **valvulopatía** valve disease
la **varicela** varicella, chicken pox
el **varón** male

el **vaso** glass
el **vegetal** vegetable
la **vejiga** bladder
la **vena** vein
el **vendaje** bandage
venir (*irregular*) to come
la **ventana** window
el **ventilador** fan
ver (*irregular*) to see
la **verdad** truth
verdadero/a true
verde green
verdoso/a greenish
la **verdura** vegetable (green)
la **vergüenza** shame
la **verruga venérea** genital wart
la **vértebra** vertebra
la **vesícula biliar** gallbladder
la **vez** time (occurrence, occasion)
la **víctima** victim
viejo/a old
el **viernes** Friday
la **vigilia** wakefulness
el **VIH** HIV
el **vino** wine
virar(se) to roll over
la **viruela** smallpox
las **viruelas locas** chicken pox
el **virus** virus
la **visita** visit

el/la **visitante** visitor
visitar to visit
la **vista** sight
la **vitamina** vitamin
la **viuda** widow
el **viudo** widower
vivir to live
vivo/a alive
volver (o–ue) to return
vomitar to vomit
el **vómito** vomit
la **voz** voice

y

y and
ya already, at last, right now
el/la **yerno/a** son-in-law, daughter-in-law
el **yeso** cast
yo I
el **yogur** yogurt

z

la **zanahoria** carrot
el **zapato** shoe
el **zika** zika
el **zumo** juice

Answer Key to *Ejercicios*

We have excluded those exercises whose responses may vary.

Chapter 1

1.1 Ejercicio (*Answers may vary slightly.*)
A. Hola. Buenos días. Buenas tardes. Buenas noches.
B. Adiós. Hasta luego.
C. Soy . . . Me llamo . . .
D. Me alegro. Lo siento.
E. Mucho gusto. Encantado/a.

1.2 Ejercicio
1. Dr. Vargas: —Buenos días. Soy el doctor Vargas.
2. Sr. Flores: —Buenos días, doctor. Soy Francisco Flores.
3. Dr. Vargas: —Mucho gusto.
4. Sr. Flores: —El gusto es mío. ¿Cómo está usted?
5. Dr. Vargas: —Muy bien, gracias, ¿y usted?
6. Sr. Flores: —Bien, bien, gracias. Doctor, le presento a mi esposa Marisol García de Flores.
7. Dr. Vargas: —Encantado.
8. Sra. Flores: —Igualmente. Usted habla español. ¿De dónde es usted?
9. Dr. Vargas: —Soy de Puerto Rico.

1.7 Ejercicio
A. El doctor Colón es neurólogo.   La doctora Palma es neuróloga.
B. El doctor Aquino es odontólogo.   La doctora Losada es odontóloga.
C. Ana es trabajadora social.   Tomás es trabajador social.
D. El señor García es consejero.   La señora Marques es consejera.
E. Leomara es farmacéutica.   Alfredo es farmacéutico.
F. El doctor Mena es psiquiatra.   La doctora Mariano es psiquiatra.
G. La doctora López es cardióloga.   El doctor López es cardiólogo.
H. La doctora Negrón es dentista.   El doctor José Peña Ortiz es dentista.

433

1.8 Ejercicio

A. la clínica	las clínicas	F. la frazada	las frazadas
B. la puerta	las puertas	G. la almohada	las almohadas
C. el monitor	los monitores	H. el doctor	los doctores
D. la cama	las camas	I. el hospital	los hospitales
E. la sábana	las sábanas		

1.9 Ejercicio

A. tú	D. usted
B. tú	E. tú
C. usted	F. usted

1.10 Ejercicio

A. él es	F. nosotros somos
B. nosotros somos	G. ellos son
C. ellos son	H. ellos son
D. ellas son	I. (la clínica) es
E. (la familia) es	J. ustedes son

1.11 Ejercicio

A. Usted necesita un enfermero.
B. Usted necesita un cardiólogo.
C. Usted necesita un endocrinólogo (un nutricionista, dietista, oftalmólogo).
D. Usted necesita un cirujano.
E. Usted necesita un oncólogo (un cirujano).
F. Usted necesita un oftalmólogo.
G. Usted necesita un radiólogo (un técnico de radiología).
H. Usted necesita un dietista (un nutricionista).
I. Usted necesita un psicólogo (un psiquiatra, un trabajador social).
J. Usted necesita un reumatólogo.
K. Usted necesita un ortopedista.
L. Usted necesita un dermatólogo.
M. Usted necesita un pediatra.
N. Usted necesita un odontólogo (un dentista).

1.18 Ejercicio

A. alto	bajo	G. corto	largo
B. delgado	gordo	H. joven	mayor, anciano
C. bajo	alto	I. largo	corto
D. pequeño	grande	J. feo	bonito, guapo
E. anciano	joven	K. gordo	delgado, flaco
F. grande	pequeño	L. bonito	feo

1.19 Ejercicio

A. Sí, es una doctora inteligente.
B. Sí, son unos estudiantes interesantes.
C. Sí, es una enfermera joven.
D. Sí, es un profesor guapo.
E. Sí, es un médico alto.
F. Sí, son unos pacientes delgados.
G. Sí, son unos doctores mayores.
H. Sí, es un neurólogo simpático.

1.20 Ejercicio

A. Pedro es feo. ¿Cómo es Estrella?   Estrella no es fea. Es bonita.
B. Marta es gorda. ¿Cómo es Juan?   Juan no es gordo. Es delgado.
C. Miguel es alto. ¿Cómo es Rosa?   Rosa no es alta. Es baja.
D. Ana es baja. ¿Cómo es Marco?   Marco no es bajo. Es alto.
E. María es mayor. ¿Cómo es José?   José no es mayor. Es joven.
F. Carlos es guapo. ¿Cómo es Ana?   Ana no es guapa. Es fea.
G. Luis es delgado. ¿Cómo es Estrella?   Estrella no es delgada. Es gorda.
H. Juana es joven. ¿Cómo es Timoteo?   Timoteo no es joven. Es anciano.

Chapter 2

2.1 Ejercicio

A. Mi mamá **está** enferma.
B. ¿**Estás** bien?
C. **Estoy** mucho mejor, gracias a Dios.
D. Mis pacientes **están** mejores.
E. Marisol y yo **estamos** preocupados por Elsita.
F. La clínica **está** en la Maple Street.
G. El odontólogo **está** en la clínica los lunes.

2.5 Ejercicio

A. **Estoy** en casa.
B. ¿Dónde **está** usted?
C. ¿**Estás** en el baño?
D. Mis hijos y yo **estamos** en la cafetería.
E. El pediatra **está** en el consultorio hoy.
F. El doctor y la enfermera **están** en la clínica con un paciente.
G. La clínica ambulatoria **está** en el primer piso.
H. **Estoy** en la segunda planta.

2.13 Ejercicio

Buenos días. Me llamo Hilda Rodríguez Portocarrero. **Soy** enfermera en el hospital Nuestra Señora de la Altagracia. El hospital **es** grande y famoso. El hospital **está** en Lima, Perú. Trabajo con la doctora Kathi Collins. La doctora Collins **es** norteamericana. Ella **está** en el hospital todos los días, pero yo no. Los sábados yo **estoy** en la clínica y los domingos **estoy** en casa. Los domingos la clínica **está** cerrada. La doctora **es** alta y delgada. Yo **soy** baja y no muy delgada. La doctora y yo **estamos** muy contentas.

2.14 Ejercicio

A. ¿De dónde **es usted**?
B. ¿Cuándo **está usted** en el hospital?
C. ¿Cuál **es** su profesión?
D. ¿Cómo **es la enfermera**?
E. ¿Cómo **está usted**?
F. ¿Quién **es la pediatra**? ¿Quién **es la doctora Marcelina Allende de Oviedo**?

2.23 Ejercicio

A. fácil
B. difícil
C. abril
D. café
E. peroné
F. sábado
G. oncólogo
H. final

Chapter 3

3.8 Ejercicio

A. Una cama es buenísima cuando tengo sueño.
B. Un carro deportivo es buenísimo cuando tengo prisa.
C. Una frazada es buenísima cuando tengo sueño.
D. Un osito de peluche es buenísimo cuando tengo miedo.
E. Una hamburguesa es buenísima cuando tengo hambre.
F. Un ventilador es buenísimo cuando tengo calor.
G. Un vaso de agua es buenísimo cuando tengo sed / calor.
H. Una discusión es buenísima cuando tengo razón.

3.20 Ejercicio

A. La rodilla no está quebrada, gracias a Dios; está torcida.
B. Los tobillos no están quebrados, gracias a Dios; están torcidos.
C. El cuello no está quebrado, gracias a Dios; está torcido.
D. Las muñecas no están quebradas, gracias a Dios; están torcidas.
E. El dedo no está quebrado, gracias a Dios; está torcido.
F. La espalda no está quebrada, gracias a Dios; está torcida.
G. El tobillo izquierdo no está quebrado, gracias a Dios; está torcido.
H. El radio derecho no está quebrado, gracias a Dios; está torcido.

3.21 Ejercicio

A. La encía está hinchada, pero no está infectada.
B. Los labios están hinchados, pero no están infectados.
C. La rodilla está hinchada, pero no está infectada.
D. Los tobillos están hinchados, pero no están infectados.
E. El dedo del pie está hinchado, pero no está infectado.
F. El codo izquierdo está hinchado, pero no está infectado.
G. La lengua está hinchada, pero no está infectada.
H. El ojo derecho está hinchado, pero no está infectado.

Chapter 4

4.1 Ejercicio

A. ¿Cuántas costillas tienes?	Tengo veinticuatro costillas.
B. ¿Cuántos dedos tienes?	Tengo diez dedos.
C. ¿Cuántas vértebras tienes?	Tengo veinticuatro vértebras.
D. ¿Cuántas orejas tienes?	Tengo dos orejas.
E. ¿Cuántos dedos de los pies tienes?	Tengo diez dedos de los pies.
F. ¿Cuántos hermanos tienes?	Tengo (#) hermanos.
G. ¿Cuántos escritorios hay en la clase?	Hay (#) escritorios en la clase.
H. ¿Cuántos solteros hay en la clase?	Hay (#) solteros en la clase.
I. ¿Cuántos libros hay en la clase?	Hay (#) libros en la clase.
J. ¿Cuántas personas con sangre del tipo O hay en la clase?	Hay (#) personas con sangre del tipo O en la clase.
K. ¿Cuántas sillas hay en la clase?	Hay (#) sillas en la clase.
L. ¿Cuántas ventanas hay en la clase?	Hay (#) ventanas en la clase.
M. ¿Cuántos vegetarianos hay en la clase?	Hay (#) vegetarianos en la clase.
N. ¿Cuántos estudiantes de enfermería hay en la clase?	Hay (#) estudiantes de enfermería en la clase.
O. ¿Cuántas personas que cumplen años en mayo hay en la clase?	Hay (#) personas que cumplen años en mayo en la clase.
P. ¿Cuántas personas que usan lentes hay en la clase?	Hay (#) personas que usan lentes en la clase.

4.2 Ejercicio

A. Su temperatura está en noventa y ocho grados.
B. Su temperatura está en ciento punto ocho grados.
C. Su temperatura está en noventa y siete punto cuatro grados.
D. Su temperatura está en ciento tres grados.
E. Su temperatura está en ciento cuatro punto dos grados.
F. Su temperatura está en noventa y ocho punto nueve grados.
G. Su temperatura está en ciento uno punto dos grados.
H. Su temperatura está en ciento punto tres grados.

4.3 Ejercicio

A. Su tensión arterial está en ciento diez sobre sesenta y ocho.

B. Su tensión arterial está en ciento sesenta y seis sobre ciento diez.

C. Su tensión arterial está en ciento treinta y cuatro sobre ochenta.

D. Su tensión arterial está en ciento veintiocho sobre setenta.

E. Su tensión arterial está en ciento veintidós sobre ochenta y cuatro.

F. Su tensión arterial está en ciento dieciocho sobre noventa y dos.

G. Su tensión arterial está en ciento seis sobre setenta y cuatro.

H. Su tensión arterial está en ciento veinte sobre ochenta.

4.11 Ejercicio

A. sus sábanas

B. su cama

C. nuestras frazadas

D. sus hijos

E. su silla

F. su consultorio

G. mi estetoscopio

4.14 Ejercicio

A. Son las tres.

B. Son las doce y quince. Son las doce y cuarto. Son las doce quince.

C. Son las diez y media. Son las diez treinta.

D. Es la una menos veinticinco. Son las doce treinta y cinco.

4.15 Ejercicio

A. Son las once menos quince de la mañana.
   Son las once menos cuarto de la mañana.
   Son las diez cuarenta y cinco de la mañana.

B. Son las seis y quince de la mañana.
   Son las seis y cuarto de la mañana.

C. Son las ocho y media de la noche.
   Son las ocho treinta de la noche.

D. Son las doce menos cinco de la noche.
   Son las once cincuenta y cinco de la noche.

E. Son las cuatro menos cuatro de la tarde.
   Son las tres cincuenta y seis de la tarde.

F. Son las seis y cinco de la tarde.

G. Es la una de la tarde.

H. Son las cinco y veintinueve de la mañana.

4.16 Ejercicio

A. Usted tiene una cita con el dentista (el odontólogo) el jueves catorce de diciembre a las tres y media de la tarde.

B. Usted tiene una cita en la clínica el martes veintidós de enero a las diez y quince (y cuarto) de la mañana.

C. Usted tiene una cita con el doctor Contreras Medina el viernes veintiocho de febrero a las siete menos quince de la tarde.

D. Su madre tiene una cita con el neurólogo, el Dr. Solano, el miércoles 30 de mayo a la una de la tarde.

Chapter 5

5.1 Ejercicio
A. mi cuñada

B. mi nieto

C. mi hermanastro

D. mi tía

E. mi primo

F. mi prima

G. mi suegra

H. mi hijastro

5.2 Ejercicio
Hola. Me llamo Arturo. Mi **papá** se llama Juan Martínez. Él tiene una **hermana** que se llama Carmen y es mi **tía**. También tiene un **hermano** que se llama Pedro y es mi **tío**. Soy el **sobrino** de mi tía Carmen y mi tío Pedro. Tío Pedro tiene dos hijos. Ellos son mis **primos**. El padre de mi padre es mi **abuelo** Javier Martínez. La esposa de mi abuelo es mi **abuela**.

5.9 Ejercicio
A. llegar a las seis

B. recetar medicina para el dolor

C. caminar en el parque

D. leer las instrucciones

E. comprar el medicamento

F. escribir una receta

G. cocinar vegetales

H. sufrir de una enfermedad.

I. cuidar a un paciente

J. necesitar una receta

K. comer una ensalada

L. vivir por cien años

5.10 Ejercicio
Me llamo Shawn. **Soy** enfermero y **trabajo** en la clínica de lunes a viernes. No **vivo** lejos de la clínica y **camino** a la clínica todos los días. La clínica **abre** a las ocho de la mañana. La doctora Valerio **trabaja** en la clínica también. Ella y yo **cuidamos** a nuestros pacientes. La doctora **examina** a los pacientes y **receta** los medicamentos. Yo **enseño** a los pacientes cómo tomar sus medicamentos. Los pacientes **compran** sus medicamentos en la farmacia y **visitan** la clínica cuando están enfermos o **necesitan** más medicamentos.

5.11 Ejercicio
A. Mi abuelo cocina vegetales para la familia.

B. Juan Miguel camina al hospital para trabajar todos los días.

C. Usted lee libros en inglés y español.

D. Los doctores recetan los medicamentos.

E. Marisol y su hermana hablan por teléfono todos los sábados.

F. Yo como mucha ensalada porque tiene fibra y muchas vitaminas.

G. Una enfermera visita a mi abuela en su casa una vez a la semana.

H. Luisito toma un vaso de agua porque tiene mucha sed.

I. Miguelina compra libros por Internet con su tarjeta de crédito.

5.12 Ejercicio

A. Sí, camino a la clase (*or*) No, no camino a la clase.

B. Llego a la clase a la(s) <hora>.

C. Sí, tomo antiácidos por la noche (*or*) No, no tomo antiácidos por la noche.

D. Trabajo de <día> a <día>.

E. Sí, abro las ventanas de mi casa en la noche (*or*) No, no abro las ventanas de mi casa en la noche.

F. Practico el español con <persona>.

G. Sí, leo el libro de español por la noche (*or*) No, no leo el libro de español por la noche.

H. Sí, bebo bebidas alcohólicas todos los días (*or*) No, no bebo bebidas alcohólicas todos los días.

I. Estudio por <número> horas los fines de semana.

J. Sí, sufro de alergias (*or*) No, no sufro de alergias.

5.17 Ejercicio

A. Aprendo español rápidamente.

B. Enseño inglés **a** mis padres.

C. Mi esposa y yo hablamos español en casa.

D. Cuido **a** mis padres en la casa.

E. Visito **a** mi mamá todas las semanas.

F. Llamo **a** mi hermana por teléfono los domingos.

G. Mi hermano come una hamburguesa al mediodía.

H. Mi tío bebe tres tazas de café por la mañana.

Chapter 6

6.1 Ejercicio

A. El acetaminofén está disponible en tableta, gragea, líquido, jarabe, inyección y forma intravenosa.

B. La leche de magnesia está disponible en suspensión.

C. El Pepto Bismol está disponible en suspensión y tabletas.

D. La Visene está disponible en gotas.

E. La insulina está disponible en inyección subcutánea.

F. El salbutamol está disponible en tabletas, jarabe, suspensión y aerosol.

G. La guaifenesina está disponible en jarabe, tabletas y cápsulas.

H. La hidrocortisona 2% está disponible en crema y ungüento.

I. La nicotina está disponible en parche, dulce, chicle (goma de masticar) y aerosol.

J. La Compazina está disponible en supositorio y tableta.

K. La vacuna para la varicela está disponible en inyección.

L. El ibuprofeno está disponible en tableta, cápsula, gragea, suspensión, gotas, inyección y forma intravenosa.

6.2 Ejercicio

A. Toma	E. toma
B. toma	F. toman
C. Tomas	G. toman
D. tomamos	

6.5 Ejercicio

A. Tome el medicamento todos los días sin falta.

B. Amoxicilina (250 mg/5 ml), tome 1 cucharadita 3 veces al día por 5 días.

C. Guaifenesina, tome 1 cucharada 4 veces al día para la congestión.

D. Salbutamol, tome 1 inhalación cada 4 a 6 horas cuando sea necesario para la fatiga.

E. Donepezilo, tome 10 mg por la boca (por vía oral) 1 vez al día (diario) por la mañana.

F. Ginkgo, tome 160 mg por la boca (por vía oral) a las 8:00 a.m. (las 8 de la mañana) y las 8:00 p.m. (las ocho de la noche).

G. Haloperidol, tome 5 mg por la boca (por vía oral) a las 8:00 p.m.

H. Acetaminofen, tome 2 tabletas cada 4 a 6 horas cuando sea necesario para el dolor.

I. Mylanta, tome 2 cucharadas al acostarse.

J. Omeprazole, tome 1 cápsula a las 8:00 a.m. (a las 8 de la mañana).

K. Isoniazid, tome 1 tableta todos los días por la mañana.

L. Fluoxetine 20 mg, tome 1 cápsula por la mañana.

M. Phenytoin 100 mg, tome 1 cápsula 3 veces al día.

N. Loperamide, tome 1 cápsula cada 2 a 3 horas cuando sea necesario para la diarrea.

6.6 Ejercicio

abrir	¡Abra!
agitar	¡Agite!
aplicar	¡Aplique!
enjuagar	¡Enjuague!
exhalar	¡Exhale!
inhalar	¡Inhale!
mantener	¡Mantenga!
oprimir	¡Oprima!
poner	¡Ponga!
quitar	¡Quite!

6.7 Ejercicio (*Answers will vary.*)

A. Acetaminofén es un analgésico. No es un antiinflamatorio no esteroide. Es para la fiebre y el dolor pero no es para la inflamación.

B. Albuterol es un aerosol. Es un broncodilatador.

C. Penicilina es una tableta. Es un antibiótico.

D. Coumadin es una tableta. Es un anticoagulante.

E. Tylenol es una tableta. Es analgésica y antipirética.

F. Diazepam es una tableta. Es un tranquilizante y un antiepiléptico (anti-convulsivo).

G. Carbamazepina es una tableta. Es un antiepiléptico (anticonvulsivo).

H. Ex-Lax es una tableta, una tableta masticable y una preparación con choco-late. Es un laxante.

I. Difenhidramina es una tableta, cápsula (gragea) o líquido. Es antihistamínico (antialérgico).

J. Ácido fólico es una tableta. Es una vitamina.

K. Pepto Bismol es una suspensión. Es un antiácido. Es un antidiarreico.

L. Robitussin DM es un jarabe. Es un expectorante y un antitusígeno.

M. Crema hidrocortisona es una crema o ungüento. Es un antialérgico. Es para la picazón.

N. Fenobarbital (*belladonna*) es una tableta, una inyección o un líquido. Es anti-convulsivo y antiepiléptico.

6.10 Ejercicio

Don Ignacio, es muy importante usar **estos** medicamentos en la manera indicada. **Esta** crema es para aliviar el dolor de la quemadura. En caso de fiebre, **estas** pas-tillas son para quitar la fiebre. Si tiene mucho dolor, **estas** pastillas son para el do-lor. **Este** jarabe es para la tos. Si está peor mañana, favor de llamar a **este** número de teléfono. Finalmente, **estas** recetas son para comprar más medicamentos.

6.13 Ejercicio

A. El doctor **le receta** un medicamento a Juan.

B. La doctora **le pregunta** su historia médica a él.

C. Yo **le escribo** una carta a la compañía de seguros.

D. La anestesióloga **me explica** el procedimiento.

E. El enfermero **les habla** español a los pacientes.

F. Usted **les compra** la medicina a sus padres.

G. La pediatra **le receta** un antibiótico para mi bebé.

6.14 Ejercicio

A. **Les** receto un medicamento a sus hijos.

B. **Le** escribo una carta a usted.

C. **Le** doy una aspirina a la paciente.

D. **Les** enseño español a los estudiantes.

E. **Le** tomo la temperatura al paciente cada cuatro horas.

F. **Le** leo el libro a usted.

G. La doctora **nos** contesta la pregunta a nosotros.

6.16 Ejercicio

A. Es importante ponérselo por la mañana.
B. No se la dé si tiene fiebre.
C. Déselo a las ocho de la noche.
D. Escríbamela.
E. No se lo tome si tiene irritación.
F. Déselo con mucha agua.

Chapter 7

7.1 Ejercicio

A. La carne de res es carne roja.
B. El pescado es del océano.
C. El mantecado es rico en calcio.
D. La avena es buena para la picazón.
E. Para consumir bacteria beneficiosa, coma yogur.
F. Para tener más fibra en la dieta, coma pan integral.
G. Para tener más vitamina A, coma zanahorias.
H. Un ingrediente principal de la ensalada es la lechuga.
I. El huevo es posible futuro madre o padre de familia.
J. Para bajar el colesterol, coma avena.

7.2 Ejercicio

A. A mí **me aburre** trabajar en una oficina.
B. A mis padres **les fascina** cuidar a su nieto.
C. A mí **me interesa** cocinar sin mucha grasa.
D. A los estudiantes **les fascina** aprender el español.
E. A nuestro profesor **le importa** hablar dos idiomas.
F. A nosotros **nos gusta** comer arroz con pollo y ensalada.

7.12 Ejercicio

A. No, no debe cocinar con manteca.
B. Sí, debe comer pollo y pescado.
C. No, no debe comer mucho coco.
D. Sí, debe tomar leche baja en grasa.
E. Sí, debe comer queso bajo en grasa.
F. No, no debe comer papas fritas.
G. Sí, debe usar aceite de maíz.
H. En vez de la carne de res, debe comer (*answers will vary*).
I. Debe quitar la piel del pollo antes de cocinar.

7.13 Ejercicio

A. No, no debe usar mucha azúcar cuando cocina.

B. Sí, debe comer ensalada.

C. No, no debe beber vino.

D. No, no debe comer muchos dulces.

E. Sí, debe comer frijoles.

F. No, no debe usar leche condensada.

G. Sí, debe tomar refrescos dietéticos.

H. Sí, debe usar azúcar artificial.

7.18 Ejercicio

A.	F	D.	C
B.	F	E.	F
C.	F	F.	F

Chapter 8

8.6 Ejercicio

A.	_____ ponerle puntos	E.	_____ examinarle la próstata
B.	_X_ escucharle el corazón	F.	_X_ escucharle los pulmones
C.	_X_ pesarle	G.	_X_ tomarle la temperatura
D.	_____ ponerle un suero	H.	_X_ sacarle sangre para un análisis

8.7 Ejercicio

A. Voy a mirarle los ojos.   __E__ Respire profundamente.

B. Voy a percutirle el pecho.   __F__ ¿Le duele cuando lo presiono?

C. Voy a mirarle la garganta.   __B__ ¡Golpecitos!

D. Voy a tocarle el cuello.   __D__ Mueva la cabeza hacia la derecha.

E. Voy a escucharle los pulmones.   __G__ Acuéstese boca arriba por favor.

F. Voy a presionarle el abdomen.   __A__ ¿Tiene problemas con la vista?

G. Voy a hacerle un electrocardiograma.   __C__ Abra la boca y diga «a-a-a-a».

H. Tenemos que examinarle los testes.   __H__ Vire la cabeza y tosa.

8.11 Ejercicio

A. ¿Qué es un angiograma?

B. ¿Qué es una supervisión Holter?

C. ¿Qué son las imágenes por resonancia magnética?

D. ¿Qué es una broncoscopia?

E. ¿Qué es una biopsia?

F. ¿Qué es un mamograma?

G. ¿Qué es la espirometría?

H. ¿Qué es una colonoscopia?

8.15 Ejercicio

A. Mamá está preparando una ensalada de fruta.

B. Estoy recetando algo para el dolor.

C. Estamos trabajando en la clínica ambulatoria hoy.

D. El cardiólogo está llegando al hospital ahora.

E. Estás mejorando.

F. La doctora está percutiendo el pecho.

Chapter 9

9.1 Ejercicio

A. Anoche mis tíos y mis primos nos **visitaron**.

B. Ellos **llegaron** a las cinco de la tarde.

C. Mis padres **cocinaron** mucha comida deliciosa.

D. Mi hermano y yo **comimos** ensalada, carne y arroz.

E. Después de comer, yo **estudié** para la clase de español.

F. En la noche mi tía **sufrió** de acidez.

G. A las ocho mi tío **compró** un antiácido para mi tía.

H. Mi tía se **tomó** el antiácido con un vaso de agua.

9.2 Ejercicio

A. ¿En qué año **nació** usted?

B. ¿A usted le **escribió** la doctora una receta nueva?

C. ¿Por cuántos años **vivieron** sus padres con usted?

D. ¿Cuántas botellas de vino **bebieron** los enfermeros en la fiesta?

E. ¿**Viste** tú el accidente ayer?

F. ¿A qué hora **saliste** tú de tu casa esta mañana?

G. ¿**Cuidaron** bien los enfermeros a tu padre en el hospital?

H. ¿**Tragó** doña María la pastilla grande sin problema?

9.7 Ejercicio

A. Ayer fue miércoles.   SER

B. La prueba de Pap fue negativa.   SER

C. La semana pasada fui a la clínica.   IR

D. Fui estudiante de medicina en el 2014.   SER

E. El enfermero fue a la cafetería para comer.   IR

F. El cirujano que me operó fue el doctor Pérez.   SER

G. Mi madre y yo fuimos al consultorio el martes. IR

H. Mis hijos fueron a Chile para visitar a sus abuelos. IR

9.8 Ejercicio

Anoche el bebé **estuvo** enfermo. Mi pobre bebé **tuvo** una fiebre alta. Su temperatura **estuvo** en cuarenta grados. Nosotros **fuimos** al hospital. El doctor que nos atendió **fue** el doctor Vargas. Yo **estuve** muy nerviosa. La enfermera le **puso** un suero. El doctor me **dijo** que **fue** una infección de los oídos y nos **recetó** un antibiótico.

9.9 Ejercicio

El tres de enero el doctor Aquino y Ana **comieron** en la casa de Javier.

El cinco de enero el doctor Aquino **visitó** a doña Mercedes en Boston.

El once de enero el doctor Aquino **trabajó** en la clínica desde las ocho hasta las cinco.

El trece de enero el doctor Aquino y don Máximo **fueron** a la clase de inglés.

El catorce de enero el doctor Aquino **consultó** con el anestesiólogo.

El quince de enero el doctor Aquino no **comió** nada, **bebió** líquidos claros y **tomó** citrato de magnesio.

El dieciséis de enero el doctor Aquino **tuvo** una colonoscopia.

El diecisiete de enero el doctor Aquino **fue** al consultorio de la doctora Muñoz Domínguez para un examen físico.

El treinta de enero el doctor Aquino **fue** de vacaciones a Venezuela.

9.12 Ejercicio

A. La biopsia fue positiva. Tenga confianza. Todo va a estar bien.

B. El análisis de sangre fue negativo. Gracias a Dios.

C. El electrocardiograma fue negativo. Gracias a Dios.

D. La prueba de tuberculosis fue positiva. Tenga confianza. Todo va a estar bien.

E. La tomografía computarizada fue negativa. Gracias a Dios.

F. La prueba del SIDA fue negativa. Gracias a Dios.

G. La prueba de Papanicolaou fue negativa. Gracias a Dios.

H. El sonograma de la vesícula biliar fue negativo. Gracias a Dios.

9.16 Ejercicio

Cuando yo **era** niño, mi familia **vivía** en Puerto Rico. Mis abuelos **vivían** con nosotros. Mi abuela **sabía** mucho de las plantas medicinales. Cuando yo **tenía** gripe, ella me **hacía** té de hojas de limón y naranja. Cuando **tenía** gases en la barriga, me **preparaba** té de anís. Mis padres no me **daban** remedios caseros. Ellos me **llevaban** a la farmacia, y el farmacéutico nos **vendía** un jarabe o una pastilla. No me **gustaban** los jarabes. **Prefería** las tisanas de mi abuelita.

9.19 Ejercicio

D. grupo de apoyo

C. placa

I. malla metálica

F. ecocardiograma

B. dieta saludable para el corazón

G. stent

A. palpitaciones

E. dolor pesado del pecho

H. electrocardiograma

Chapter 10

10.2 Ejercicio

A. La tuberculosis del pulmón es **una bacteria**.

B. La piel amarillenta es un síntoma de **hepatitis**.

C. Los pacientes que sufren de **epilepsia** tienen convulsiones.

D. Los pacientes con hiperglucemia padecen de **diabetes**.

E. Los tobillos hinchados son un síntoma de **insuficiencia cardíaca**.

F. Si un tumor es **maligno**, el paciente tiene cáncer.

G. La fatiga, o falta de aire, es un síntoma del **asma**.

H. Un análisis de esputo puede confirmar un diagnóstico de **tuberculosis**.

I. La causa principal de la enfermedad valvular del corazón es **la fiebre reumática**.

10.8 Ejercicio

A. Mi hermano **ha tenido** piojos.

B. Yo **he sufrido** de bronquitis crónica.

C. ¿**Has puesto** tú la vacuna de la hepatitis B?

D. Mis padres **han comprado** sus medicamentos.

E. Mi hermano y yo **hemos consultado** con un urólogo.

F. El doctor me **ha hecho** el examen rectal digital de la próstata.

10.14 Ejercicio

Dra. Ávila: ¿Sufre usted de **alguna** enfermedad?

Doña Rosa: No, no sufro de **ninguna** enfermedad.

Dra. Ávila: ¿Toma usted **algún** medicamento?

Doña Rosa: No tomo **ningún** medicamento.

Dra. Ávila: ¿Es usted alérgica a **algún** alimento?

Doña Rosa: No soy alérgica a **ningún** alimento.

Dra. Ávila: En su familia, ¿**alguien** ha tenido cáncer?

Doña Rosa: No, en mi familia **nadie** ha tenido cáncer.

Dra. Ávila: ¿Hay **alguien** en la casa para ayudarla?

Doña Rosa: Vivo sola. No hay **nadie** más en casa.

10.20 Ejercicio

A. Los hombres deben hacerse autoexamen de **los testículos**.

B. La histerectomía es una cirugía para sacar **el útero**.

C. La orina empieza en **los riñones** y pasa a **la vejiga**.

D. **El pulmón** es el órgano de la respiración.

E. La parte del tubo digestivo que llega al estómago es **el esófago**.

    F. Un óvulo sale de **un ovario** y entra en la trompa de Falopio.

    G. **El hígado** es el órgano más grande en el cuerpo.

    H. **La amígdala** es parte del sistema linfático.

    I. La colecistectomía es cuando sacan **la vesícula biliar**.

10.21 Ejercicio

    A. la artroscopia

    B. la cirugía ambulatoria

    C. la nefrectomía

    D. la laparoscopia

    E. la cirugía exploratoria

10.26 Ejercicio

A. Los antibióticos curan los virus.	Falso
B. La influenza es contagiosa.	Verdadero
C. Hay vacuna para curar la pandemia de gripe.	Falso
D. La gripe no causa dolores musculares.	Falso
E. Todos los pacientes se mejoran sin complicación.	Falso

Chapter 11

11.1 Ejercicio

Mi madre tiene los tobillos hinchados y dificultad para respirar. El cardiólogo dice que la va a **internar** para un ecograma y una cateterización cardíaca. Si todo va bien, le va a **dar de alta** en dos días. Ella está en la sala de emergencias y no quiere **quedarse interna** pero el cardiólogo dice que el corazón es el músculo más importante del cuerpo y hay que cuidarlo.

11.4 Ejercicio

Buenos días. Me llamo Juan y mi esposa se llama Melania. Yo **me levanto** a las cinco de la mañana y **me baño**. Melania **se levanta** a las cinco y media y **se baña**. Yo **me afeito** mientras Melania **se seca** el cabello. Después, nosotros **nos vestimos**, **desayunamos** y **salimos** de la casa a las siete.

11.13 Ejercicio

    A. Se me rompió un hueso.

    B. Se me olvidó ponerme la insulina.

    C. Se te fracturó el dedo.

    D. Se te quemó la mano.

    E. ¿Se le perdió la receta?

    F. Se me hincharon los tobillos.

11.14 Ejercicio

    A. ¿**Puede** usted dormirse sin tomar una pastilla para dormir?

    B. ¿Cuánto tiempo hace que usted no **duerme** bien?

C. ¿Cuántas horas **durmió** usted anoche?

D. ¿**Puede** usted abrir la botella?

E. ¿**Puede** usted tragar la pastilla grande sin problema?

F. ¿**Puede** usted llegar mañana a las siete de la mañana?

G. La enfermera dijo que usted no **durmió** bien anoche. ¿Tiene sueño?

11.19 Ejercicio

A. Si tomo mucho café me siento **agitado**.

B. Cuando estoy resfriado me siento **molesto**.

C. Cuando trabajo mucho llego a la casa muy **agotado**.

D. Estoy **ansioso** cuando tengo una cita con el odontólogo.

E. Me pongo **agobiado** cuando hay mucho trabajo y poco tiempo.

F. Me siento muy **soñoliento** cuando paso la noche sin dormir bien.

G. Cuando tengo dolor de cabeza y tomo un calmante me siento **aliviado**.

Chapter 12

12.1 Ejercicio

A. ¿Quién es / Cómo se llama su ginecólogo?

B. ¿Cuándo comenzó su último período?

C. ¿Cuánto tiempo duran sus períodos?

D. ¿Son regulares sus períodos?

E. ¿Le duelen sus períodos?

F. ¿Cuándo fue su última prueba de Pap(anicolaou)?

G. ¿Cuándo fue su último ultrasonido?

H. ¿Cuánto tiempo hace que no tiene la menstruación?

I. ¿Ha subido de peso?

J. ¿Usa drogas? ¿Fuma?

12.9 Ejercicio

A. La **episiotomía** es una incisión en la vulva para facilitar el parto del feto.

B. La **operación cesárea** es necesaria cuando el parto vaginal no es posible.

C. La **placenta** es un órgano que está entre la superficie interior del útero y el cordón umbilical.

D. Cuando no hay **dilatación del útero** se usa medicamento para adelantar el parto.

E. El embarazo **ectópico** es un embarazo anormal porque el óvulo fertilizado no está en el útero.

F. El **parto prematuro** es un parto antes de treinta y siete semanas de embarazo.

12.11 Ejercicio

A. No hagas la cita para hoy. Haz la cita para mañana.

B. Sal temprano de la casa. No salgas tarde.

C. Ve al consultorio. No vayas al hospital.

D. No bañes al bebé hoy. Baña al bebé mañana.

E. No te bañes hoy. Báñate mañana.

F. Ponte la bata del hospital. No te pongas ropa interior.

G. No comas nada después de las once. Come bien mañana.

12.12 Ejercicio

A. ¡No te preocupes!

B. ¡Relájate!

C. ¡No comas nada!

D. Si tienes sed, ¡come pedacitos de hielo!

E. ¡Empuja!

F. ¡No empujes!

G. ¡Respira!

H. ¡No respires!

12.13 Ejercicio

A. ¡Muévate!

B. ¡Levántate!

C. ¡Vírate!

D. ¡Báñate hoy!

E. ¡Come!

F. ¡Acuéstate!

G. ¡Levanta el brazo!

H. ¡Respira!

A. ¡No te muevas!

B. ¡No te levantes!

C. ¡No te vires!

D. ¡No te bañes hoy!

E. ¡No comas!

F. ¡No te acuestes!

G. ¡No levantes el brazo!

H. ¡No respires!

Illustration Credits

Karrie McCarter provided digital bone images.

The comic strips that appear on pages 177 and 270 are © 2007 Baldo Partnership. Dist. by Universal Uclick. Reprinted with permission. All rights reserved.

The comics that appear on pages 55 and 252 are courtesy of humorist Pepe Angonoa and used with permission.

The illustration *Mi Plato* that appears on page 188 is a public domain resource provided by the United States Department of Agriculture.

The illustration *El plato de buen comer* that appears on page 189 is a public resource of La Secretaría de Salud of Mexico (Norma oficial mexicana NOM-043-SSA2-2005).

The zika cycle illustration on page 284 is adapted from a public domain resource provided by the United States Center for Disease Control.

Truth-Function of Aiken, South Carolina, provided the companion video still shots that appear throughout the book.

Dr. Jorge Amarante, Nutriólogo Clínico, shot the photos of his daughter Naura on pages 185 and 186 and the self-portrait that appears on page 25.

Otoniel Acevedo Medina took the photos of a newborn physical exam on page 225 and a pregnant woman on page 368.

Sarah E. Bartley contributed the sonogram and the photo of the author's grandsons on pages 123 and 364.

The following photos were downloaded from Thinkstock: woman with headache on page 64; woman with cold on page 66; blood draw on page 229; water boiling on page 287; woman with head scarf on page 289; breast exam on page 290; nurse and patient on page 322; surgery on pages 301 and 323; woman shampooing on page 328; woman with towel on page 329; man with poor hygiene on page 329; burned arm on page 332; cocaine user on page 353; and breastfeeding on page 375.

Frank Dlugoleski of DartZ Business Solutions LLC created the icons that distinguish goals and classroom activities and the following drawings: nurses, page 6; clinic, page 8; nurses, page 9; specialists, page 12; body forms, page 20; hot water bottle, page 37; bedside, page 38; pain scale, pages 38, 40, and 88; elevator bank, page 42; man soaking feet, page 62; head and head and body, pages 71 and 73; skeleton front and back, pages 74 and 75; muscles, pages 77 and 78; broken bones, page 86; two men on telephone, page 102; clock faces, page 108; family trees, pages 125 and 127; action words, page 132; Alfredo and Mercedes, page 141; medication forms, page 151; *sarpullido*, page 166; pill reminder, page 175; breakfast foods, page 191; fruits and vegetables, page 194; physical exam, page 223; multiple signs, page 237; emergency room patients, page 258; hip replacements, page 261; cardiovascular disease, page 262; cardiac rehabilitation, page 265; heart attack, page 266; *visita al doctor*, page 268; measles and mumps, page 281; cycle of zika infection, page 284; various internal organs, page 322; morning routine, page 330; teeth, page 336; dental treatments, page 337; dental hygiene, page 339; and feeling states, page 343.

Robert O. Chase created the remaining drawings and illustrations and took the following photographs: Dr. Cordova, page 15; woman with pot, page 20; elderly man, page 20; woman with head scarf, page 20; pyramid, page 29; sign at Tlatelolco, page 30; grandparents and child, page 30; hospital signage, pages 44, 50, and 53; man mixing concrete, page 57; sutured arm and leg, page 82; women hugging, page 90; blood pressure, page 101; family, page 118; three generations of women, page 124; birthday party, page 144; men at pharmacy, page 150; IV bag, page 151; pharmacy, page 164; various pictures of herbs, fruits, and vegetables, pages 177, 187, 197, 198, 207, and 210; hospital signs, pages 217 and 222; doctor suturing boy, page 225; photo of clinic sign, page 230; CT scan, page 232; throat exam, page 235; ambulances, pages 245 and 250; herbs and cacti, pages 271 and 272; hospitalized woman, page 321; mother bathing baby, page 326; elderly woman, page 346; aloe, page 355; *chamán*, page 356; family, page 363; infant, page 370; and man with baby, page 384.

Index